DERM

FACTS

DERM

FACTS

Hunter H. Sams, MD
Resident, Division of Dermatology
Vanderbilt University School of Medicine
Nashville, Tennessee

Publisher: HANLEY & BELFUS
                  Medical Publishers
                  210 South 13th Street
                  Philadelphia, PA 19107
                  (215) 546-7293, 800-962-1892
                  FAX (215) 790-9330
                  Web site: http://www.hanleyandbelfus.com

Note to the reader: Although the information in this book has been carefully reviewed for correctness of dosage and indications, neither the authors nor the editors nor the publisher can accept any legal responsibility for any errors or omissions that may be made. Neither the publisher nor the editors make any warranty, expressed or implied, with respect to the material contained herein. Before prescribing any drug, the reader must review the manufacturer's current product information (package inserts) for accepted indications, absolute dosage recommendations, and other information pertinent to the safe and effective use of the product described.

Library of Congress Cataloging-in-Publication Data

Sams, Hunter.
    Derm facts / written by Hunter Sams.
      p.; cm.
    ISBN 1-56053-482-6 (alk. paper)
    1. Dermatology—Handbooks, manuals, etc. 2 Skin—Diseases—Handbooks, manuals,
    etc. I. Title.
      [DNLM: 1. Skin Diseases—Handbooks. WR 39 S193d 2001]
    RL74 .S225 2001
    616.5—dc21

DERM FACTS   ISBN 1-56053-482-6

Last digit is the print number: 9   8   7   6   5   4   3   2   1

Dedication

To two gentlemen dermatologists, Wiley M. Sams and W. Mitchell Sams, Jr., whose legacy is my pride.

To my wife Sharon, whose support was instrumental in the development of this book.

Contents

Acknowledgments

As a compilation of details, *Derm Facts* has been gleaned from multiple sources by innumerable outstanding authors and researchers.

Particularly important is the influence of three outstanding dermatologists:

Alan S. Boyd, MD contributed information, compiled over many years, in "Associations" and particularly in "Dermatopathology."

Lloyd E. King, Jr., MD, PhD provided opportunity and encouragement to develop a "peripheral brain."

W. Mitchell Sams, Jr., MD influenced my decision to pursue dermatology, my love of writing, and provided the genes to make it happen.

Introduction

This book is intended as a portable, accessible, "peripheral brain" of dermatologic information. Its concise, alphabetical, table-based format is designed to provide easy access to a wealth of useful derm facts. In the left-hand column of each section are signs, symptoms, conditions, or medications, and on the right is the associated condition or explanation intended to inform, jog the memory, give clues, and hopefully to provide insight. More common or more strongly associated topics in the right-hand columns are in bold. Purposefully omitted were a complete differential diagnosis and specific medication information.

Additions, corrections, and comments are welcome.

Abbreviations Used in Derm Facts

Ab	antibody
ACE	angiotensin converting enzyme
AD	autosomal dominant
AFX	atypical fibroxanthoma
AIDS	acquired immunodeficiency syndrome
AK	actinic keratosis
AKA	also known as
ALHE	angiolymphoid hyperplasia with eosinophilia
AML	acute myelogenous leukemia
ANCA	anti-neutrophilic cytoplasmic antibodies
aq.	aqueous
AR	autosomal recessive
ASA	acetylsalicylic acid
AV	arterio-venous
AVM	arterio-venous malformation
BCC	basal cell carcinoma
BP	bullous pemphigoid
cAMP	cyclic adenosine monophosphate
cGMP	cyclic guanine monophosphate
CAD	coronary artery disease
CHF	congestive heart failure
CIE	congenital ichthyosiform erythroderma
CLL	chronic lymphocytic leukemia
CMC	chronic mucocutaneous candidiasis
CML	chronic myelogenous leukemia
CMV	cytomegalovirus
CNCH	chondrodermatitis nodularis chronicus helices
CNS	central nervous system
CP	cicatricial pemphigoid
CTCL	cutaneous T cell lymphoma
CV	cardiovascular
CVA	cerebrovascular accident
d.	disease
DEB	dystrophic epidermolysis bullosa
DFSP	dermatofibrosarcoma protuberans
DIC	disseminated intravascular coagulation
DIF	direct immunofluorescence

Abbreviations Used in Derm Facts

DIP	Distal interphalangeal
DLE	discoid lupus erythematosus
DM	diabetes mellitus
DNA	deoxyribonucleic acid
DSAP	disseminated superficial actinic porokeratosis
EAC	erythema annulare centrifugum
EB	epidermolysis bullosa
EBA	epidermolysis bullosa acquisita
EBV	Epstein-Barr virus
EED	erythema elevatum diutinum
EHK	epidermolytic hyperkeratosis
EM	electron microscopy
esp.	especially
FTT	failure to thrive
GI	gastrointestinal
GU	genitourinary
GVH	graft versus host
H/A	headache
HAV	hepatitis A virus
HBV	hepatitis B virus
HCV	hepatitis C virus
HDL	high density lipoprotein
HIV	human immunodeficiency virus
HPV	human papilloma virus
HSM	hepatosplenomegaly
HSV	herpes simplex virus
HTLV	human T-lymphocyte virus
IBD	inflammatory bowel disease
IF	immunofluorescence
IIF	indirect immunofluorescence
IgA	immunoglobulin A
IgE	immunoglobulin E
IgG	immunoglobulin G
IgM	immunoglobulin M
ILVEN	inflamed linear verrucous epidermal nevus
IP	incontinentia pigmenti
IUGR	intra-uterine growth retardation

Abbreviations Used in Derm Facts

JEB	junctional epidermolysis bullosa
JXG	juvenile xanthogranuloma
KA	keratoacanthoma
LDL	low density lipoprotein
LE	lupus erythematosus
LFT	liver function test
LGV	lymphogranuloma venereum
LP	lichen planus
LPP	large plaque parapsoriasis
LSC	lichen simplex chronicus
MCV	molluscum contagiosum virus
MEN	multiple endocrine neoplasia
MI	myocardial infarction
MR	mental retardation
NLD	necrobiosis lipoidica diabeticorum
NSAIDs	non-steroidal anti-inflammatory drugs
N/V	nausea/vomiting
NXG	necrobiotic xanthogranuloma
OCD	obsessive compulsive disorder
OCPs	oral contraceptive pills
PABA	*para*-aminobenzoic acid
PAN	polyarteritis nodosa
PCN	penicillin
PCT	porphyria cutanea tarda
PED	palmoplantar ectodermal dysplasia
pet.	petroleum
PG	pyoderma gangrenosum
PIP	proximal interphalangeal
PLC	pityriasis lichenoides chronica
PLEVA	pityriasis lichenoides et varioliformis acuta
PMLE	polymorphous light eruption
PPK	palmoplantar keratoderma
PRP	pityriasis rubra pilaris
PSS	progressive systemic sclerosis
PUPPP	pruritic & urticarial papules & plaques of pregnancy
PUVA	psoralen + ultraviolet A light
PXE	pseudoxanthoma elasticum

Abbreviations Used in Derm Facts

RA	rheumatoid arthritis
RF	rheumatoid factor
RNA	ribonucleic acid
ROM	range of motion
RR	red reflex
RSV	respiratory syncytial virus
s.	syndrome
SCC	squamous cell carcinoma
SCIDs	severe combined immunodeficiency syndrome
SCLE	subacute cutaneous lupus erythematosus
SK	seborrheic keratosis
SLE	systemic lupus erythematosus
SM	splenomegaly
sol.	solution
SPP	small plaque parapsoriasis
SSSS	staphylococcal scalded skin syndrome
TCN	tetracycline
TEN	toxic epidermal necrolysis
TMEP	telangiectasia macularis eruptiva perstans
TSS	toxic shock syndrome
URI	upper respiratory infection
XLD	X-linked dominant
XLR	X-linked recessive

Advocacy, Registry, and Support Groups

American Autoimmune Related Diseases Association, Inc. (AARDA) (**Lupus**) 22100 Gratiot Ave. East Detroit, MI 48021 810-776-3900 800598-4668 fax # 810-776-3903 aarda@aol.com www.aarda.org

Alliance of Genetic Support Groups 35 Wisconsin Circle, Suite 440 Chevy Chase, MD 20815 301-652-5553 fax # 301-654-0171 Joan Weiss, Ex. Dir.

American Hair Loss Council (**Alopecia**) 30 Grassy Plain Road Bethel, CT 06801 888-873-9719 www.ahlc.org

American **Porphyria** Foundation PO Box 22712 Houston, TX 77227 713-266-9617 fax # 713-871-1788 porphyrus@juno.com www.enterprise.net/apf Desiree Lyon, Ex. Dir.

American Skin Association, Inc. 150 East 58th Street, 33rd Floor New York, NY 10155-0002 212-753-8260 fax # 212-688-6547 AmericanSkin@compuserve.com Joyce Weidler

Association for Children with **Russell-Silver Syndrome** 22 Hoyt St. Madison, NJ 07940 201-377-4531 201-822-2715 Jodi G. Zwain, Ex. Dir.

Ataxia-Telangiectasia Children's Project 668 S. Military Trail Deerfield Beach, FL 33442 954-481-6611 800-543-5728 fax 954-725-1153 info@atcp.org www.atcp.org

Basal Cell Carcinoma Nevus Syndrome/Gorlin Syndrome Home Page www.hometown. aol.com/gorlinadvocate/skinindex.html gorlinadvocate@aol.com

Beckwith-Wiedemann Support Network 3206 Braeburn Circle Ann Arbor, MI 48108 313-973-0263 800-837-2976 fax # 313-973-9721 Susan Fettes, Ex. Dir.

Bloom's Syndrome Registry Laboratory of Human Genetics New York Blood Center 310 East 67th St. New York, NY 10021 212-570-3075 fax # 212-570-3195 James L. German III, MD

Chronic Granulomatous Disease Association 2616 Monterey Road San Marino, CA 91108-1646 818-441-4118 Mary A. Hurley

Cornelia de Lange Syndrome Foundation 60 Dyer Ave. Collinsville, CT 06022 800-223-8355 203-693-0159 fax # 203-693-6819 Julie A. Mairano, Ex. Dir.

Dermatitis Herpetiformis Gluten Intolerance Group of North America 15110 10th Avenue, SW Suite A Seattle, WA 98166 206-246-6652 fax # 206-246-6531 gig@accessone.com www.gluten.net Cynthia Kupper

Ehlers-Danlos National Foundation 6399 Wilshire Blvd. Suite 510 Los Angeles, CA 90048 323-651-3038 fax # 323-651-1366 EDNFboard@aol.com www.ednf.org Linda Neumann-Potash

Epidermolysis Bullosa Research Association of America (DEBRA) 40 Rector Street, 14th Floor New York, NY 10006 212-513-4090 fax # 212-513-4099 debraorg@erols.com www.debra.org Miriam Feder, Exec. Dir.

Erythropoietic Protoporphyria Research and Education Fund (EPPREF) Channing Laboratory 181 Longwood Ave. Boston, MA 02115-5804 617-525-2249 fax 617-731-1541 mmmathroth @bics.bwh.harvard.edu www.BWH.partners.org/EPPREF

Familial Polyposis Registry (**Gardner Syndrome**) Cleveland Clinic Foundation Dept. of Colorectal Surgery Cleveland, OH 44195 216-444-6470 fax # 216-445-8627 James Church, MD Exec. Dir.

Foundation for **Ichthyosis** & Related Skin Types (FIRST) 650 N. Cannon Avenue, Suite 17 Lansdale, PA 19446 800-545-3286 215-631-1411 fax # 215-631-1413 info@scalyskin.org www.scalyskin.org Jean Pickford, Exec. Dir.

Genetic Alliance 4301 Connecticut Ave., NW, #404 Washington, DC 20008-2304 202-966-5557 800-336-GENE Fax 202-966-8553 www.geneticalliance.org

Advocacy, Registry, and Support Groups

Gluten Intolerance Group of North America (GIG) (**dermatitis herpetiformis**) 15110 10th Ave. SW Suite A Seattle, WA 98166-1820 (206)2466531 gig@accessone.com www.gluten.net

Hereditary Hemorrhagic Telangiectasia Foundation International PO Box 8087 New Haven, CT 06530 410-357-9932 800-448-6389 fax # 410-357-9932 hhinfo@hht.org www.hht.org Rita Van Bergejik, Ex. Dir.

Hermansky-Pudlak Syndrome Network, Inc. (HPS Network) One South Road Oyster Bay, NY 11771-1905 516-922-3440 800-789-9477 Fax 516-922-4022

Histiocytosis Association of America 302 N. Broadway Pitman, NJ 08017 609-589-6606 800-548-2758 609-589-6614 histiocyte@aol.com www.histio.org

Incontinentia Pigmenti Support Network 34929 Elm Wayne, MI 48184

International **Fibrodysplasia Ossificans Progressiva** Association (IFOPA) PO Box 196217 Winter Springs, FL 32719-6217 407-365-4194 ifopa@vol.com www.med.upenn.edu/ortho/fop

International **Progeria** Registry NY State Institute for Basic Research 1050 Forest Hill Rd. Staten Island, NY 10314 718-494-5333 fax # 718-494-1026

Klippel-Trenaunay Support Group 5404 Dundee Rd. Edina, MN 55436 952-925-2596 fax # 952-925-4708 jvessey@uswest.net

Lupus Foundation of America, Inc. 1300 Piccard Drive, Suite 200 Rockville, MD 20850-4303 301-670-9292 800-558-0121 fax # 301-670-9486 lfanatl@aol.com www.lupus.org/lupus Deb Blom, Interim Exec. Dir. Duane Peters, Dir. of Communications & Advocacy

National **Alopecia Areata** Foundation 710 C Street, Suite 11 San Rafael, CA 94901 415-456-4644 fax # 415-456-4274 naaf@compuserve.com www.alopeciaareata.com Vicki Kalabokes, Exec. Dir.

National Association for **Pseudoxanthoma Elasticum** 3500 East 12th Avenue Denver, CO 80206 303-355-3866 fax # 303-355-3859 pxenape@estreet.com www.ttuhsc.edu/pages/nape Al Ferrari, President

National Association for **Pseudoxanthoma Elasticum** 3500 East 12th Ave. Denver, CO 80206 303-355-3866 fax # 303-355-3859 pxenape@estreet.com www.napxe.org Carolyn Freedman, Ex. Dir.

National Ataxia Foundation (**Ataxia-Telangiectasia**) 2600 Fernbrook Lane, Suite 119 Plymouth, MN 55447-4752 763-553-0020 fax # 763-553-0167 naf@mr.net www.ataxia.org

National **Eczema** Association for Science & Education (NEASE) 1220 SW Morrison St., Suite 433 Portland, OR 97205 503-228-4430 800-818-7546 fax # 503-224-3363 nease@teleport.com www.eczema-assn.org Robert O. McAlister, Ph.D., Exec. Dir.

National Foundation for **Ectodermal Dysplasias** 410 E. Main Street PO Box 114 Mascoutah, IL 62258-0114 618-566-2020 fax # 618-566-4718 nfed4@aol.com www.nfed.org Mary Kaye Richter, Exec. Dir.

National Incontinentia Pigmenti Foundation (NIPF) 30 East 72nd St., 16th Floor New York, NY 10021 212-452-1231 fax # 212-452-1406 nipf@pipeline.com

National **Lymphatic & Venous Diseases** Foundation, Inc. 255 Commandants Way Chelsea, MA 02150 617-889-2103 800-301-2103

National **Lymphedema** Network Latham Square 1611 Telegraph Ave., Suite 1111 Oakland, CA 94612-2138 510-208-3200 800-541-3259 fax# 510-208-3110 www.lymphnet.org

National **Marfan** Foundation 382 Main Street Port Washington, NY 11050 516-883-8712 800-862-7326 fax # 516-883-8040 staff@marfan.org www.marfan.org Carolyn Levering, Exec. Dir.

Advocacy, Registry, and Support Groups

National **Neurofibromatosis** Foundation (NNFF) 95 Pine St., 16th Floor New York, NY 10005 212-344-NNFF   800-323-7938   fax # 212-747-0004   TDD:212-344-NNFF   NNFF@aol.com www.nf.org

National Organization for **Albinism** & Hypopigmentation (NOAH) PO Box 959 E. Hampstead, NH   03826-0959   603-887-2310   800-473-2310   Fax 603-887-2310   noah@albinism.org www.albinism.org

National Organization for Rare Disorders, Inc. PO Box 8923 New Fairfield, CT 06812-8923 203-746-6518   800-999-6673   Fax 203-746-6481 www.rarediseases.org

National **Pemphigus** Foundation   P.O. Box 9606   Berkeley, CA 94709-0606   510-527-4970   fax # 510-527-8497

PVnews@aol.com   www.pemphigus.org   Janet Segall

National **Psoriasis** Foundation   6600 SW 92nd Ave., Suite 300   Portland, OR 97223-7195   503-244-7404 800-723-9166   fax # 503-245-0626   getinfo@npfusa.org   www.psoriasis.org   Gail Zimmerman, Exec. Dir.

National Registry for **Ichthyosis** & Related Disorders   University of Washington, Dept. of Dermatology Box 356524 Seattle, WA 98195-6524   800-595-1266 ichreg@u.washington.edu

National **Tuberous Sclerosis** Association, Inc. (NTSA)   8181 Professional Place, Suite 110 Landover, MD 20785   800-225-6872   301-459-9888   fax # 301-459-0394   ntsa@ntsa.org www.ntsa.org Vicky Whittemore

National **Vitiligo** Foundation 611 South Fleishel Ave. Tyler, TX 75701 903-531-0074 fax # 903-525-1234 vitiligo@trimofran.org www.vitiligofoundation.org Shannon Ruesewald, Exec. Dir.

National **Vulvodynia** Association   P.O. Box 4491 Silver Spring, MD 20914-4491 301-299-0775 fax # 301-299-3999   matenva@graphcom.com   www.nva.org   Phyllis Mate, Exec. Dir.

Neurofibromatosis, Inc. 8855 Annapolis Rd., #110 Lanham, MD 20706-2924   301-577-8984 800-942-6825 fax # 301-577-0016   TDD 410-461-5213 NFInc1@aol.com www.nfinc.org

Nevus Network   PO Box 1981 Woodbridge, VA 22193 703-492-0253 405-377-3403 nevus-net@bigfoot.com www.nevusnetwork.org

Nevus Outreach, Inc. 1616 Alpha Street Lansing, MI 48910 877-426-3887 517-487-2306 fax # 515-684-0953 info@nevus.org   www.nevus.org   Kevin Williams, President

Osteogenesis Imperfecta Foundation 5005 W. Laurel St., Suite 210 Tampa, FL 33607   813-282-1161   813-287-8214   Vonnie H. Coleman, Ex. Dir.

Proteus Syndrome Foundation (PSF) 6235 Whetstone Dr. Colorado Springs, CO 80918 719-264-8445 abscit@aol.com www.proteus-syndrome.org

PXE International, Inc. (**Pseudoxanthoma Elasticum**) 23 Mountain St. Sharon, MA 02067   781-784-3817   fax # 781-784-6672   STerry@pxe.org   www.pxe.org   Ms. Sharon Terry, President

Rubinstein-Taybi Parent Contact Group PO Box 146 Smith Center, KS 66967 913-697-2984

Scleroderma Foundation 89 Newbury Street Suite 201 Danvers, MA 01923-1075 978-750-4499 800-422-1113   Helpline: 800-722-HOPE   fax # 978-750-9902   sfinfo@scleroderma.org   scle-rofed@aol.com   www.scleroderma.org   Karl Kastorf, Exec. Dir.

Scleroderma Research Foundation   Pueblo Medical Commons 2320 Bath Street, Suite 307 Santa Barbara, CA 93105   805-563-1164   fax # 805-563-2402   srfsure@srfcure.org   www.srfcure.org Sharon Monsky

Share & Care (**Cockayne Syndrome**) Network, Inc. PO Box 552 Stanleytown, VA 24168-0552 540-629-2369   fax # 540-647-3739   cockayne@kimbanet.com   www.kimbanet.com/cockayne

Advocacy, Registry, and Support Groups

Sjögren's Syndrome Foundation   333 N. Broadway, Suite 2000   Jericho, NY 11753   516-933-6365   fax # 516-933-6368   ssf@idt.net   www.sjogrens.com   Alexis Stegemann, Exec. Dir.

Sturge-Weber Foundation   PO Box 418   Mt. Freedom, NJ 07970-0418   973-895-4445   800-627-5482   fax # 973-895-4846   swf@sturge-weber.com   info@sturge-weber.com   www.sturge-weber.com   Karen Ball, Exec. Dir.

Xeroderma Pigmentosum Registry   UMD New Jersey Medical School Department of Pathology Medical Science Building, Room C-520   185 S. Orange Ave. Newark,NJ   07103-2714   201-982-6255   fax # 201-982-7293

Xeroderma Pigmentosum Society   PO Box 4759   Poughkeepsie, NY 12602   518-851-2612   fax # 518-851-2612   xps@xps.org   www.xps.org   Caren Mahar

Allergies and Sensitizers

airborne contact	poison ivy-oak-sumac (burning), pollen, ragweed
allergens, common	balsam of Peru, benzocaine, cosmetics, ethylenediamine hydrochloride, mercurochrome, mercaptobenzothiazole, neomycin, nickel, perfumes, poison ivy, poison oak, potassium dichromate, thimerosal
antibiotic allergy	neomycin, penicillin, streptomycin
antibiotic patch-test series	ampicillin 5% aq., bacitracin 20% in pet., chloramphenicol 5% in pet., clindamycin 1% aq., erythromycin 5% in pet., furacin 0.2% in pet., garamycin 20% in pet., lincomycin 1% aq., mafenide 5% in pet., neomycin 20% in pet. nystatin 100,000 units/mL in alcohol, penicillin 100,000 units/ml, polymxin B 3% in pet., sodium fusidate 2% in pet., streptomycin 2.5% aq. sol., sulfanilamide 5% in pet., tetracycline 5% in pet., tetracycline 5% in pet., tobramycin 20% in pet.
arsenic containing	Asiatic pills, DeValagin's solution, Donovan's solution, Fowler's solution
black-rubber mix containing	boots, cane tip, eyeglass holder, gloves (black rubber), knee-high stocking rubber ring, money counters, scuba mask, shoes, squash ball, tires, truncheon, underwear elastic, wind surfing boards
carba mix containing	1,3-diphenylguanidine, diethydithiocarbamate, dibutyldithiocarbamate (natural rubber latex in shoes)
cement dermatitis	cobalt, **dichromate**, nickel
cheilitis, allergic	carrots, coffee, menthol, orange peel
Compositae **family**	see *sesquiterpene lactone containing plants*
corticosteroid classes, based on cross-reactivity	**Class A**: hydrocortisone, hydrocortisone with C17 or C21 acetate ester, methylprednisolone +/- acetate, prednisone, prednisolone +/- acetate, tixocortol pivalate **Class B**: amcinonide, budesonide, desonide, flucinonide, fluocinolone acetonide, halcinonide, triamcinolone **Class C**: betamethasone (not valerate), betamethasone & disodium phosphate, desoxymethasone, dexamethasone & disodium phosphate, flucortolone **Class D**: aclomethasone dipropionate, betamethasone valerate & dipropionate, clobetasol propionate & butyrate, fluocortolone hexanoate & pivalate, hydrocortisone-17 butyrate, hydrocortisone butyrate & valerate, prenicarbate
corticosteroids, paraben-free	Dermolate anti-itch cream, Dermolate scalp itch lotion, Hytone cream, Rhulicort cream & lotion
cosmetic ingredients	fragrance, lanolin, Quaternium 15
douche sensitizers	benzethonium chloride, eucalyptus oil, methyl salicylate, oxyquinoline, perfumes, phenylmercuric acetate, thymol
eczema, delayed & urticaria	see *urticaria & delayed eczema*
eczematous contact dermatitis	alcohol, balsam of Peru, benzoic acid, cinnamic acid, cinnamic aldehyde, cobalt chloride, sodium benzoate, sorbic acid
elderly, common sensitizers	dichromates, nickel, paraphenylenediamine, poison ivy, poison oak, poison sumac, ragweed, rubber

Allergies and Sensitizers

eyeglass frame dermatitis	azo dyes, beeswax-turpentine mixture, butyl acrylate, cellulose acetate, cellulose propionate, epoxy resin, ethyl acetate, ethylene blycol, ethylene oxide, nickel, *p*-tert-butylphenol, phenyl salicylate, resorcinol monobenzoate, tricresyl phosphate, triphenyl phosphate
eyelid dermatitis	cosmetics, nail polish (toluene sulfonamide/formaldehyde resin)
formaldehyde-containing	**apparel**: anti-wrinkle, anti-static, chamois, chlorine resistant, mildew resistant, moth-proof finish, permanent press, screen prints, suede, wash & wear, waterproof finish cements & pastes, cleaning fluids, dry cleaning, **cosmetics**: bath oil, bubble bath, fingernail polish, shampoo, wave sets, fixatives embalming fluid **medications**: anhidrotics, contraceptives, denatured alcohol, methenamine, mouthwashes, orthopedic casts, renal dialysis, tanning agents, wart removers **other**: antiperspirants, paints, polishes, preservatives phenolic resins & urea plastics (buttons, jewelry, adhesives, footwear) photographic plates and chemicals smoke from burning charcoal, cigarettes, cigars, coal, wood toxoids & vaccines
fragrance	cinnamic alcohol, cinnamic aldehyde
hairdressers	*para*-phenylenediamine, nickel, glyceryl monothioglycolate, formaldehyde, hair dyes, perfumes, rubber gloves
hand dermatitis; foods	corn, fruit juice, pineapple, wet foods
histamines	beefsteak, cheese, chicken liver, eggplant, spinach, tomatoes, wine (red)
hypersensitivity reactions	**Type I (IgE-dependent)**: anaphylaxis, IgE mast cell degranulation; pruritus, urticaria **Type II (cytotoxic)**: hapten binding to tissue proteins, drug-antibody complex formation **Type III (immune complex)**: drug-antibody conjugates enter circulation; serum sickness, immune complex vasculitis, occurs 7-10 days after exposure **Type IV (cell-mediated, delayed hypersensitivity)**: T-lymphocyte mediated with release of lymphokines; allergic contact dermatitis
jewelry	nickel
leather	chromates
lemon, orange peel	limonene
leukoderma, contact	butylcatechol, *para*-tertiary butylphenol, phenolic detergents
mercaptobenzothiazole-containing	adhesives, black tires, cleansers, detergents, fungicides, greases, photographic film emulsion, rubber, rubberized fabrics (bras & girdles), shoes, veterinarian medicaments
metals	chromium, nickel

Allergies and Sensitizers

nail polish	toluene sulfonamide/formaldehyde resin
neomycin cross-reactors	butirosin, gentamicin, kanamycin, paromomycin, spectinomycin, streptomycin, tobramycin
neomycin-sensitive	use betadine, Bactroban, ilotycin
paraphenylenediamine	coloring agent to dye hair; frequent cause of contact dermatitis in hairdresser's hands
patch test (standard)	**Hermal; medications**: benzocaine, neomycin sulfate **preservatives**: imidazolidinyl urea, quaternium-15, formaldehyde **rubber compounds**: thiuram mix, mercaptobenzothiazole, carba mix, black rubber IPPD, mercapto mix **vehicle**: lanolin alcohol **metals**: nickel sulfate, potassium dichromate **fragrances**: cinnamic aldehyde, balsam of Peru **resins**: epoxy, *p-tert*-butylphenol formaldehyde, colophony **miscellaneous**: ethylenediamine dihydrochloride, *p*-phenylenediamine **T.R.U.E.; medication**: quinoline mix, caine mix, neomycin sulfate **preservatives**: paraben mix, Cl Me isothiasolinone, thimerosal, quaternium-15, formaldehyde **rubber compounds**: thiuram mix, mercaptobenzothiazole, carba mix, black rubber PPD mix, mercapto mix **vehicles**: wood alcohol **metals**: cobalt chloride, nickel sulfate, potassium dichromate **fragrances**: fragrance mix, balsam of Peru **resins**: epoxy, *p-tert*-butylphenol formaldehyde, colophony **miscellaneous**: ethylenediamine dihydrochloride, *p*-phenylenediamine
patch test grading	**?**; doubtful reaction manifested by faint erythema **+1**; weak positive reaction manifested by infiltrated erythema with possible papules **+2**; strong reaction showing papules & vesicles **+3**; extreme reaction with confluent bullae
photoallergic dermatitis	**antibiotic/antifungal**: bithionol, fenticlor, jadit, multifungin, salicylanilides (halogenated) **fragrances**: 6-methylcoumarin, musk ambrette **medications**: chlorpromazine, piroxicam, promethazine, sulfanilamide **miscellaneous**: plants of the *Compositae* family, diphenhydramine, psoralen, sandalwood, stilbenes, sulfonylureas, thiazides **sunscreens**: benzophenone, digalloyltrioleate, PABA esters
phototoxic	**coal-tar**: acridine, anthracene, phenanthrene **drugs**: phenothiazines, sulfonamides **dyes**: acridine orange, acriflavine, anthraquinone, dibromofluorescein, eosin, methylene blue, neutral red, rose bengal, toluidine blue **furocoumarins**: psoralen, 8-methoxypsoralen, 4,5,8-trimethylpsoralen
phytophotodermatitis-causing	*Compositae*: milfoil, stinking mayweed, yarrow *Moraceae*: figs *Papilionaceae*: psoralen *Rutaceae*: bergamot, bitter orange, burning bush, fraxinella, gas plant, lemon, lime, Persian lime *Umbelliferae*: angelica, carrot, chervil (wild), cow parsley, dill, fennel, giant hogweed, lovage, masterwort, parsnip

Allergies and Sensitizers

plastic	acrylic nails, resins (epoxy & formaldehyde), nail lacquer
poison ivy, oak	catechols, urushiol (Rhus plants) see *Toxicodendron*
preservatives in food	benzoic acid, calcium propionate, citric acid, monoglycerol citrate, parabens, polysorbate, quaiac gum, sodium benzoate, sodium bisulfite, sorbic acid
rhus-containing	Brazilian pepper, cashews, gingko tree, Indian marking nut, poison ivy, poison oak, poison sumac, Japanese lacquer tree, mango, rengas tree
rosacea (avoid)	**activity/emotions**: anxiety, **exercise, stress** **beverages: alcohol** (esp. beer, bourbon, champagne, gin, red wine, vodka), **hot drinks** (all kinds) **foods**: avocados, bananas, broad leaf beans and pods (navy, lima, pea), cheese (except cottage cheese), chocolate, citrus fruits, eggplant, figs, foods high in histamine, liver, plums (red), raisins, sour cream, soy sauce, **spicy foods**, spinach, thermally hot foods, tomatoes, vanilla, vinegar, yeast extract, yogurt **medications**: vasodilators, topical steroids **medical conditions**: chronic cough, menopause **skin care products**: acetone, fragrances, hydro-alcohol, witch hazel **temperatures**: hot baths, hot tubs, overheating, saunas **weather: cold weather, hot weather**, humidity, strong winds, **sun**
sensitized to: may be sensitive to/flares with	**benzocaine**: azo dyes, PAS, procaine, sulfa **ethylenediamine**: tripelennamine/pyribenzamine, pyrilamine/Triaminic, piperazine, hydroxyzine groups (aminophylline, Merthiolate, Mycolog) **formaldehyde**: methenamine **iodine**: contrast agents, SSKI **neomycin**: aminoglycosides **PABA**: azo dyes, PAS, procaine, sulfa poison ivy: mangoes **PPD**: azo dyes, PAS, procaine, sulfa **thiuram**: disulfiram
sensitizers, topical that may provoke reaction upon systemic administration	balsam of Peru, caladryl, chlorobutanol, cobalt, diphenhydramine, disulfiram, ethylenediamine hydrochloride, ethyl aminobenzoate, formaldehyde, halogenated hydroxyquinolones, hydrazine hydrobromide, iodine, mercurials (organic & inorganic), metallic mercury, neomycin, paraphenylenediamine, resorcinol, thiamin, thiram
sensitizers; topical that may sensitize & related medications that may produce contact-type dermatitis	alcohol: alcoholic beverages aminophylline suppositories: ethylenediamine antihistamine ammoniated mercury: organic & inorganic mercurials, mercury amalgam antistine drops: ethylenediamine antihistamines arnica (tincture): elixir terpene hydrate balsam of Peru: benzoin inhalation Benadryl; dramamine benzocaine: *see para-amino compounds* bismark brown: *see para-amino compounds* disphenol A: diethylstilbestrol caladryl cream: benadryl, dramamine chlorobutanol: chloralhydrate chloroquin: atabrine cobalt chloride: vitamin B12 epoxy amine hardener: ethylenediamine antihistamine, aminophylline ethylenediamine hydrochloride: ethylenediamine antihistamines formaldehyde: urotropin, mandelamine, urised glyceryl PABA

sensitizers *(continued)*	*see para-amino compounds* halogenated hydroxyquinolines: vioform, dioquin hydralizine hydrochloride: isoniazid, apresoline, nardil iodine: iodides, iodinated organic compounds mercurochrome: *see mercury* mercury:mercurial diuretics, calomel, mercury amalgam methylene blue: phenothiazines neomycin sulfate: streptomycin, kanamycin, framycetin, paranomycin orange peel oil: elixir terpene hydrate para-amino compounds: PABA, azo dyes, Dymelor, Orinase, Diabinese, sulfonamides, Diuril, Hydrodiuril, Saluron, renese, para-aminosalicylic acid phenothiazine: phenergan quinilor compound: vioform, dioquin resorcin: hexylresorcinal thiram, disulfram: antabuse triethylenetetramine: ethylenediamine antihistamine, aminophylline turpentine-cardamon flavor: elixir terpene hydrate
sesquiterpene lactone containing plants	arnica, artichoke, bitterweed, boneset, broomweed, burdock, burrobrush, capeweed, chamomile, champaca, chicory, chrysanthemum, cocklebur, cosmos, costus, cottonthistle, encelia, feverfew, fireweed, fleabane, guayule, hempweed, ironweed, laurel oil, leafcup, lettuce, liverwort, marguerite, marigold, marsh elder, oxeye, pyrethrum, ragweed, sagebrush, sneezeweed, sowthistle, starthistle, stinkwort, sunflower, tansy, tulip tree, whitewood, wormwood, yarrow
shoe dermatitis	mercaptobenzothiazole, tetraethylthiuram, potassium dichromate, *para*-tertiary butylphenol formaldehyde
spermicide sensitizers	hexylresorcinol, nonoxyl, oxyquinoline sulfate, phenylmercuric acitate, phenylmercuric borate, quinine hydrochloride
spices; eczematous dermatitis	capsicum, cayenne pepper, cinnamon, cloves, laurel, mace, nutmeg, vanilla
sunscreens	PABA
systemic dermatitis	alcohol, aminophylline, azo dyes, benzocaine, calomel, chloral hydrate, cinnamon, diphenhydramine, doxylamine, dramamine, ethylenediamine (Phenergan), formaldehyde, hydralazine, hydrazine, iodine, isoniazid, mandelamine, mercurials, methenamine, Nardil, neomycin, oral hypoglycemic agents, PABA, *para*-phenylenediamine, p-aminosalicylic acid, penicillin, phenothiazines, procaine, potassium iodide, procainamide, quinine, quinidine, resorcinol, saccharin, silvadene, streptomycin, sulfonamides, thiamin, thiuram, vitamin B12
textiles	azo dyes
thiuram-containing	disinfectants, fungicides, germicides, insecticides, latex preservative, lubricating oils, neoprene, neoprene adhesives, pesticides, polyolefin plastics, putty, repellents, rubber vulcanization accelerators, shampoo, soap
***Toxicodendron* plants**	poison ivy (*Toxicodendron radicans*), poison oak (*Toxicodendron quercifolium*), poison oak (*Toxicodendron diversiloba*), poison sumac (*Toxicodendron vernix*) **relatives**: black varnish tree, Brazilian pepper, cashew nut tree, el litre tree, ginko tree, Japanese lacquer tree, mango, marking nut tree (India), pepeo tree, rengas tree

Allergies and Sensitizers

ulcers, agents may cause sensitization	ethylenediamine hydrochloride, lanolin, neomycin, nitrofurazone, paraben preservatives, Vitamin E creams
urticaria	**cholinergic**: emotional stress, exercise, heat **foods**: bananas, caffeine, cheese, chocolate, citrus, coffee, cow milk, eggs, fish, grapes, mushrooms, nuts, pork, shellfish, strawberries, tomatoes, vegetables, wheat, yeast fermentation (alcohol) **fungus**: dermatophytes, **candidiasis** **infection**: dental, sinus, tonsillar, gallbladder, GI, GU **inhalants**: pollens, mold, feather down, smoke, volatile chemicals, animal dander, spores, aerosols, dust **injectants**: blood, insect stings, vaccines **insects**: bedbugs, mites, fleas **medications**: amidopyrine, antibiotics, **aspirin**, atropine, cocaine, codeine, ibuprofen, indomethacin, mefanamic acid, morphine, **penicillin**, phenylbutazone, pilocarpine, polymyxin B, quinine, sodium benzoate, sulindac, tartrazine (FDA yellow dye, No. 5), thiamin **parasites**: amebiasis, *Ancylostoma, Ascaris, Echinococcus, Fasciola*, Filariae, giardiasis, malaria, *Schistosoma, Strongyloides, Trichinella, Toxocara* **physical**: cold, heat, pressure, solar, vibration, water **viral**: hepatitis B, infectious mononucleosis, coxsackie
urticaria & delayed eczema	acrylic acid, ammonium persulfate, benzocaine, castor bean, cinnamic aldehyde, endive, epoxy resin, latex, lemon perfume, lettuce, nickel, rhodium, platinum, rubber, sorbic acid, teak, vinyl pyridine
urticaria, cold	cryoglobulinemia, cryofibrinogenemia, cold hemolysins, syphilis, connective tissue d., hematopoietic malignancy
urticaria, contact	**animals**: arthropods, cockroach, dander, guinea pig, hair, jellyfish, saliva (dog, rat) **antibiotics**: bacitracin, cephalosporin, chloramphenicol, gentamicin, neomycin, penicillin, rifamycin, streptomycin **chemicals**: acrylic monomer, aliphatic polyamine, aminophenazone, aminothiazole, ammonia, ammonium persulfate, balsam of Peru, benzaldehyde, benzoic acid, benzophenone, butyl-hydroxytoluene, camphor, $CaOCl_2$, cassia oil, cetyl alcohol, cinnamic acid, cinnamic aldehyde, clioquinol, cobalt chloride, diethyltoluamide, dimethylsulfoxide, diphenylcyclopropenone, epoxy resin, ethyl aminobenzoate, lanolin, lindane, formaldehyde, menthol, monoamylamine, NaOCl, parabens (ethyl, methyl), polyethylene glycol 3-400, polysorbate, phenyl mercuric propionate, p-aminodiphhenylamine, platinum salts, salicylic acid, sorbic acid, stearyl alcohol, sulfur dioxide, terpinyl acetate, vanillin, vinyl pyridine, vitamin E oil, xylene **medications**: *see medication section* **cosmetics**: nail polish, hair spray, perfumes **foods**: apricot pit, apple, bean, beer, buckwheat flour, caraway seed, carrot, cucumber pickle, egg, endive, fish, flour, garlic, kiwi, lettuce, litchi, maize, mango, meat (chicken, lamb, turkey, beef, liver, pork), milk, mustard, peach, peanut, potato, rice, salami casing (mold), shellfish, soybean, spices, strawberry, tomato, watermelon **other**: serum (horse, tetanus), rhus, rubber **plants**: cactus, marine plants, nettles

Allergies and Sensitizers

urticaria, contact (*continued*)	**textiles**: silk, wool **wood**: exotic woods
urticaria, immediate (foods)	**fruits**: apple, kiwi, peach, strawberry **meats**: beef, calf liver, lamb, pork, turkey **miscellaneous**: beer, cheese, egg, flour, milk, salad dressing (sorbic acid) **seafood**: codfish, lobster, prawns, shrimp **vegetables**: bean, carrot, lettuce, onion, parsley, parsnip, potato, rice, tomato
urticaria, non-allergic contact	acetic acid, alcohol, balsam of Peru, benzoic acid, caterpillar hair, cinnamic acid, cinnamic aldehyde, cobalt chloride, dimethyl sulfoxide, insect stings, methyl nicotinate, moths, nicotinic acid ester, sodium benzoate, sorbic acid
vegetables, eczematous dermatitis	artichoke, asparagus, carrot, celery, chicory, chives, corn, cucumber, endive, garlic, horseradish, leek, lettuce, onion
vitiligo, contact	**chemicals**: diisoprophyl fluorophosphate, hydroquinione, mercaptoamines, *p*-cresol, *p*-isopropylcathechol, *p*-methylcatechol, *p*-nonylphenol, *p*-octylphenol, *p-tert*-amylphenol, *p-tert*-butylcatechol, *p-tert*-butylphenol, physostigmine, thio-TEPA **other**: adhesive tape, germicidal phenolic detergents, latex glue, rubber products, shoes, wristwatch straps

Diseases or Signs and Their Associations

Disease or Sign	Association
acanthosis nigricans	acrochordons, acromegaly, Addison's d., Bloom's s., cancer (gastric), Crouzon's s., Cushing's d., diabetes mellitus, drugs, gonadal d., hyperandrogenic states, hyperinsulinism, hyperthyroidism, hypogonadism with insulin resistance, hypothyroidism, **insulin resistance**, Lawrence-Seip s., **obesity**, polycystic ovary s., pituitary extract therapy, pituitary tumor, pinealoma, polycystic ovary s., Rabson-Mendenhall s., Rud's s., Seip-Lawrence s., thyroid d., tripe palm, Wilson's d.
acanthosis nigricans, malignant	**adenocarcinoma** (bowel, breast, gallbladder, **gastric**), Hodgkin's lymphoma, liver, lung, mycosis fungoides, ovaries, prostate
acne	calcinosis cutis, chronic granulomatous d., hypopigmentation, hyperpigmentation, keloid scars, SAPHO s.
acne necrotica miliaris	professional persons, stress
acne venenata	asbestos, chlorinated aromatic hydrocarbons, cosmetics, crude petrolatum, cutting oil, DDT, heavy coal tar distillates, steroids
acquired perforating disorder	chronic active hepatitis, chronic renal failure, **diabetes**, hypothyroidism, internal malignancy, liver failure
acroangiodermatitis	AVM, chronic venous insufficiency
actinic elastosis	actinic purpura, colloid milium, nodular elastosis, poikiloderma of Civatte, stellate spontaneous pseudoscars
acute myelogenous leukemia	neutrophilic eccrine hidradenitis, Sweet's s.
acute necrotizing ulcerative gingivitis	fatigue, HIV, poor oral hygiene, smoking, stress
Addison's d.	adrenal hemorrhage, amyloidosis, cytomegalovirus, histoplasmosis, Hodgkin's lymphoma, metastatic carcinoma, pituitary gland dysfunction, primary adrenal gland failure, sarcoidosis, tuberculosis, vitiligo
adenoma	Muir-Torre s.
adenoma sebaceum	*see angiofibroma*
AIDS	*see HIV infection*
alcoholism/ETOH consumption	**dermatologic**: flushing, furuncles, leukoplakia, nail changes, nummular eczema, oral carcinoma, griseofulvin intolerance, hyperpigmentation, lichenoid dermatitis, oral changes, palmar erythema, pruritus, psoriasis, pyoderma vegetans, telangiectasia, unilateral nevoid telangiectasia, urticaria **endocrine**: hypogonadism, hyperestrogenism, PCT, pseudo-Cushing's s. **exacerbated diseases**: discoid eczema, psoriasis, rosacea **infections**: erysipelas, *Vibrio vulnificus* sepsis, acquired purpura fulminans, pancreatitis, subcutaneous fat necrosis **nutritional**: marasmus, kwashiorkor, pellagra, riboflavin (B2) deficiency, scurvy, zinc deficiency **other**: coagulopathy, Cullen's sign, Dupuytren's contracture, Grey-Turner's sign, Madelung's d.

Diseases or Signs and Their Associations

Disease or Sign	Association
alopecia areata	*see hair section*
amyloidosis	familial Mediterranean fever, Muckle-Wells s.
amyloidosis, lichen	Chinese, connective tissue d., eczema (associated with celiac d.), HIV, MEN 2A, Naegeli-Franceschetti-Jadassohn s., pachyonychia congenita, PUVA, radiodermatitis, Riehl's melanosis, SLE
amyloidosis, macular	Asians, connective tissue d., eczema (associated with celiac d.), MEN 2A, Middle Easterners, Naegeli-Franceschetti-Jadassohn s., nostalgia paresthetica, pachyonychia congenita, primary biliary cirrhosis, PUVA, radiodermatitis, Riehl's melanosis, scleroderma, SLE, South Americans
amyloidosis, nodular	paraproteinemia, proteinuria
amyloidosis, primary	multiple myeloma (15%)
amyloidosis, secondary	actinic keratosis, Addison's d., annular elastolytic giant cell granuloma, BCC, Bowen's d., CTCL, cylindroma, dermatofibroma, dystrophic epidermolysis bullosa, hidradenitis suppurativa, junctional nevus, lepromatous leprosy, osteomyelitis, pilomatrixoma, porokeratosis, PUVA treated, RA, seborrheic keratosis, syphilis, tuberculosis
amyloidosis, secondary systemic	**autoimmune**: ankylosing spondylitis, Behçet's s., IBD, RA, Reiter's s., Sjögren's s., SLE **dermatologic**: acne, burns, EB panniculitis, ectodermal dysplasia, hidradenitis suppurativa, leprosy, psoriasis, venous ulcer **other**: bronchiectasis, Castleman's d., cystic fibrosis, diabetes mellitus, Hodgkin's d., infections (recurrent)
anetoderma	AIDS, elastin abnormalities, familial, immunologic defects
angioedema	hypocomplementemic urticarial vasculitis s., urticarial vasculitis
angiofibroma	adenoma sebaceum, Bourneville's s., fibrous papules of the nose, oral fibromas, pearly penile papules, perifollicular fibromas, tuberous sclerosis, Vogt triad
angiokeratoma circumscriptum	cavernous hemangioma, Cobb's s., Klippel-Trenaunay-Weber s., nevus flammeus
angiokeratoma of Fordyce	hernia, lymphogranuloma venereum, prostatitis, thrombophlebitis, variocele
angiokeratomas	Fabry's d., fucosidosis, Klippel-Trenaunay-Weber s., sialidosis
angiolymphoid hyperplasia with eosinophilia	regional LAD, peripheral eosinophilia
angiotensin converting enzyme (ACE) elevations	berylliosis, chronic inflammatory d., diabetes mellitus, Gaucher's d., leprosy, malignant histiocytosis, *Mycobacterium avium intracellulare* infection, sarcoid, silicosis, tuberculosis
annulus migrans	acropustulosis, generalized pustular psoriasis, Reiter's s.
aplasia cutis congenita	4p-syndrome, 13-trisomy s., Adams-Oliver s., Bart's s., ectodermal dysplasia, oculo-cerebro-cutaneous s.

Diseases or Signs and Their Associations

Disease or Sign	Association
arthritis mutilans	multicentric reticulohistiocytosis, psoriasis
asthma	IgA deficiency s.
ataxia telangiectasia	carcinoma (biliary, gastric, ovarian), leukemia, lymphoma
atopic dermatitis (*see also eczema*)	acne (decreased), allergic rhinitis (>15%), anhidrotic ectodermal dysplasia, asthma, cataracts, chronic granulomatous d., conjunctivitis, eczema herpeticum, exfoliative erythroderma, geographic tongue, growth retardation, **ichthyosis vulgaris**, keratosis pilaris, Netherton's d., pityriasis alba, secondary infections, urticaria, **xerosis** (>50%) **rare associated diseases**: acrodermatitis enteropathica, agammaglobulinemia, ahistidinemia, ataxia telangiectasia, hyper IgE s., IgA deficiency s., IgM deficiency s., phenylketonuria, tyrosinemia, Wiskott-Aldrich s., X-linked agammaglobulinemia (Bruton's)
atopy	allergic rhinitis, **asthma**, cheilitis, conjunctivitis, Dennie-Morgan lines, geographic tongue, ichthyosis vulgaris, IgA deficiency s., **keratosis pilaris**, Netherton's s., Staphylococcal infections, urticaria, viral infections (molluscum, HSV), white dermatographism, xerosis
atrophoderma (follicular)	Bazex's s., chondrodysplasia punctata
atrophoderma vermiculatum	birefringent hairs, Eisenmenger complex, epidermal cysts, folliculitis decalvans, intra-auricular septal defect, mongolism, Rombo s.
basal cell carcinoma	arsenic exposure (arsenic keratoses), amputation stumps, BCC nevus s., Basex s., Bowen's d., dermatofibroma, DLE, dermatofibroma, epidermolysis bullosa, epidermal nevus, gummas, Hermansky-Pudlak s., hidradenitis suppurativa, **immunosuppression**, leg ulcers, **light skin color**, linear epidermal nevi, linear unilateral basal cell nevus s., lupus vulgaris, Merkel cell ca., Muir-Torre s., nevus sebaceous of Jadassohn (5-7%), onchocerciasis, porokeratosis, radiotherapy, Rasmussen s., Rombo s., Rothmund-Thomson s., trauma, stasis dermatitis, **sun exposure**, vaccination scars, wire rimmed glasses, xeroderma pigmentosa
basal cell epithelioma	porokeratosis of Mibelli
Bazex's s.	cancer of upper respiratory system; tongue, pharynx, esophagus, lung
Becker's nevus	developmental defects (spina bifida, breast hypoplasia, limb asymmetry), smooth muscle hamartoma
biliary cirrhosis	hyperpigmentation, jaundice, lichen planus, nail clubbing, nodular xanthoma, palmar xanthoma, pruritus, sarcoid, tuberous xanthoma
birth, lesions presenting at	acrogeria, acrokeratosis verruciformis, aggressive infantile fibromatosis, aplasia cutis, ash leaf macule, blue rubber bleb nevus s., congenital self-healing reticulohistiocytoma, congenital total lipodystrophy, cutis marmorata telangiectatica congenita, diffuse and macular atrophic dermatosis, endovascular papillary angioendothelioma of childhood (Dabska tumor), epidermolysis bullosa (Koebner), erythema toxicum neonatorum, fibrous hamartoma of infancy, fibro-

Diseases or Signs and Their Associations

Disease or Sign	Association
	matosis colli, follicular atrophoderma, generalized congenital fibromatosis, hemangiomas, herpes gestationis, incontinentia pigmenti, infantile myofibromatosis, inflammatory linear verrucous epidermal nevus, infundibulofolliculitis, juvenile hyaline fibromatosis, juvenile xanthogranuloma, lymphangiomas of the alveolar ridges in neonates, mastocytoma, multiple lentigines s., nevus comedonicus, nevus lipomatosus cutaneous superficialis (Hoffman-Zurhelle), Peutz-Jeghers s., piebaldism, pili torti, pseudoainhum, self-healing reticulohistiocytosis, stiff skin s., smooth muscle hamartoma, transient neonatal pustular melanosis, verrucous nevus, Waardenburg's s., white forelock, white sponge nevus
Birt-Hogg-Dube s.	adenoma (colon), pulmonary cysts, renal tumors, spontaneous pneumothorax
Bloom's s.	adenocarcinoma (sigmoid colon), leukemia, lymphoma, lymphosarcoma, SCC
Bowen's d.	porokeratosis of Mibelli
bromhidrosis	thiabendazole administration
bullous pemphigoid	amyotrophic lateral sclerosis, diabetes mellitus, LE, myasthenia gravis, pernicious anemia, polymyositis, RA, thyroiditis, ulcerative colitis
calcinosis cutis	PACK s.
cancer	**breast**: ataxia-telangiectasia carriers, Cowden's s., Peutz-Jeghers s. **esophagus**: Howel-Evans' s. **gastrointestinal**: acanthosis nigricans, Cronkhite-Canada s., dermatomyositis, familial atypical multiple mole melanoma s., Muir-Torre s., Peutz-Jeghers s. **pancreas**: familial atypical multiple mole melanoma s., Peutz-Jeghers s. **pulmonary**: Langerhan's cell histiocytosis **renal**: von Hippel-Lindau d. **thyroid**: Gardner's s., Sipple's s.
candidiasis, chronic mucocutaneous	adrenal abnormalities, AIDS, biotin dependent carboxylase deficiency, common variable immunodeficiency, dental enamel dysplasia s., diabetes mellitus, DiGeorge's s., EEC s., hyper IgE s., hypogammaglobulinemia, hypoparathyroidism, hypothyroidism, immunodeficiency, iron deficiency, myasthenia gravis, myeloperoxidase deficiency, Nezelof's s., parathyroid, polyendocrinopathy, severe combined immunodeficiency s., thymoma, vitiligo
carcinoid s., precipitated by	avocados, cheese, chocolate, eating, eggplant, emotional stress, EtOH, hot beverages/foods, pressure (on the tumor), red plums, tomatoes, Valsalva maneuver, walnuts
Castleman's d.	HHV-8 (in HIV), POEMS s.
cellulitis	burns, eczema, edema, prior surgery, radiation therapy, tinea pedis
Chediak-Higashi s.	lymphoma

Diseases or Signs and Their Associations

Disease or Sign	Association
cheilitis granulomatosa	Crohn's d., Melkersson-Rosenthal s., sarcoidosis
chilblains	angiokeratoma of Mibelli, chronic myelomonocytic leukemia
chloracne	erythema nodosum, exposure (chlorinated phenols, cutting oil, dioxin, electrical insulation, fungicide, herbicide, insecticide, wood preservative), palmar & plantar hyperhidrosis, porphyric changes
cirrhosis, biliary	PACK s.
cirrhosis, hepatic	hemochromatosis, lichen planus, porphyria cutanea tarda, SLE
coloboma	Goltz's s., whistling face s.
Cowden's d.	breast cancer (30%), fibrocystic breast disease, GI polyps (35%), neurologic disease, ovarian cysts, thyroid cancer (5%)
Crohn's d.	epidermolysis bullosa acquisita, erythema multiforme, **erythema nodosum**, exfoliative dermatitis, false + Kveim test, herpes zoster, IgA deficiency, lichen nitidus, LE, necrotizing vasculitis, palmar erythema, polyarteritis nodosa, psoriasis, pustular response to trauma, **pyoderma gangrenosum**, Reiter's s., Stevens-Johnson s., striae, subcorneal pustular dermatosis, urticaria, vitiligo, zinc deficiency
Crouzon's s.	acanthosis nigricans
cryoglobulinemia, essential mixed	**autoimmune**: Behçet's d., hypersensitivity vasculitis, RA, Sjögren's s., SLE **lymphoproliferative**: CLL, lymphoma, multiple myeloma, Waldenstrom's macroglobulinemia **infectious**: cytomegalovirus, HBV, **HCV**, mononucleosis, subacute bacterial endocarditis, toxoplasmosis
CTCL	Hodgkin's d., large cell lymphoma, leukemia, myeloma, paraproteinemia
Cushing's s.	acanthosis nigricans, acne, alopecia, ecchymoses, hirsutism, McCune-Albright s., NAME s.
cutis marmorata, persistent	DeLang s., Down s., Trisomy 18
cutis verticis gyrata	acromegaly, Apert's s., acanthosis nigricans, amyloidosis, leukemia, myxedema, pachydermoperiostosis, Rosenthal-Kloepfer s., syphilis, Touraine-Solente-Golae s., tuberous sclerosis
cylindroma	Ancell-Spiegler s., Brooke-Spiegler s., trichoepitheliomas
Darier's d.	affective disorders, **bone cysts**, depression, epilepsy, encephalopathy, Kaposi's varicelliform eruption, mental retardation, renal agenesis, **retinitis pigmentosa**, salivary gland obstruction, schizophrenia, testicular agenesis **exacerbation**: lithium, sweating, trauma, UVB light
delusion of parasitosis	cerebral atherosclerosis, CVA, drug abuse, endocrinopathies, hemodialysis, medications, pellagra, vitamin B_{12} deficiency

Diseases or Signs and Their Associations

Disease or Sign	Association
dermatitis herpetiformis	Addison's d., diabetes mellitus, gluten sensitivity enteropathy, **intestinal lymphoma**, iodide sensitivity, LE, RA, thyroid disease, ulcerative colitis
dermatofibromas, multiple	myasthenia gravis, SLE
dermatomyositis	**cancer** (breast, bronchogenic, **ovary**, cervix, gastrointestinal, penile, non-melanoma skin), panniculitis (lobular), Raynaud's phenomenon, sclerodactyly
dermatophytosis, chronic	atopic dermatitis, corticosteroids, Cushing's d., diabetes mellitus, immunodeficiency, lymphoma
diabetes insipidus	eosinophilic granuloma of bone, Hand Schüller Christian d., xan thoma disseminatum
diabetes mellitus	**dermatologic**: acanthosis nigricans, alopecia areata, anhidrosis, atrophie blanche, bullous pemphigoid, central papillary atrophy, cherry angiomas, clear cell syringoma, dermatitis herpetiformis, dermatographism, diabetic bullae (bullosis diabeticorum), diabetic dermopathy (shin spot), Dunnigan s., EBA, erythrasma (women), erythromelalgia, finger pebbling, foot ulcers, leg ulcers, lichen planus, localized bullous pemphigoid, furuncles/carbuncles, granuloma annulare, hyperhidrosis, knuckle pads, Kyrle's d., lichen planus, necrobiosis lipoidica diabeticorum, necrotizing fasciitis, PXE, palmar/plantar fibromatosis, plane xanthoma, plantar fibromatosis, porphyria cutanea tarda, pruritus vulvae, reacting perforating collagenosis, reticulated erythematous mucinosis, scleredema, seborrheic dermatitis, skin tags, skin thickening, tendinous xanthoma, thrush, vitiligo, Werner's s., xanthoma disseminatum, yellow skin **infectious**: botryomycosis, chronic mucocutaneous candidiasis, chronic paronychia, crusted scabies, erosa interdigitalis blastomycetica, Fournier's gangrene, malignant external otitis (Pseudomonas), paronychia (Candida), vaginal candidiasis, *Vibrio vulnificus*, zygomycosis **nails**: paronychia, Beau's line, leukonychia, onychauxis, onychogryphosis, onycholysis, onychomadesis, onychomycosis, pterygium, pterygium inversum unguis, Rosenau's depressions, splinter hemorrhages, telangiectasias, Terry's nails, yellow nail s. **systemic**: ataxia telangiectasia, Achard-Thiers s., IgA deficiency, metageria, POEMS s., pangeria (Werner's s.), Prader-Willi s. **other**: glossodynia, gustatory sweating, Lawrence-Seip s., malum perforans pedis, night blindness, non-thrombocytopenic purpura, orodynia, partial lipodystrophy, pathologic gustatory sweating, penile fibromatosis (Peyronie's d.), perleche, premature aging, rubeosis, subcutaneous fat necrosis, Talwin addiction, total lipodystrophy
dialysis	polyarteritis nodosa, pruritus
Dowling-Degos' d.	hidradenitis suppurativa, Kitamura's reticulate acropigmentation

Diseases or Signs and Their Associations

Disease or Sign	Association
Down s.	alopecia areata, angular chelitis, atrophoderma vermiculata, chelitis, elastosis perforans serpiginosa, geographic tongue, hepatitis B, leukemia, lymphoma, macroglossia, scabies (crusted), perforating collagenosis, scabies, scrotal tongue, syringoma (eruptive)
DSAP	immunosuppressive therapy, p53, phototherapy for psoriasis, SCC
Dupuytren's d.	alcoholism, diabetes, liver disease, seizure disorders, smoking
dyskeratosis congenita	Hodgkin's d., leukemia, leukoplakia, nail dystrophy, rectal adenocarcinoma, SCC
dystrophic epidermolysis bullosa	absent nails, caries, failure to thrive, melanoma, milia, pseudo-syndactyly, SCC, sepsis, scarring, scarring alopecia
EB-recessive dystrophic	SCC
eczema	ataxia telangiectasia, atopic dermatitis, Bruton's x-linked agamma-globulinemia, cardio-facio-cutaneous s., chronic granulomatous d., Dubokowitz's s., episodic lymphopenia with lymphocytotoxin, house dust mite infestation, hyper IgE s., IgA deficiency, IgM deficiency, Leiner's d., Letterer-Siwe d., leukocyte alkaline phosphatase deficiency, lymphopenic aggamaglobulinemia, phenylketonuria, protein calorie deficiency, Wiskott-Aldrich s., x-linked agammaglobu-linemia, x-linked immunodeficiency with elevated IgM
eczema craquele	Hodgkin's d., myxedema, stomach adenocarcinoma, zinc deficiency
eczema herpeticum	**atopic dermatitis**, burns, contact dermatitis (chronic irritant), congenital ichthyosiform erythroderma, Darier's d., Hailey-Hailey d., ichthyosis vulgaris, impetigo, mycosis fungoides, pemphigus foliaceus, pemphigus vulgaris, seborrheic dermatitis, Wiskott-Aldrich s.
elastosis perforans serpiginosa	argyria, **Down s., Ehlers-Danlos s., Marfan s.,** morphea, **osteogenesis imperfecta, pseudoxanthoma elasticum**, Rothmund-Thomson s., systemic sclerosis
elephantiasis	chromomycosis, filariasis, schistosomiasis
endocarditis	reactive angioendotheliomatosis, proliferating angioendotheliomatosis, lupus erythematosus
eosinophilic fasciitis	myeloproliferative disorders
epidermal cysts	Gardner's s.
epidermal nevus	BCC, SCC, syringocystadenoma papilliferum
epidermolysis bullosa acquisita	bronchial cancer, **inflammatory bowel d.**, lymphoma, multiple myeloma
epilepsy	juvenile xanthogranuloma, Vogt triad
eruptive xanthomas	chronic pancreatitis, hypertriglyceridemia
erysipelas	burns, eczema, edema, prior surgery, radiation therapy, tinea pedis
erythema ab igne	Merkel cell carcinoma, SCC

Diseases or Signs and Their Associations

Disease or Sign	Association
erythema annulare centrifugum	ascaris, autoimmune disease, blood dyscrasia, *Candida*, carcinoma, dermatophyte infection, drug sensitivity, Epstein-Barr virus, hypereosinophilic s., *Penicillium* mold sensitivity
erythema elevatum diutinum	dermatitis herpetiformis, HIV, IgA myeloma, myelodysplasia, prostate carcinoma, RA, streptococcal infection
erythema gyratum repens	**dermatologic**: ichthyosis (16%), palmar-plantar keratoderma (10%) **malignancy**: carcinoma (84%; bladder, breast, cervix, esophagus, lung, prostate, stomach), multiple myeloma
erythema multiforme	**infectious**: adenovirus, coccidioidomycosis, coxsackievirus B5, hepatitis A virus, herpes zoster, histoplasmosis, **HSV**, infectious mononucleosis, milker's nodule, mycobacteria, ***Mycoplasma pneumoniae***, orf, psittacosis, septicemia (gram negative), *Streptococcus*, tuberculosis, tularemia, *Yersinia* **other**: acute GVHD, contact dermatitis, drugs, leukemia (acute), x-ray therapy
erythema nodosum	**bacterial**: *Campylobacter jejuni*, *Chlamydia*, leishmaniasis, leptospirosis, *Streptococcus*, toxoplasmosis, tuberculosis, Whipple's d., *Yersinia* **drugs**: estrogens, OCPs, sulfones **fungal**; blastomycosis, coccidioidomycosis, histoplasmosis, *Trichophyton* **malignancy**: Hodgkin's d., leukemia, post-radiated pelvic cancer **miscellaneous**: Behçet's s., Crohn's d. (2-15%), IBD, Lofgren's s., pregnancy, ulcerative colitis (4-10%), sarcoidosis **viral**: cat-scratch, HSV, mononucleosis, lymphogranuloma venereum, ornithosis, psittacosis
erythermalgia (secondary)	cutaneous vasculitis, drugs, hypertension, RA, SLE
erythromelalgia	gout, heavy metal poisoning, lupus erythematosus, occlusive vascular d., polycythemia vera, neurological d., thrombocytopenia
exfoliate erythroderma	see *signs & symptoms* section
familial Mediterranean fever	erysipeloid eruption, Henoch-Schönlein purpura, renal amyloidosis, urticaria, vasculitic nodules
Fanconi's s.	leukemia, SCC of mucocutaneous junction
fibrofolliculomas	Birt-Hogg-Dube s.
fibromas	Gardner's s.
follicular atrophoderma	atrophoderma vermiculata, Bazex's s., Conradi's d., keratosis follicularis spinulosa atrophicans, keratosis palmoplantaris disseminata, keratosis pilaris rubra facei, ulerythema oophyrogenes
follicular mucinosis	mycosis fungoides, systemic lymphoma
folliculitis, perforating	acanthosis nigricans, arteriosclerosis, psoriasis
gammopathy	angioimmunoblastic lymphadenopathy, diffuse plane xanthomatosis, erythema elevatum diutinum, necrobiotic xanthogranuloma, papular

Diseases or Signs and Their Associations

Disease or Sign	Association
	mucinosis, plane xanthoma, scleromyxedema, scleredema, subcorneal pustular dermatosis
Gardner's s.	cancer (colon, GI)
geographic tongue	see glossitis, benign migratory
glaucoma	Behçet's d., nevus of Ota, Sturge-Weber s., Vogt-Koyanagi-Harada s.
glomerulonephritis	congenital lues, phenol, lepromatous leprosy, nephritogenic strains of Group A streptococcus, secondary lues, Henoch-Schönlein purpura, varicella
glossitis, benign migratory	AIDS, asthma, atopy, **Down s.**, eczema, hay fever, HLA-Cw6, LP, **normal persons**, oral lithium treatment, **psoriasis**
granuloma annulare (generalized)	carbohydrate intolerance, diabetes mellitus, HIV
granulomatous slack skin	Hodgkin's d.
Grover's d.	adhesive tape, allergic contact dermatitis, atopic dermatitis, eczema, PRP, pityriasis versicolor, pemphigus foliaceus
Hailey-Hailey d.	allergic contact dermatitis, SCC
Hashimoto's thyroiditis	lupus erythematosus, PSS, Sjögren's s., hypothyroidism
hematopoietic ulcers	congenital hemolytic anemia, Cooley's anemia (thalassemia major), cryofibrinogenemia, cryoglobulinemia, macroglobulinemia, polycythemia vera, sickle cell anemia, thrombocytopenic purpura
Henoch-Schönlein purpura	antiphospholipid syndrome, Behçet's disease, Berger d. (IgA glomerulonephritis), cancer (colon, bronchial, prostatic), cryoglobulinemia, drugs (ampicillin, penicillin, erythromycin, quinidine, quinine) familial Mediterranean fever, hematologic malignancies, hepatitis C, influenza vaccination, lymphoma, monoclonal gammopathy, *Mycoplasma pneumoniae,* PAN, pregnancy, rheumatoid arthritis, SLE, **URI** (Group A streptococcus, B-hemolytic streptococcus)
hepatitis	bedbug bites, Chediak-Higashi s., Down s. (more susceptible), X-linked agammaglobulinemia, generalized pustular psoriasis, pyoderma gangrenosum, lichen planus, ketoconazole treatment (rare), *Vibrio vulnificus* infection, secondary lues, benign cutaneous polyarteritis nodosa, polyarteritis nodosa, urticaria, SLE, Wegener's granulomatosis
hepatitis B	asymptomatic erythematous eruption (chronic), dermatomyositis-like, erythema nodosum, essential mixed cryoglobulinemia, leukocytoclastic vasculitis, LP, Gianotti-Crosti s., polyarteritis nodosa, pyoderma gangrenosum, serum sickness-like, urticaria
hepatitis C	erythema multiforme, leukocytoclastic vasculitis, lichen planus, lymphocytic salivary gland infiltration, mixed cryoglobulinemia (36-45%), polyarteritis nodosa, porphyria cutanea tarda,
hepatitis, chronic active	lichen planus, SLE
herpes gestationis	hydatiform moles, germ cell tumors

Diseases or Signs and Their Associations

Disease or Sign	Association
herpes simplex, generalized	leukemia, lymphoma, mycosis fungoides
herpes simplex, recurrent	erythema multiforme
herpes zoster	AIDS, corticosteroids, Hodgkin's disease, immunosuppressive drugs, increasing age
herpes zoster, disseminated	leukemia, lymphoma
hidradenitis suppurativa	acne (severe), amyloidosis (secondary), anemia, chronic granulomatous d., interstitial keratitis, hypoproteinemia, obesity
HIV infection	**infectious**: bacillary angiomatosis, candidiasis, condyloma, cryptococcus, cytomegalovirus, *Demodex*, dermatophyte, oral hairy leukoplakia, herpes simplex, histoplasmosis, HIV exanthem, human papillomavirus, Kaposi's sarcoma, leprosy, molluscum contagiosum, *Mycobacterium avium*-intracellulare, Penicillinosis, *Pityrosporum*, scabies (crusted), *Pneumocystis carinii* (cutaneous), PRP, *Staphylococcus aureus* infection, Syphilis, tinea versicolor, toxoplasmosis, tuberculosis, varicella zoster **miscellaneous**: alopecia areata, aphthous ulcers, drug reactions, eosinophilic folliculitis, GA, gingival hypertrophy, hyperalgesic pseudothrombophlebitis, periorbital ecchymosis, photosensitivity (acquired), PCT, premature graying (poliosis), trichomegaly (acquired), vitiligo **neoplastic**: BCC, extramedullary plasmacytoma, lymphoma, SCC **papulosquamous**: balanitis circinata, exfoliative erythroderma, ichthyosis (acquired), keratoderma blennorrhagicum, pityriasis rubra pilaris, psoriasis, Reiter's s., seborrheic dermatitis, thrombocytopenic purpura, xerosis **vascular**: EED, hyperallergic pseudothrombophlebitis, lymphomatoid granulomatosis, telangiectasia, TTP, vasculitis
Hodgkin's d.	Addison's d., exfoliative dermatitis, granulomatous slack skin, herpes zoster, mycosis fungoides, pruritus, urticaria
hypereosinophilic s.	dermatographism, EAC, erythroderma, Raynaud's phenomenon, T-cell lymphoma, vasculitis
hypertrichosis lanuginosa	acanthosis nigricans-like, anorexia nervosa, cancer (bladder, breast, colon, gallbladder, lung, ovarian, pancreas, rectum, uterine), carcinoid, CLL, drugs, follicular hyperkeratosis, glossitis, ichthyosis, lymphoma, nail pitting, palmar-plantar keratoses, subungual epidermal hyperplasia
ichthyosis hystrix	aminoaciduria, anaphylaxis (to food), asthma, atopic diathesis, epilepsy, IgE elevation, impaired cellular immunity, mental retardation, skeletal abnormalities
ichthyosis vulgaris	atopic dermatitis (50%), cardio-facio-cutaneous s., hypohidrosis with heat intolerance (rare), keratosis pilaris
ichthyosis, acquired	**malignancies**: carcinoma (breast, cervix, colon, lung), carcinomatosis, **Hodgkin's d.**, lymphoma (10%), Kaposi's sarcoma, leiomyosar-

Diseases or Signs and Their Associations

Disease or Sign	Association
	coma, multiple myeloma, mycosis fungoides, rhabdomyosarcoma **infectious**: AIDS, HIV, HTLV-II, lepromatous leprosy **systemic**: dermatomyositis, eosinophilic fasciitis, essential fatty acid deficiency, hemochromatosis, hyperthyroidism hypothyroidism, Kwashiorkor, malabsorption, malnutrition, mixed connective tissue d., renal failure (chronic), sarcoidosis, SLE **other**; DEB (Cockayne-Touraine), drugs, xeroderma pigmentosa
ichthyosis, recessive X-linked	asymptomatic corneal opacities (50% adults), cryptorchidism (25%), testicular cancer
id reaction	contact allergy, fungal infection, stasis dermatitis
ILVEN	congenital skeletal deformities, internal organ malformations
immunodeficiency	alopecia, eczema, skin infection, lupus erythematosus-like
impetigo herpetiformis	hypoparathyroidism, hypocalcemia
infantile acropustulosis	scabies
inflammatory bowel d.	annular erythema, aphthous ulcers, bowel associated dermatosis-arthritis s., clubbing, cutaneous Crohn's d., epidermolysis bullosa, erythema nodosum, erythema multiforme, fistulae, granuloma, lichen planus, malnutrition, metastatic Crohn's d., pyoderma gangrenosum, urticaria, vasculitis, vitiligo
juvenile xanthogranuloma	neurofibromatosis type 1, Niemann-Pick d., seizures, urticaria pigmentosis
Kaposi's sarcoma	AIDS, angioimmunoblastic LAD with dysproteinemia
Kawasaki d.	Asians
keloids	acne, acromegaly, blacks, hyperthyroidism, pregnancy, Rubinstein-Taybi s.
keratoacanthoma	exposure to pitch & tar, HPV-16 & 37, organ transplant, smoking, sun exposure, Muir-Torre's s., xeroderma pigmentosum
keratoconjunctivitis sicca	PACK s.
keratoderma	dyskeratosis congenita, ectodermal defects, hidrotic ectodermal dysplasia, Huriez s., KID s., pachyonychia congenita (type II),
keratoderma, acquired	AIDS, dermatophyte infections, diabetes mellitus, myxedema
keratoderma, palmar and plantar	Jackson-Sertoli s. (limited plantar), PRP, psoriasis, Reiter's s., Richner-Hanhart s., Saezary s., Steijlen's s.
keratopathy	chloroquine ingestion, congenital lues
keratosis pilaris	atopic dermatitis, ichthyosis vulgaris, keratosis pilaris rubra facei
Koebner's phenomenon in psoriasis	**endogenous**: dermatitis, furuncles, lichen planus, lymphangitis, miliaria, PR, vitiligo, zoster **exogenous**: abrasions, acupuncture, irritants, chemical burns, burns, contusions, electrodesiccation, excoriation, fellatio, freezing, incision, laceration, pressure, radiation, rubbing, scrapes, scratches, shaving, skin grafts, surgery, tape, tattoos, vaccinations

Diseases or Signs and Their Associations

Disease or Sign	Association
Kyrle's d.	congestive heart failure, diabetes mellitus, hepatic insufficiency, renal disease
lentigines (disorders)	Peutz-Jeghers s., LEOPARD s., lentiginosis with cardiocutaneous myxomas, Touraine's centrofacial lentiginosis, Tay's s., Soto's s., Ruvalcaba-Myhre-Smith s.
leukemia	ataxia telangiectasia, Bloom's s., Bruton's X-linked agammaglobulinemia, bullous pyoderma gangrenosum, Cockayne's s., Down s., ecthyma gangrenosa, erythromelalgia, gangrene, Langerhan's cell histiocytosis, scabies (crusted), pernio, Sweet's s., urticaria, zygomycosis
leukemia (acute granulocytic)	cutaneous extramedullary hematopoiesis, neutrophilic hidradenitis, pyoderma gangrenosum (bullous hemorrhagic), Sweet's s.
leukonychia	acrokeratosis verruciformis, alopecia areata, anemia, cachectic state, carcinoid s., cirrhosis, congenital, cryoglobulinemia, Darier's d., dyshidrosis, erythema multiforme, exfoliative dermatitis, fungi, gout, Hodgkin's d., hypoalbuminemia, hypocalcemia, Kawasaki s., lead poisoning, LEOPARD s., leprosy, leukonychia striata semilunaris, malaria, pachyonychia congenita, pellagra, rickettsial infection, sickle cell anemia, sulfonamides, syphilis, tuberculosis, trauma, trichinosis, ulcerative colitis, zinc deficiency
leukopenia	chickenpox, leishmaniasis, measles, RMSF, rubella, SLE
lichen planus	amebiasis, bladder infections, chronic active hepatitis, HBV, **HCV**, HSV-2, primary biliary cirrhosis (usually post-penicillamine therapy), syphilis, ulcerative colitis
lichen sclerosis	alopecia areata, *Borrelia burgdorferi*, diabetes mellitus, morphea, pernicious anemia, SCC, thyroid d., vitiligo
lichen simplex chronicus (secondary)	atopic dermatitis, lichen planus, seborrheic dermatitis, stasis dermatitis, tinea corporis, xerosis
lichen spinulosis	arsphenamine, gold, HIV, Hodgkin's d., lichen scrofulosorum, mycotic id reactions, seborrheic dermatitis, syphilis, thallium
lipodermoid tumors	epidermal nevus s.
lipomas	Dercum's d., proteus s.
livedo	atrophie blanche, cutaneous polyarteritis nodosa, DLE, polyarteritis nodosa, PSS, rheumatoid arthritis, secondary syphilis, SLE
livedo reticularis	arterial or air emboli, arteriosclerosis, arteritis, collagen vascular disease, cryoglobulinemia, decompression sickness, DMF, dermatomyositis, dysproteinemia, hypercalcemia, hyperparathyroidism, meningococcemia, PAN, pancreatitis, pheochromocytoma, pneumococcal sepsis, polycythemia vera, primary or vascular disease, RA, rheumatic fever, scleroderma, SLE, syphilis, thrombocytopenic purpura, tuberculosis
Lofgren's s.	pulmonary infections, sarcoidosis

Diseases or Signs and Their Associations

Disease or Sign	Association
lupus erythematosus	dermatofibroma, xeroderma pigmentosa
lupus erythematosus, neonatal	anemia, cholestatic liver disease (10%), heart block (50%), leukopenia, pneumonitis, skin disease (50%), splenomegaly, thrombocytopenia (10%)
lupus vulgaris	BCC, SCC
lymphedema	cellulitis (recurrent), congenital, postoperative, post-radiation, malignant infiltration
lymphoma	Duncan's d., hidradenitis suppurativa, hyperpigmentation, Langerhan's cell histiocytosis, Louis-Bar s., perioral dermatitis, psoriasis, reticulated erythematous mucinosis, toxic shock s.
lymphomatoid papulosis	10-20% develop MF or Hodgkin's lymphoma
Maffucci's s.	pancreatic cancer, chondrosarcoma, sarcoma
medulloblastoma	Gorlin's s.
melanoma, poor prognosis	age > 50, **disseminated disease**, increased mitotic activity, microscopic satellites, location (head, neck, trunk, hands, feet), males, ulceration
melasma	cosmetics, endocrine disease, female, hepatic disease, Hispanic, neuroleptic medications, nutrition, OCPs, ovarian dysfunction, parasitosis, pregnancy, thyroid disease
meningococcemia	children < 5, military recruits, patients with complement deficiency
milia formation	acne, bullous lichen planus, congenital, dermabrasion, epidermolysis bullosa, herpes zoster, porphyria cutanea tarda, Rombo s., second degree burn, scar, sweat retention s., topical steroids
Mondor's d.	breast cancer, breast surgery, excessive physical strain, infection, RA, trauma
monilethrix	cataracts, keratosis pilaris, nail anomalies, physical retardation, syndactyly, teeth anomalies
mononucleosis	Duncan's d.
Muir-Torre s.	colon, endometrium, GI, laryngeal cancer
multiple myeloma	alopecia, amyloidosis (primary), angioedema, cryoglobulinemia, ichthyosiform dermatitis, leukocytoclastic vasculitis, necrobiotic xanthogranuloma, petechiae, POEMS s., plane xanthoma, pruritus, purpura, pyoderma gangrenosum, Raynaud's, scleredema, scleromyxedema, subcorneal pustular dermatosis, Sweet's s.
multiple sclerosis	erythromelalgia, pruritus
myasthenia gravis	basaloid follicular hamartomas, chronic mucocutaneous candidiasis with thymoma, lichen planus, pemphigus erythematosus, SLE, trichoepithelioma
mycosis fungoides	actinic reticuloid, alopecia mucinosa, IgM deficiency, lymphomatoid granulomatosis, lymphomatoid papulosis, lymphomatoid pityriasis lichenoides

Diseases or Signs and Their Associations

Disease or Sign	Association
necrobiosis lipoidica	diabetes mellitus (66%)
necrolytic migratory erythema	glucagonoma (90%)
Netherton's s.	ichthyosis linearis circumflexa, lamellar ichthyosis, pili torti, trichorrhexis invaginata, trichorrhexis nodosa
neurofibromatosis I	**endocrine**: acromegaly, cretinism, diabetes, gynecomastia, hyperparathyroidism, hyperthyroidism, hypothyroidism multiple endocrine adenomatosis, pheochromocytoma, precocious puberty, **neoplasms**: acoustic neuroma, AML, astrocytoma, CML, ependymoma, fibrosarcoma, glioma (optic nerve), nephroblastoma, neurofibrosarcoma, ocular melanoma, rhabdomyosarcoma, schwannoma **neurological**: deafness, exophthalmos, macrocephaly, mental retardation, seizures, speech impediments **skeletal**: kyphosis, pseudoarthrosis, scoliosis, short stature
neurofibromatosis type II	central neurofibromatosis; bilateral acoustic neuromas
neuroma, mucosal	Sipple's s.
neutrophilic eccrine hidradenitis	**AML** (100%), breast cancer, chemotherapy (myelomonocytic leukemia), GU tumors, Hodgkin's d., HIV, lung cancer, non-Hodgkin's lymphoma, osteosarcoma, teratoma, testicular carcinoma
nevi	NAME s.
nevi, blue	cardiac myxoma, LAMB s., lentigines, nodular mastocytosis
nevi, connective tissue	Buschke-Ollendorff s., elastosis perforans serpiginosa, pseudoxanthoma elasticum
nevi, elastin	Buschke-Ollendorff s., elastosis perforans serpiginosa, isolated, pseudoxanthoma elasticum
nevi, linear epidermal	proteus s.
nevoid basal cell s.	astrocytoma, craniopharyngioma, fibrosarcoma, medulloblastoma, meningioma
nevus anemicus	neurofibromatosis
nevus comedonicus	BCC, benign eccrine tumors, follicular tumors, trichilemmal cyst
nevus flammeus	Klippel-Trenaunay-Weber s., Sturge-Weber s.
nevus of Ota	intracranial melanoma, meningeal melanoma
nevus sebaceous	BCC, sebaceous carcinoma, syringocystadenoma papilliferum, syringoma, trichilemmoma
nevus, halo	dysplastic nevi, melanoma, pernicious anemia, poliosis, vitiligo (20%), Vogt-Koyanagi-Harada s.
ochronosis	alkaptonuria
oral cancer	alcoholism, betel nut, iron deficiency, reverse smoking, smoking, syphilitic glossitis, wine

Diseases or Signs and Their Associations

Disease or Sign	Association
osteolysis	acne fulminans, juvenile hyaline fibromatosis, PSS, systemic nodular panniculitis (Weber-Christian), xanthoma disseminatum
osteoma cutis	Albright's s., basal cell epithelioma, dermatomyositis, inflammatory diseases, intradermal nevi, mixed tumor of the skin, primary from childhood, scars, scleroderma
osteomyelitis	congenital syphilis, diabetic foot ulcer, mycetoma (Madura foot), secondary syphilis, tertiary lues
osteoporosis	progeria
otitis media	Langerhan's cell histiocytosis
pachyonychia congenita	Schäfer's s.
Paget's d.	breast cancer (95%)
Paget's d., extramammary	carcinoma-breast, colon, genitourinary (10%), sweat gland carcinoma (10%)
panniculitis	**infectious:** actinomycosis, blastomycosis, *Campylobacter* colitis, cat scratch d., *Chlamydia*, chromomycosis, coccidioidomycosis, cryptococcosis, gonorrhea, histoplasmosis, leprosy, lymphogranuloma inguinale, mononucleosis, mycetoma, ornithosis, *Salmonella*, *Shigella*, sporotrichosis, streptococcal, syphilis, trichophytosis, tuberculosis, *Yersinia* **other**: Behçet's d., carcinoma, Crohn's d., drugs, erythema nodosum, fasciitis with eosinophilia, Hodgkin's d., leukemia, necrobiosis lipoidica, OCPs, periarteritis nodosa, pregnancy, sarcoidosis, sarcoma, Sweet's s., ulcerative colitis
papillomas, multiple (perioral and mucous membrane)	Goltz s.
papular mucinosis	eosinophilia-myalgia s., neurologic abnormalities, polyarthritis, proximal myopathy
parakeratosis, shoulder	parakeratotic aggregations at follicular infundibula; seborrheic dermatitis
paronychia	acrodermatitis enteropathica, enchondroma, histiocytosis X, mucocutaneous candidiasis, multicentric reticulohistiocytosis, occupations, pemphigus, progressive systemic sclerosis, psoriasis, Reiter's s., retinoids, Rubinstein-Taybi s., Stevens-Johnson s., SLE, yellow nail s.
pellagra	alcoholism, carcinoid, corn diet, drugs, eating disorder, GI bypass surgery, Hartnup d.
pemphigus erythematosus	bronchial carcinoma, LE, myasthenia gravis with malignant thymoma
pemphigus foliaceus	**precipitating factors**: emotional stress, fatigue, heat, menstruation, sunlight
pemphigus vulgaris	Ashkenazi Jews, colon cancer, Hodgkin's d., Kaposi's sarcoma, lymphoma, myasthenia gravis, thymoma (<5%)

Diseases or Signs and Their Associations

Disease or Sign	Association
pemphigus, paraneoplastic	breast cancer, CLL, Castleman's d., non-Hodgkin's **lymphoma** (90%), thymoma, spindle cell neoplasms, Waldenstrom's macroglobulinemia
peptic ulcer d.	telangiectasia macularis eruptive perstans
pernio	Northern Europeans, myelomonocytic leukemia (elderly)
Peutz-Jeghers s.	GI cancer
pheochromocytoma	neurofibromatosis, Sipple's s., von Hippel-Lindau s.
piebaldism	heterochromia irides, Hirschsprung's d., MR, osteopathia striata, Woolf's s., Ziprowski-Margolis s.
pityriasis amantacea	psoriasis, seborrheic dermatitis
pityriasis lichenoides	HIV, streptococcal pharyngitis, *Toxoplasma gondii*
pityriasis rubra pilaris	HIV
Pityrosporum ovale	achromia parasitica, confluent & reticulated papillomatosis of Gougerot & Carteaud, obstructive dacryocystitis, seborrheic dermatitis, **pityriasis versicolor**
Plummer-Vinson s.	SCC (mouth, pharynx, esophagus) 10%
poikiloderma vasculare atrophicans	acrodermatitis chronica atrophicans, arsenism, dyskeratosis congenita, Fanconi's s., Kindler's s., large plaque parapsoriasis, lupus erythematosus, poikiloderma congenitale, Werner's s., xeroderma pigmentosum
polyarteritis nodosa	allergic hyposensitization, drug reaction, familial Mediterranean fever, hairy cell leukemia, **HBV** (chronic), HIV, inflammatory bowel disease, lymphoreticular malignancies, methamphetamine abuse, mixed cryoglobulinemia, parvovirus B19, post-infectious serous otitis, post-streptococcal B infection, RA, SLE, trichinosis
polycystic ovaries	Stein-Leventhal s.
polymyositis	Sjögren's s.
pompholyx (dyshidrotic eczema)	atopy, nickel allergy (26%)
porokeratosis of Mibelli	BCC, Bowen's d., SCC
porphyria cutanea tarda	carcinomatosis, cirrhosis, diabetes mellitus, drugs, **EtOH, HCV,** hemochromatosis, **hepatoma, HIV,** Hodgkin's d., lupus erythematosus, lymphoma, polychlorinated aromatic hydrocarbons, reticuloendotheliomatosis
progressive systemic sclerosis	dysphagia, esophageal stricture, hypothyroidism, pericarditis, pulmonary fibrosis, Raynaud's phenomenon, Sjögren's s.
pseudolymphoma, B-cell	borreliosis
pseudolymphoma, T-cell	allergic contact dermatitis, drug allergy (phenytoin)
pseudoporphyria	see *Skin Diseases and Medications*

Diseases or Signs and Their Associations

Disease or Sign	Association
pseudoxanthoma elasticum	angioid streaks (85%), elastosis perforans serpiginosa
pseudoxanthoma elasticum, perforating	angioid streaks of eye (rare), hypertension, obesity
psoriasis	antimalarials, Crohn's d. (1.6x), diabetes, eczema, gouty arthritis, heart failure, HIV, hypertension, IBD, lichen planus, lichen simplex chronicus, obesity, oropharyngeal infections, seborrheic dermatitis, smoking, stress, ulcerative colitis (3.8x) **reduced incidence**: allergic contact dermatitis, atopic dermatitis, bacterial & viral skin infections, urticaria
psoriasis, erythrodermic	antimalarials, B-blockers, corticosteroids, infection, lithium, NSAIDs, phototoxic erythema
psoriasis, guttate	β-hemolytic streptococcal (*S. pyogenes*) throat infection (up to 85%), drug eruption
psoriasis, pustular (von Zumbusch)	arthropathy, HLA-B27, hypoalbuminemia (with 2° hypocalcemia), infections, lithium, OCPs, **pregnancy, steroid withdrawal**
psoriatic arthritis, juvenile	chronic anterior uveitis
psychocutaneous dermatoses	alopecia areata, automutilation, dermatitis artefacta, dermatothlasia, dysmorphic disorder, factitial syndromes, lichen simplex chronicus, neurotic excoriation, prurigo nodularis, psychogenic pruritus, psychogenic purpura, telogen effluvium trichotillomania, trigeminal trophic s.
pustular eruption	acetaminophen, amoxicillin, ampicillin, calcium channel blockers, carbamazepine, cefaclor, erythromycin, imipenam, nifedipine, ofloxacin, penicillin, quinidine
pustulosis palmaris et plantaris	heavy smokers, high humidity & temperature, thyroid abnormalities, tonsillitis
pyoderma gangrenosum	chronic active hepatitis, **IBD** (Crohn's d.-16%, ulcerative colitis-15%), **leukemia** (10%), immunodeficiency, monoclonal gammopathy, myelofibrosis, myeloid metaplasia, myeloma, paraproteinemia, polycythemia vera, primary biliary cirrhosis, **RA**, sarcoid, SLE, Takayasu's arteritis
pyoderma gangrenosum, bullous hemorrhagic	myelogenous leukemia (80%)
pyoderma vegetans	ulcerative colitis
pyogenic granuloma	pregnancy
pyostomatitis vegetans	50-70% associated with IBD
radiodermatitis	BCC, fibrosarcoma, malignant fibrous histiocytoma, SCC
Raynaud's phenomenon	**connective tissue:** CREST s., dermatomyositis, mixed connective tissue d., PACK s., **PSS**, rheumatoid arthritis, scleroderma, Sjögren's s., SLE **hematologic:** cold agglutinins, cryoglobulinemia, dysproteinemia, multiple myeloma, panarteritis nodosa, paroxysmal hemoglobinuria,

Diseases or Signs and Their Associations

Disease or Sign	Association
	thrombosis, thrombotic thrombocytopenic purpura, Wegener's granulomatosis **medicine:** β-adrenergic blockers, cancer chemotherapy, ergots, heavy metal **miscellaneous:** bowel bypass s., electrical shock, endocarditis (subacute bacterial), hypereosinophilic s., pilomatrixoma **neurologic:** carpal tunnel s., cervical rib s., CNS disease, multiple sclerosis, shoulder girdle compression s., thoracic outlet s. **occupational:** occupational trauma, pneumatic hammer use, vibrating machinery, vinyl chloride exposure **systemic:** carcinoma, cirrhosis, hypothyroidism, lymphosarcoma, malaria, morphea (generalized) **vascular**; arterial embolism, arteriosclerosis obliterans, Buerger's d., coronary artery d.
reticular erythematous mucinosis	carcinoma (colon, breast), diabetes mellitus, hyperthyroidism, hypothyroidism, thrombocytopenic purpura
rheumatoid arthritis	bullous pemphigoid, cicatricial pemphigoid, dermatitis herpetiformis, epidermolysis bullosa acquisita, erythema elevatum diutinum, Felty's s. (1%), livedo vasculitis, nail ridging & beading, pemphigus foliaceus, pemphigus vulgaris, pyoderma gangrenosum, Sjögren's s., subcorneal pustular dermatosis, yellow nail s.
sarcoidosis	Addison's d., carcinoma, cataracts, glaucoma, Heerfordt s., Lofgren's s., papilledema, thyroid d., uveitis, vitiligo
sarcomas	Maffucci's s.
scabies, crusted (Norwegian)	leukemia, lymphoma
schizophrenia	acrocyanosis
scleredema	DM with CAD, monoclonal gammopathy, multiple myeloma, streptococcal infection
scleroderma	Sjögren's s., Werner's s.
seborrheic dermatitis (*see also eczema*)	AIDS, denervation, diabetes mellitus, HIV infection, Leiner's d., neuroleptic drugs, Parkinson's d., seizures, sprue
seborrheic keratoses	Hermansky-Pudlak s.
serum sickness	antithymocyte globulin, streptokinase
serum sickness-like	penicillin, sulfa
sickle cell anemia	leg ulcers, melanosis (legs)
Sjögren's s.	B-cell lymphoma (44x), hypereosinophilic s., necrotizing vasculitis, polyarteritis nodosa, polymyositis, RA, Raynaud's phenomenon, scleroderma, SLE, Sweet's s.
Sjögren's s., secondary	cirrhosis (primary biliary), Hashimoto's thyroiditis, hepatitis (chronic active), polyarteritis nodosa, polymyositis, RA, scleroderma, SLE

Diseases or Signs and Their Associations

Disease or Sign	Association
skin tags	obesity, pregnancy
Sneddon-Wilkinson d.	apudoma, CD30 + anaplastic large cell lymphoma, Crohn's d., hyperthyroidism, **IgA paraproteinemia, IgA myeloma**, IgG paraproteinemia, Mycoplasma pneumoniae infection, non-small cell lung carcinoma, pyoderma gangrenosum, RA, ulcerative colitis
spider nevus	alcoholism, chronic liver d., estrogens, OCPs, pregnancy, RA, thyrotoxicosis
spindle cell tumors	Danoff s.
squamous cell carcinoma	**dermatologic**: acrodermatitis chronica atrophicans, acrokeratosis verruciformis, actinic keratosis, balanitis xerotica obliterans, cheilitis glandularis, chronic sinus tract, cutaneous horn, discoid lupus erythematosus, DSAP, dyskeratosis congenita, dystrophic epidermolysis bullosa, epidermal inclusion cyst, epidermal nevus, epidermodysplasia verruciformis, epidermolysis bullosa, epidermal inclusion cyst, epidermal nevus, erosive lichen planus (?), erythroplakia, hidradenitis suppurativa, leg ulcers, leukoplakia, lichen planus (chronic oral, hypertrophic), lichen sclerosis, **light skin color**, linear porokeratosis, luetic interstitial glossitis, lupus vulgaris, necrobiosis lipoidica, nevus sebaceous, perifolliculitis capitis abscendens et suffodiens, porokeratosis of Mibelli, PSS, rhinoscleroma, seborrheic keratosis, speckled leukoplakia, submucosal fibrosis, tropical ulcer, tylosis, wart, warty dyskeratoma, xeroderma pigmentosa, Zinsser-Engman-Cole s. **exposure**: arsenic keratosis, betel nut chewing, burn wounds, mineral oils, nicotine stomatitis, paraffin, radiation dermatitis, radiotherapy, radon contaminated rings, snuff dipping, **sun**, thermal burns, thermal keratosis **infectious**: condyloma acuminata, granuloma inguinale, oral florid papillomatosis, osteomyelitis, yaws ulcers (tertiary disease) **neoplastic**: Bowen's d., erythroplasia of Queyrat, Merkel cell carcinoma, Paget's d., proliferating pilar tumor **other**: Fanconi's d., Hermansky-Pudlak s., Huriez s. (dorsal hands), KID s., Plummer-Vinson s., Rothmund-Thomson s.
squamous cell carcinoma, oral	betel nut chewing, dyskeratosis congenita, EtOH, tobacco use
stasis dermatitis	autoeczematization, lichen simplex chronicus
status cosmeticus	benzoic acid, bronopol, cinnamic acid, dowicil 200, formaldehyde, fragrance, lactic acid, nonionic emulsifiers, propylene glycol, quaternary ammonium compounds, sodium lauryl sulfate, sorbic acid, sunscreen agents, urea
Stevens-Johnson s.	*see erythema multiforme*
striae distensae	Marfan s.
subcorneal pustular dermatosis	monoclonal gammopathies, myeloma, pyoderma gangrenosum

Diseases or Signs and Their Associations

Disease or Sign	Association
subcutaneous fat necrosis	pancreatic carcinoma, pancreatitis, pancreatic pseudocyst
Sweet's s.	adenocarcinoma (breast, prostate, rectum), ALL, **AML** (10-20%), Behçet's d., CLL, CML, erythema nodosum, IBD, LE, leukemia (hairy cell), lymphoma, monoclonal gammopathy, myelodysplastic s., myeloma, pregnancy, RA, Sjögren's s., sarcoidosis, carcinoma (gastric, ovarian , testes), URI, vaccinations
syringoma, eruptive	Down s.
systemic lupus erythematosus	anticardiolipin Ab s., IgA deficiency s., Sjögren's s.
telogen effluvium	heparin, OCPs
temporal arteritis	polymyalgia rheumatica (50%)
thrombocytopenia	Kasabach-Merritt s., Letterer-Siwe d., SLE, strawberry angiomas, Wiskott-Aldrich s.
thrush (adults)	advanced cancer, AIDS, broad spectrum antibiotics, cytotoxic therapy, **dentures**, diabetes mellitus, hematologic malignancy, radiation, systemic corticosteroids, thymoma
thymoma	chronic mucocutaneous candidiasis, Good's s., lichen planus (esp. oral), myasthenia gravis, pemphigus erythematosus, pemphigoid, SLE
thyroiditis	chronic mucocutaneous candidiasis, IgA deficiency, IgM deficiency
tinea versicolor	Cushing's d., diabetes mellitus, herpes gestationis, ichthyosis, immunosuppression, malnutrition, OCPs, pregnancy, systemic steroids
toxic epidermal necrolysis	Crohn's d., GVH, HIV infection, leukemia, lymphoma, SLE. See *Medications*
trichoepitheliomas	Brooke-Spiegler s.
tuberous sclerosis	cardiac rhabdomyoma, cystic fibromatosis (lung), pheochromocytoma, renal hamartoma, sarcoma
ulcerative colitis	erythema nodosum, IgA deficiency, lichen planus, oral aphthae, pyoderma gangrenosum, pyodermite vegetante of Hallopeau, rheumatoid arthritis, vesiculopustular eruption
ulcers	chromate workers, congenital sensory neuropathy, malum perforans pedia, neuropathies
ulcers, lower extremity	abdominal surgery, CHF, diabetes insipidus, diabetes mellitus, hypogonadism, injury, Klinefelter's s., prolidase deficiency, sickle cell d. thrombophlebitis
unilateral nevoid telangiectasia	chronic alcoholic liver d. (men), cirrhosis, congenital, estrogen herapy, idiopathic, pregnancy
urticaria (*see allergy section*)	amebiasis, bullous pemphigoid, carcinoma, cold hemolysins, contactants, cryoglobulins, dermatomyositis, drugs, erythema multiforme, EPP (solar urticaria), foods, inhalants, internal disease, juvenile RA, leukemia, lymphoma, physical factors, polymyositis, psy-

Diseases or Signs and Their Associations

Disease or Sign	Association
	chogenic, rheumatic fever, Henoch-Schönlein s., serum sickness, SLE, Sjögren's s., TEN, vasculitis (necrotizing)
vasculitis	bacterial endocarditis, bowel-bypass s., mixed cryoglobulinemia, photocopy paper fumes **antigens**: endogenous antigens (DNA, RF binding to IgG), foods, food additives, infections (hepatitis A, B, C), medications (allopurinol, aminopenicillins, hydantoins, penicillin, propylthiouracil, pyrazolones, sulfonamides, thiazides), proteins (serum sickness), tumor antigens (lymphoreticular or hematopoietic)
vasculitis, cutaneous small vessel	adult T-cell leukemia, AIDS, Behçet's d., bowel bypass s., cancer (breast, colon, head and neck, lung, prostate, renal), cryoglobulinemia, cystic fibrosis, HIV, Hodgkin's d., hyperglobulinemic states, lymphosarcoma, multiple myeloma, mycosis fungoides, primary biliary cirrhosis, RA, Sjögren's s., SLE, ulcerative colitis
vasculitis, leukocytoclastic	**drugs & chemicals**: allopurinol, aspirin, herbicides, insecticides, iodides, penicillin, petroleum products, phenacetin, propylthiouracil, quinidine, sulfonamides **infections**: candidiasis, cytomegalovirus, hepatitis (A, B, C), histoplasmosis, influenza, mononucleosis, *Mycobacterium tuberculosis*, streptococcus B **malignancy**: CLL, hairy cell leukemia, histiocytic lymphoma, Hodgkin's d., multiple myeloma, solid tumors **systemic disease**: biliary cirrhosis, chronic active hepatitis, hemolytic anemia, mixed cryoglobulinemia, ulcerative colitis
vasculitis, nodular	large calves, livedo, tuberculosis
vasculitis, urticarial	EBV, fluoxetine, HBV, HCV, IgA multiple myeloma, IgM gammopathy, infectious mononucleosis, metastatic testicular teratoma, mixed cryoglobulins, relapsing polychondritis, Schnitzler's s., serum sickness, Sjögren's s., SLE (especially in hypocomplementemic)
vesicobullous eruption of chronic inflammatory d.	AIDS (with mycobacterial infection), Behçet's d., myeloproliferative disease, RA (severe), Sweet's s., ulcerative colitis
vitiligo	**dermatologic**: alopecia areata, atopic dermatitis, balanitis xerotica obliterans, halo nevus, Kaposi's sarcoma, leukotrichia, lichen planus, lichen sclerosis, lichen simplex, malignant melanoma, morphea, premature gray hair, progressive systemic scleroderma, psoriasis, Vogt-Koyanagi s. **systemic**: Addison's d. (2%), AIDS, asthma, ataxia telangiectasia, auditory defects (congenital), biliary cirrhosis, Bourneville's s., candidiasis (mucocutaneous), common variable immunodeficiency s., diabetes mellitus, Down s., GI malignancy, hypoparathyroidism, IgA deficiency, infection, inflammatory bowel disease, **iritis**, lymphoma, Maffucci's s., myasthenia gravis, pernicious anemia, RA, stress, sunburn, Tay's s., trauma **thyroid d.**: Graves' d., hyperthyroidism, hypothyroidism, thyroiditis, toxic goiter

Diseases or Signs and Their Associations

Disease or Sign	Association
vitiligo, facial	Alezzandrini's s.
vitiligo, universal	multiple endocrine neoplasia s.
Von Hippel-Lindau d.	hypernephroma, pheochromocytoma
warty dyskeratoma	immunosuppressive therapy, tobacco chewing
Werner's s.	fibrosarcoma, leiomyosarcoma, meningioma
Wiskott-Aldrich s.	astrocytoma, leiomyosarcoma, leukemia, lymphosarcoma, reticulum cell sarcoma
xanthelasma	apo-E2 phenotype, atherosclerosis, cerebrotendinous xanthomatosis, familial dysbetalipoproteinemia type III, familial hypercholesterolemia, hepatic cholestasis, hyperapobetalipoproteinemia, **normolipemic** (50%), polygenic hypercholesterolemia, β-sitosterolemia, sporadic hypercholesterolemia
xanthoma disseminatum	diabetes insipidus (33%)
xanthoma striatum palmare	biliary cirrhosis, diabetes mellitus, hyperlipoproteinemia type III & IV
xanthoma, diffuse plane	cryoglobulinemia, eosinophilic granulomatosis, leukemia, lymphoma, monoclonal gammopathy, **multiple myeloma, paraproteinemia**, rheumatoid arthritis
xanthoma, eruptive	**diabetes mellitus, estrogen, EtOH,** familial hyperlipoproteinemia type V, familial hypertriglyceridemia, hypothyroidism, isotretinoin, lipoprotein lipase deficiency, myxedema, nephrotic s., pancreatitis, Von Giercke's d.
xanthoma, intertriginous	homozygous familial hypercholesterolemia (pathognomonic)
xanthoma, palmar crease	familial dysbetalipoproteinemia type III (pathognomonic)
xanthoma, tendinous	β-sitosterolemia, cerebrotendinous xanthomatosis, diabetes mellitus, heterozygous familial hypercholesterolemia, homozygous familial hypercholesterolemia, hyperapobetalipoproteinemia, myxedema, obstructive liver d.
xanthoma, tuberous	hyperlipoproteinemia type II & III
xanthomas	atherosclerosis, biliary disease, CTCL, diabetes mellitus, hypothyroidism, leukemia, lymphedema, lymphoma, multiple myeloma, pancreatitis, renal disease
xeroderma pigmentosum	AK, BCC, lacrimation, leukemia, melanoma, mental retardation, neurological disease, photophobia, SCC

Autoantibodies

ANA

Collagen Vascular Disease	% Positive ANA
CREST (Limited systemic sclerosis)	85-90
Dermatomyositis (adult)	≈70-80
Dermatomyositis (child)	≈20
Discoid LE	≈10
Drug induced subacute cutaneous LE	≈75
Drug-induced SLE	>95
Generalized systemic sclerosis	≈90-95
Neonatal LE	>95
Normal individuals	≈5
Sjögren's syndrome	≈70-80
Subacute cutaneous LE (SCLE)	>70
Systemic lupus erythematosus (SLE)	>95

ANA Patterns	Antibody-producing Pattern and Related Skin Disorders
Centromeric	**Anti-centromere**: generalized systemic sclerosis (20%), CREST (50-70%)
Cytoplasmic	**Anti-Ro/SS-A**: SLE (40%), SCLE (75%), drug-induced SCLE (>80%), neonatal LE (>95%), Sjogren's syndrome (50-80%) **Anti-tRNA synthetases** (anti-Jo-1): dermatomyositis(<20%) **Anti-mitochondrial**: primary biliary cirrhosis (>90%)
Nuclear; diffuse (homogenous smooth)	**Anti-double strand DNA**: specific for SLE (60%) **Anti-histone**: drug induced SLE (>95%)
Nuclear; rim (peripheral)	**Anti-nuclear pore**, anti-lamin: SLE (rare) anti-dsDNA
Nuclear; speckled (particulate)	**Anti-Ro/SS-A**: SLE (40%), SCLE (75%), drug induced SCLE (>80%), neonatal LE (>95%), Sjögren's syndrome (50-80%) **La/SS-B**: same as Ro/SS-A **Anti-U$_1$RNP**: SLE (35%), mixed connective tissue disease (>95%) **Anti-Scl 70** (DNA topoisomerase 1): generalized systemic sclerosis (33%), CREST (18%) **Anti-Sm**: specific for SLE (25-40%)
Nucleolar	**Anti-nucleolar** (anti-RNA polymerase): generalized systemic sclerosis (40-50%), CREST (<20%)

Source: Daniel McCauliffe, MD

Basic Science

Antigens

bullous pemphigoid	bullous pemphigoid antigen-1, 230 kDd; bullous pemphigoid antigen-2, 180 kDa
cicatricial pemphigoid	bullous pemphigoid antigen-2
EBA	α chain of type VII collagen (290 kDa)
EB, dystrophic	type VII collagen
EB, generalized atrophic benign	bullous pemphigoid antigen-2, laminin
EB, junctional-pyloric atresia	integrin $\alpha 6\ \beta 4$
EB, junctional-lethal	laminin 5 α_3, β_3, γ_2
EB simplex recessive with muscular dystrophy	plectin
EB simplex recessive-Koebner	keratin 14
EB, simplex	keratins 5, 14
EBA	type VII collagen (anchoring fibrils)
herpes gestationis	bullous pemphigoid antigen-2
ichthyosis vulgaris	profilaggrin?
lamellar ichthyosis	keratinocyte-specific transglutaminase
pemphigus foliaceus	desmoglein-1 (a cadherin) 160 kd
pemphigus vulgaris	desmoglein-3 (a cadherin) 130 kd

Chromosomes

1	dysplastic nevus s., xeroderma pigmentosa
1p	Ehlers-Danlos type VI, erythrokeratoderma viriabilis, erythrokeratoderma with ataxia
1q	Chediak-Higashi s. (CHS), EB-junctional-Herlitz (LAMB3, LAMC2), familial cold urticaria, PCT, porphyria variegata (PPOX), Vohwinkel s. (LOR)
2	acrokeratoelastoidosis, kappa light chain, elastin molecule
2p	Carney/LAMB/NAME s. (2p16)
2q	Cockayne s.-XP-B (ERCC3), EB-pyloric atresia (ITGA6), Ehlers-Danlos IV (COL3A1) (2q31), lamellar ichthyosis, Waardenburg's s. type I (2q35,), Waardenburg's s. type III (2q35 PAX-3), wrinkly skin s. (WSS, 2q32), xeroderma pigmentosum-complement group B (ERCC3, XPB) (2q21)
3p	EB-dystrophic dominant (3p21.3, COL3A1), EB-pretibial type (3p21.3), EB-Bart type (3p21.3), Hailey-Hailey d. (3q21-q24), Marfan s. type II (3p25-p24.2), Muir-Torre s. (3p21.3), von Hippel-Lindau s. (3p26-p25), Waardenburg's s. type II (3p14.1-p12.3, MITF), XP-C (3p25, XPC)
3q	Hailey-Hailey d.
4p	chondrodysplasia punctata (4p16-p14), Ellis-van Creveld s. (4p16)

Basic Science

Chromosomes

4q	piebaldism (C-KIT), sclerotylosis
5q	Gardner's s. (APC)
6	HLA-A,B,C,DR,DP,DQ,E,F,G, C3 and C4, β2 microglobulin, TNFα and TNFβ
6p	hemochromatosis
7	Ehlers-Danlos type IV (arthrochalasis multiplex congenita), pro alpha 2 (I) gene
7p	arginosuccinic aciduria
7q	EEC s. (7q11.2-q21.3), Ehlers-Danlos s. type VII (7q22.1)
8	Rothmund-Thomson s.
8p	Pfeiffer s. (8p12-p11.2), Werner s. (8p12-11.2, WER)
8q	EB-Ogna (8q24), EB-muscular dystrophy (8q24, PLEC)
9	hereditary coproporphyria
9p	albinism 3 (TRP1), blue rubber bleb nevus s. (TIE2), melanoma (9p21, CDKN2), trichoepithelioma-familial
9q	basal cell nevus s. (9q22.3, PTC), Ehlers-Danlos I, II (COL5A1), familial keratoacanthomas, hypomelanosis of Ito (9q33-qter), nail-patella s., tuberous sclerosis 1 (TSC1), XP-A (XPAC)
10p	Refsum's d. (10pter-p11.2)
10q	Apert's s. (10q26), congenital erythropoietic porphyria (10q25.2-q26.3), Cowden d. (PTEN, MMAC1), EB-junctional-GAB (10q24.3, BPAG2), Hermansky-Pudlak (HPS)
11	acute intermittent porphyria, EB-dystrophic
11p	Beckwith-Wiedemann s. (11pter-p15.4), XP-E (DDB)
11q	albinism-tyrosinase negative & positive (11q14-q21, TYR), ataxia telangiectasia (11q22.3), atopy (11q12-q13), hereditary angioedema (11q11-q13.1, C1NH), Papillion-Lefevre s., porphyria-acute intermittent (11q24.1-q24.2)
12q	Darier's d. (12q23-q24.1), EB-simplex, epidermolytic hyperkeratosis, non-epidermolytic palmoplantar hyperkeratosis, ichthyosis bullosa of Siemens (12q11-q13), monilethrix (12q13), multiple lipomatosis (12q15), pachyonychia congenita (12q12-q14), white sponge nevus (12p11.2-q11)
13q	XP-G (13q33, ERCC5), hidrotic ectodermal dysplasia
14	ataxia telangiectasia, heavy chain
14q	lamellar ichthyosis (TGM1)
15q	albinism-tyrosinase positive (15q11.2-q12), Bloom's s. (15q26.1), hypomelanosis of Ito (15q11-q13), Marfan s. (15q21.1), tyrosinemia type I (15q23-q25)
16p	Rubinstein-Taybi s. (16q13.3), tuberous sclerosis-2 (TSC2)
16q	cylindroma, tyrosinemia II- Richner-Hanhart s. (TAT)
17p	Sjogren-Larson s. (FALDH)
17q	EB-simplex, epidermolytic hyperkeratosis (generalized/palmoplantar) (17q12-q21), pachyonychia congenita, white sponge nevus, neurofibromatosis 1 (17q11.2, NF1), tylosis, EB-junctional (ITGB4)

Basic Science

Chromosomes

18p	hereditary multiple leiomyomata (18p11.32)
18q	EB-junctional (18q11.2, LAMA3), palmoplantar keratoderma, striae, erythropoietic protoporphyria (18q21.3, FCE)
19p	acanthosis nigricans, C3 deficiency, Peutz-Jeghers s. (19p13.3)
19q	XP-D (19q13.2-q13.3)
20q	McCune-Albright s. (20q13.2), SCID with ADA deficiency (20q13.11)
21	CR3 deficiency
21q	leukocyte adhesion deficiency (21q22.3)
22	lambda light chain
22q	DiGeorge s. (22q11), neurofibromatosis II (22q12.2)
X	hypomelanosis of Ito, incontinentia pigmenti type I, Menkes s.
Xp	Gorlin-Goltz s. ichthyosis-recessive X-linked (Xp22.32, STS), incontinentia pigmenti-1, Kallmann s. (Xp22.3), keratosis follicularis spinulosa decalvans (Xp22.2-p22.13), ocular albinism, Partington s. (Xp22-p21), Wiskott-Aldrich s. (Xp11.23-p11.22)
Xq	Alport s. (Xq 22), anhidrotic ectodermal dysplasia (EDA), congenital generalized hypertrichosis, dyskeratosis congenita (Xq28), Fabry's d. (Xq22), incontinentia pigmenti-2 (Xq28), Menkes s. (Xq12-q13)

Chromosomes and Disease, Alphabetized

a	acanthosis nigricans (19p), acrokeratoelastoidosis (2), acute intermittent porphyria (11), albinism 3 (TRP1) (9p), albinism-tyrosinase negative & positive (11q, TYR), albinism-tyrosinase positive (15q), anhidrotic ectodermal dysplasia (Xq, EDA), arginosuccinic aciduria (7p), ataxia telangiectasia (14),
b	β2 microglobulin (6), BCC (patched), basal cell nevus s. (9q, PTC) (), Bloom's s. (15q26.1), blue rubber bleb nevus s. (9p, TIE2)
c	C3 deficiency (19p), CR3 deficiency (21), Chediak-Higashi s. (CHS) (1q42.1-42.2), Cockayne s.-XP-B (10q11, ERCC3), congenital generalized hypertrichosis (Xq), Cowden d. (10q22-q23, PTEN, MMAC1), cylindroma (16q),
d	Darier's d. (12q23-24.1), dysplastic nevus s. (1)
e	EB-dystrophic (COL3A1) (3p21.3), EB-dystrophic (11), EB-junctional (1q25-q31, LAMB3, LAMC2), EB-junctional-GAB (10q, BPAG2), EB-junctional (17q, ITGB4), EB-junctional (18q, LAMA3), EB-muscular dystrophy (8q, PLEC), EB-Ogna (8q), EB-pretibial type (3p21.3), EB-pyloric atresia (2q, ITGA6), EB-simplex (12q), EB-simplex (17q), Ehlers-Danlos IV (2q, COL3A1), Ehlers-Danlos I, II (9q, COL5A1), Ehlers-Danlos type IV (arthrochalasis multiplex congenita) (7), Ehlers-Danlos type VI (1p36.3-p36.2), elastin molecule (2), epidermolytic hyperkeratosis (12q), epidermolytic hyperkeratosis (generalized/palmoplantar) (17q), erythropoietic protoporphyria (18q21.3, FCE), erythrokeratoderma viriabilis (1p34-35), erythrokeratoderma with ataxia (1p34-35)
f	familial cold urticaria (1q), familial keratoacanthomas (9q),

Basic Science

Chromosomes and Disease, Alphabetized

g	Gardner's s. (5q, APC),
h	Hailey-Hailey d. (3q21-24), heavy chain (14), hemochromatosis (6p), hereditary angioedema (11p, C1NH), hereditary coproporphyria (9), HLA-A,B,C,DR,DP,DQ,E,F,G, C3 & C4 (6), Hermansky-Pudlak (10q23.1-q23.3, HPS), hidrotic ectodermal dysplasia (13q), hypomelanosis of Ito (15q11-q13)
i	ichthyosis bullosa of Siemens (12q), incontinentia pigmenti type I (Xp11), incontinentia pigmenti-2 (Xq28), ichthyosis vulgaris (1q21,FLG)
k	κ light chain (2)
l	λ light chain (22), lamellar ichthyosis (2q), lamellar ichthyosis (14q, TGM1)
m	Marfan s. type II (3p25-p24.2), melanoma (9p, CDKN2), Menkes s. (X-MKN/ATP7A), monilethrix (12q13), Muir-Torre s. (3p21.3)
n	nail-patella s. (9q34.1), neurofibromatosis 1 (17q11.2, NF1), neurofibromatosis II (22), non-epidermolytic palmoplantar hyperkeratosis (12q)
o	ocular albinism (Xp), Osler-Rendu-Weber s. 2 (12q11-q14)
p	pachyonychia congenita (12q12-q14), pachyonychia congenita (17q), palmoplantar keratoderma (18q), Papillion-Lefevre s. (11q), PCT (1q), Peutz-Jeghers s. (19p13.3), piebaldism (4q12, C-KIT), porphyria variegata (1q22, PPOX), pro-α-2 (I) gene (7), porphyria-congenital erythropoietic (10q25.2-q26.3), psoriasis susceptibility (17q)
r	recessive X-linked ichthyosis (Xp, STS), Rubinstein-Taybi s. (16p13.3)
s	sclerotylosis (4q), Sjogren-Larson s. (17p11.2, FALDH), striae (18q)
t	TNF-α & β (6), trichoepithelioma-familial (9p), tuberous sclerosis 1 (9q34, TSC1), tuberous sclerosis-2 (16p13.3, TSC2), tylosis (17q), tyrosinemia II [Richner-Hanhart s.] (16q, TAT)
v	Vohwinkel s. (1q21, LOR), von Hippel-Lindau s. (3p26-p25)
w	Waardenburg's s. 1 (2q35, PAX-3), Waardenburg's s. 2 (3p & 13q, MITF), Watson s. (17q11.2), Werner s. (8p, WER), white sponge nevus (12p11.2-q11, 17q21-q22)
x	xeroderma pigmentosa (1), XP-A (9q, XPAC), XP-C (3p25, XPC), XP-D (19q), XP-E (11p, DDB), XP-F (16p13.13-p13.2), XP-G (13q33, ERCC5)

Collagen

Type	Chain composition	Tissue	Disease
I	$[\alpha 1(I)]_2 \alpha 2(I)$	bone, skin, tendon	Ehlers-Danlos type 7A, 7B
I-trimer	$[\alpha 1(I)]_3$	skin, tumors	
II	$[\alpha 1(II)]_3$	cartilage	
III	$[\alpha 1(III)]_3$	fetal skin, blood vessels, GI tract	Ehlers-Danlos type 4
IV	$[\alpha 1(IV)]_2 \alpha 2(IV)$	basement membrane	

Basic Science

Collagen

Type	Chain composition	Tissue	Disease
V	$[\alpha1(V)]_2\alpha2(V)$; $[\alpha1(V)]_3$	all	Ehlers-Danlos type 2
VI	$\alpha1(VI)$ $(2\alpha VI)$ $\alpha3(VI)$	all	
VII	$[\alpha1(VII)]_3$	anchoring fibrils	
VIII	$[\alpha1(VIII)]_3$	endothelial cells	
IX	$\alpha1(IX)$ $\alpha2(IX)$ $\alpha3(IX)$	cartilage	
X	$[\alpha1(X)]_3$	hypertrophic cartilage	
XI	$\alpha1(XI)$ $\alpha2(XI)$ $\alpha3(XI)$	cartilage	
XII	$[\alpha1(XII)]_3$	cornea, ligaments, perichondrium, periosteum, tendons	
XIII	$[\alpha1(XIII)]_3$	all	
XIV	$[\alpha1(XIV)]_3$	cornea, skin, tendons	
XV	unknown	basement membrane	
XVI	$[\alpha1(XVI)]_3$	cartilage, internal organs, skin	
XVII	$[\alpha1(XVII)]_3$	hemidesmosomes	
XVIII	unknown	basement membrane	
XIX	unknown	basement membrane	

Cytokines

basic FGF, acidic FGF	macrophages, endothelial cells	angiogenesis & fibroblast **proliferation**
CSF-1	multiple cells	macrophage activation, granulation tissue formation
EGF		epidermal growth & differentiation, wound healing, keratinocyte migration via $\alpha2$ integrins
IFN-γ	produced by Th1 cells	inhibits IgE synthesis, down-regulates Th2 responses
IL-1	produce by neutrophils, keratinocyte derived	express growth factors, T & B cell activation, chemotaxis, ICAM-1 induction, pyrogen
IL-1 sources	astrocytes, B-cells, corneal cells, dendritic cells, endothelial cells, fibroblasts, keratinocytes, Langerhan's cells, macrophages, melanoma cells, mesangial cells, neutrophils, OKM 1+ LGL	
IL-2		stimulates T lymphocytes

Basic Science

IL-3	keratinocyte derived	stimulates proliferation
IL-4	secreted by Th2 cells	synthesis of IgE, accumulation of eosinophils
IL-5	secreted by Th2 cells	synthesis of IgE, accumulation of eosinophils
IL-6	secreted by Th2 cells, keratinocyte derived	synthesis of IgE, accumulation of eosinophils
Insulin-like GF-I	fibroblasts; epidermal cells	reepithelialization and granulation tissue formation, induces TGF-α autocrine proliferation of keratinocytes
keratinocyte GF	fibroblasts	keratinocyte motility and proliferation
PDGF	platelets, macrophages, epidermal cells	fibroblast proliferation and chemoattraction, macrophage chemoattraction and activation, mediates vasoconstriction
PGE$_2$	produced by monocytes	inhibits Th1 cell derived IFN-γ
TGF-α, heparin-binding EGF	platelets	epidermal and mesenchymal regeneration, pleiotropic cell motility and proliferation
TGF-β1 and β2	platelets, macrophages	epidermal cell motility, chemotaxis of macrophages and fibroblasts, extracellular matrix synthesis and remodeling
TGF-β3	macrophages	anti-scarring effects
TNF-β	neutrophils	expression of growth factors

Enzyme	Action
ALA dehydratase	converts D-aminolevulinic acid to porphobilinogen; ALA dehydratase deficiency porphyria
cholesterol sulfate	inhibits normal desquamation of stratum corneum cells
coproporphyrinogen oxidase	converts coproporphyrinogen III oxidase to harderoporphyrinogen; hereditary coproporphyria
ferrochelatase	converts protoporphyrin to heme; erythropoietic protoporphyria
glucose-6-phosphate dehydrogenase	oxidoreductase class enzyme, first enzyme in the pentose phosphate shunt of glucose metabolism, absence may lead to increased hemolysis (e.g. for patients on dapsone)
homogentisic acid oxidase	lack leads to endogenous ochronosis (alkaptonuria)

Basic Science

Enzyme	Action
porphobilinogen deaminase	Converts porphobilinogen to hydroxymethylbilane; acute intermittent porphyria
protoporphyrinogen oxidase	converts protoporphyrinogen oxidase to protoporphyrin IX; variegate porphyria
steroid sulfatase	converts cholesterol sulfate to cholesterol; absent in recessive X-linked ichthyosis
uroporphyrinogen decarboxylase	converts uroporphyrinogen I to coproporphyrinogen I, converts uroporphyrinogen III to 7-carboxyl porphyrinogen III; porphyria cutanea tarda, hepatoerythropoietic porphyria
uroporphyrinogen II cosynthase	converts hydroxymethylbilane to uroporphyrinogen; congenital erythropoietic porphyria

Human Leukocyte Antigens (HLA): Increased Incidence

alopecia areata	DQB1*03 (DQ3), DRB1 (DR11) severe; DRB1*0401 (DR4), DQB1*0301 (DQ7)
Behçet's s.	B5, B51, B52
dermatitis herpetiformis	B8, DR3, DQw2
epidermolysis bullosa acquisita	DR2
erythema multiforme	B35, B62
erythema multiforme (herpes-associated)	DQB1*0301, DQw3, Bw62, B35, DR53, DR4
Hailey-Hailey d.	B16
herpes gestationis	DR3, DR4
lichen planus	DQw1, DR2, DR1, DR10, DRw9, Bw61/DRw9
linear IgA	B8
mycosis fungoides	DR5, DQB1*03
pemphigus foliaceus	DRB1*0102, DR1, DQw1, DR4,DQw3, DQB*0301
pemphigus vulgaris	Dw10/DR4, Dw10, DR4, DRw6, DQB1.3
pityriasis rosea	DR
psoriasis, pustular	B27
psoriasis	Cw6 (9-15x), B13, B17, Bw57
psoriatic arthritis	B27, B39, DQw3
Reiter's s.	B27 (80%)
Sezary s.	DQB1*0502
Sjögren's s.	DQw2, DR3
systemic lupus erythematosus	homozygous C4A+DR2, DR2, DR3

Basic Science

Human Leukocyte Antigens (HLA): Increased Incidence

systemic sclerosis	DQA2, C4AQ0
Unna-Thost d.	12q11-13
urticaria, chronic idiopathic	DR4, DRB4 53, DQ8, DQA 3011/12
vitiligo	A30, Cw6, Cw7, DQw3, DR4, DR6
Vogt-Koyanagi-Harada s.	Dw15, DQw3, DR4, DRw53

Keratin   Location and/or Associated Condition

Keratin	Location and/or Associated Condition
K1	structural keratin, suprabasal epidermal keratinocytes, palmoplantar suprabasal keratinocytes; non-epidermolytic palmoplantar keratoderma, epidermolytic hyperkeratosis
K2e	epidermal granular layer
K2e	ichthyosis bullosa of Siemens
K3	cornea
K4	non-keratinizing stratified squamous epithelia; white sponge nevus
K5	basal layer "mitotic" keratinocytes; epidermolysis bullosa simplex
K6	proliferation, keratoderma (epidermolytic)
K6a	outer root sheath, hyperproliferative keratinocytes, oral epithelium; pachyonychia congenita-Jadassohn-Lewandowsky type (type 1)
K6b	nail bed, myoepithelium, inflammation
K7	transformed cells
K8	simple epithelia
K9	palmar-plantar specific protein keratoderma (nonepidermolytic)
K10	structural keratin, epidermal granular layer; epidermolytic hyperkeratosis
K11	
K12	cornea
K13	white sponge nevus
K14	basal layer "mitotic" keratinocytes
K15	basal layer of non-keratinizing epithelia
K16	outer root sheath, hyperproliferative keratinocytes, oral epithelium; proliferation keratoderma (epidermolytic), pachyonychia congenita-Jadassohn-Lewandowsky type (type 1)
K17	nail bed, myoepithelium, inflammation; pachyonychia congenita (Jackson-Lawler-type 2), PRP
K18	simple epithelia
K19	bulge cells, simple epithelia
K20	Merkel cells
K21	intestinal epithelium

Basic Science

Proteins/ Amino Acids	Location, Condition, or Action
citrulline	keratotic BCC, inner root sheath, hair medulla, keratolinin
cysteine	involucrin
desmoglein 1	pemphigus foliaceous
desmoglein 3	pemphigus vulgaris
elastin	dermis; pseudoxanthoma elasticum
fibrillin	elastic microfibril of lower BMZ & dermis; Marfan's s.
filaggrin	binds keratinocytes
histidine	filaggrin, profilaggrin
involucrin	differentiation
keratolinin	differentiation
loricrin	differentiation
profilaggrin	processed to filaggrin; absent in ichthyosis vulgaris

Derm Definitions

Primary Skin Lesions

abscess	same as furuncle
boil	same as furuncle
bulla	elevated defined lesion $>/= 1$ cm^2 containing serous fluid
carbuncle	coalescing furuncles
furuncle	a pustule > 1 cm^2
macule	flat, non-palpable change in skin color, < 1 cm^2
mass	synonymous with tumor, but better term since it does not imply malignancy
nodule	large papule > 1 cm^2 extending into dermis
papule	elevated solid lesion < 1 cm^2
pustule	elevated purulent containing lesion
tumor	an elevated firm mass larger than a nodule
vesicle	elevated defined lesion < 1 cm^2 containing serous fluid
wheal	a raised transient irregularly shaped lesion due to edema

Secondary Findings

crust	dried serum, sebum, blood, or pus on eschars or ulcers surface
cyst	closed cavity lined by epithelium
ecchymoses	large purpura
erosion	moist, demarcated depressed area; loss of epidermis
excoriation	superficial linear abrasion of the epidermis from scratching
exudate	fluid, cells & cellular debris resulting from inflammation
fissure	linear split through epidermis into the dermis
hardening	thickened skin with hypo- or hyperpigmentation from prolonged irritant exposure
infarct	necrosis resulting from occlusion of blood vessels
iris	annular bulls-eye lesion
lichenification	epidermal thickening on an elevated plaque with accentuated skin markings, usually from chronic rubbing or scratching
livedo	lace-like pattern
maculosquamous	macule with fine superficial scale; not thick enough to be a plaque
necrosis	cellular death (skin cells)
papulosquamous	papules with fine superficial scale
petechiae	pinpoint purpura
plaque	raised flat lesion formed from a confluence of papules or nodules

Derm Definitions

Secondary Findings

poikiloderma	combination of atrophy, pigmentary change & telangiectasia
purpura	discoloration from bleeding into skin or mucous membrane
scale	sloughed epidermal cells in sheets; white, tan, yellow, or silver cuticular (thin, relatively large flakes), exfoliative (large, peeling sheets), follicular (keratotic plugs, spines, filament, or lichenoid scales), granular (like small grains), hystrix-like (quill-like), ichthyosiform (fish scale-like), keratotic (composed of horny masses), lamellar (thin, relatively large flakes), membranous (large, peeling sheets), pityriasiform (bran-like), psoriasiform (brittle plates in loose layers)
scar	fibrous tissue replacement of skin at site of injury or ulcer
sclerosis	induration, hardening from inflammation & increased connective tissue formation
sinus	communicating tract through the skin, frequently draining
stellate	star-like
sugillation	swollen bruises from injury
ulcer	depressed exudative lesion with loss of both epidermis & part or all of dermis
vegetation	multiple closely spaced projections in a papule or plaque

Configuration

acuminate	pointed
annular	ring-shaped
arciform	arc-shaped
asymmetrical	distributed unilaterally
atrophy	wasting of the epidermis leading to thin, transparent, or dermis leading to depression
confluent	merging together
corymbiform	grouped arrangement with central large lesion & surrounding small lesions
diffuse	widely distributed
discoid	coin-like
discrete	separate from other lesions
ecchymosis	collection of extravascular blood in dermis or subcutaneous tissue caused by trauma & resulting in a macular lesion
generalized	distributed diffusely
group	cluster of lesions

Derm Definitions

Configuration

guttate	drop-like
gyrate	ring-spiral shape
hematoma	localized, deep collection of blood beneath the subcutaneous tissue
herpetiform	clusters of vesicles
iris lesion	concentric rings; bulls-eye
keloid	benign overgrowth of connective tissue following skin injury
linear	in a line
localized	limited areas of involvement which are defined clearly
nummular	coin-like
petechiae	purplish hemorrhagic pinpoint lesions
poikilodermatous	poorly marginated patches with telangiectasia and hyper- and hypopigmented areas
polymorphous	occurring in several different forms
punctate	pointed or dotted
purpura	irregular, large macule with varied color; dark purple to brownish-yellow
reticular	lacy, network pattern
satellite	single lesion in close proximity to large group
serpiginous	snake-like
solitary	single lesion
striae	depressed bands of thin white shiny skin
symmetrical	even, bilateral involvement
telangiectasia	permanent dilatation of capillary vessels in the skin; form branching, fine, red lines
zosteriform	band-like distribution in a dermatomal distribution

Source: John Zic, MD

Dermatopathology Signs & Their Diseases, Definitions, Associations

abscess, intraepidermal	blastomycosis, bromoderma, incontinentia pigmenti, iododerma, pemphigus vegetans
acantholysis	acantholytic dyskeratotic epidermal nevus, BCC, GVH (acute), persistent acantholytic dermatosis, solitary dyskeratosis, transient acantholytic dermatosis
acantholysis, primary	Darier's d., Grover's d., Hailey-Hailey d., herpesvirus infection, pemphigus foliaceus, pemphigus vulgaris, staphylococcal scalded skin s., warty dyskeratoma
acantholysis, secondary	actinic keratosis, impetigo, SCC (adenoid dyskeratotic), subcorneal pustular dermatosis, viral vesicles
acantholytic dyskeratosis	Darier's d., warty dyskeratoma
adnexae, decreased	morphea, necrobiosis lipoidica diabeticorum, PSS, radiodermatitis
adrenoleukodystrophy	vacuolated eccrine secretory coils
amyloid deposits	amyloidosis, BCC, Bowen's disease, nevi, pilomatrixoma, porokeratosis, SCC, SK
amyloid ring	ring around lipocytes; primary amyloidosis
annulate lamellae	EM finding; intracytoplasmic membrane composed of parallel cisternae with dilation of their edges; apocrine gland cells (normal), apocrine hidrocystoma, eccrine porocarcinoma, liposarcoma, malignant mesenchymal tumor, melanoma, rhabdomyosarcoma
apoptotic bodies	*see colloid bodies*
apoptotic cells	EM, fixed drug eruption, GVH, lichen nitidus, lichenoid tissue reaction, LP, lues (secondary), LE, Merkel cell carcinoma, paraneoplastic pemphigus, phototoxicity, poikiloderma
asteroid bodies	stellate eosinophilic inclusions of collagen in macrophages or multinucleated giant cells; actinic granuloma, actinomycosis, coccidioidomycosis, elastolytic annular granuloma, leprosy, lobomycosis (asteroid body-like), NLD, sarcoid, sporotrichosis, tuberculosis
azurophilic granules, giant	giant primary granules within neutrophils; Chediak-Higashi d.
Azzopardi phenomenon	DNA-encrusted intratumoral blood vessels; oat cell metastases (from lung)
B cells, cancers	CLL, follicular lymphoma, mantle zone lymphoma, small lymphocytic lymphoma
B cells, decreased	lymphopenic agammaglobulinemia, SCIDS, thymoma with immunodeficiency, X-linked agammaglobulinemia
ball & claw	elongated rete ridges on sides of infiltrate; lichen nitidus
ballooning degeneration of epidermis	intracellular edema; epidermolytic hyperkeratosis, herpes simplex, smallpox, variola, varicella, verruca
banana bodies	EM finding; banana shaped lipid vacuoles in Schwann cells; lipogranulomatosis (Farber's d.)
basophils	contact dermatitis, incontinentia pigmenti

bean bag cells	histiocytes after phagocytosis of lymphocytes, erythrocytes, platelets; cytophagic histiocytic panniculitis
Birbeck granules	EM finding; tennis racquet-shaped bodies; Langerhan's cells & congenital self healing reticulohistiocytosis, histiocytosis X, reticulum cell sarcoma, monocytic & hairy cell leukemia (some)
birds eye cells	koilocytes; flat warts
birefringence	amyloidosis, collagen, gout, hair, silica, uric acid crystals
bramble bush elastic fibers	penicillamine-induced elastic fibers
broad based budding	blastomycosis
bullae, hemorrhagic	bullous amyloidosis, EBA, erysipelas, gas gangrene, lichen sclerosis, PCT
calcification	cutaneous cartilage tumor, cutaneous endometriosis/endosalpingosis, epidermal inclusion cyst, penile fibromatosis (Peyronie's d.), peripheral giant cell granuloma, peripheral ossifying fibroma, infantile fibromatosis (congenital fibromatosis), infarcted lipomas, lupus profundus, microcystic carcinoma, minor salivary gland calculus, pancreatic fat necrosis, pilomatrixoma, pseudotumor of Ehlers-Danlos s., PXE, sclerema neonatorum, synovial sarcoma, trichilemmal cyst, trichoepithelioma (desmoplastic)
capillaritis	familial pigmented purpuric eruption, gravitational purpura, purpura annularis telangiectoides (Majocchi's d.), lichen aureus, pigmented purpuric lichenoid dermatosis of Gougerot & Blum, itching purpura of Doucas & Kapetanakis, Schamberg's d.
cartilage	aponeurotic fibromatosis, branchial cleft cyst, cutaneous cartilage tumor, epithelioid sarcoma, extra-skeletal chondrosarcoma, fibrosarcoma, giant congenital nevus, mixed tumor (chondroid syringoma), proliferative myositis, schwannoma (malignant)
caseation necrosis	dermal collagen degeneration; lupus miliaris disseminatous facei, tertiary syphilis, tuberculosis
caterpillar bodies	PAS-positive globules on roof of blister containing basement membrane, degenerating keratinocytes and colloid bodies; PCT
cauliflower fibrils	see *collagen flowers*
CEA+	epithelioid sarcoma, granular cell tumor, intraepidermal epithelioma, Paget's d., signet ring cell carcinoma, syringocystadenoma papilliferum
cells, two types	clear cell hidradenoma, cylindroma, eccrine spiradenoma
cementasome body	see *Odland body*
ceroid-like macrophage inclusions	Hermansky-Pudlak s.
Charcot Leyden crystals	protein found in granules of eosinophils
cholesterol crystals	xanthoma cells, necrobiotic xanthogranuloma, pilar cysts
cholesterol granulomas	thymic cysts

Dermatopathology Signs & Their Diseases, Definitions, Associations

cholesterolosis	erythema elevatum diutinum, North American blastomycosis
church spire appearance	marked papillomatosis with suprapapillary thinning of epidermis; acrokeratosis verruciformis of Hopf, erythrokeratoderma viriabilis
civatte bodies	*see colloid bodies*
clear cells	balloon cell nevus, BCC, clear cell acrospiroma, clear cell hidradenoma, clear cell sarcoma, congenital nevi (early age), eccrine carcinoma, deep & penetrating nevus, malignant acrospiroma, renal cell carcinoma, trichilemmoma, SCC, sebaceous carcinoma, syringoma, white sponge nevus
cleavage, intra-epidermal	eczematous dermatitis, epidermolysis bullosa simplex, epidermolytic hyperkeratosis, EM, friction blister, herpes simplex, herpes zoster, incontinentia pigmenti, miliaria rubra, variola
cleavage, lamina densa	dystrophic epidermolysis bullosa, EM, lichen sclerosis, PCT
cleavage, lamina lucida	BP, cicatricial pemphigoid, dermatitis herpetiformis, heat, herpes gestationis, junctional epidermolysis bullosa, liquid nitrogen, PCT, pseudoporphyria, suction blister
cleavage, subcorneal	bullous diabeticorum, bullous impetigo, epidermolysis bullosa simplex, erythema toxicum neonatorum, friction blister, miliaria crystallina, pemphigus erythematosus, pemphigus foliaceus, SSSS, subcorneal pustular dermatosis
cleavage, subepidermal	BP, cicatricial pemphigoid, DH, EM, herpes gestationis, lichen planus, lichen sclerosis et atrophicus, linear IgA dermatosis, lupus erythematosus, PCT, urticaria pigmentosa
cleavage, supra-basal	Darier's d., Hailey-Hailey d., pemphigus vegetans, pemphigus vulgaris, transient acantholytic dermatosis
coat sleeve infiltrate	dense lymphocytic infiltrate around blood vessels of papillary & upper reticular dermis; EAC
collagen flowers	abnormal collagen fibril aggregates creating a flower-like appearance on cross section; Buschke-Olendorf s., cutis laxa, Ehlers-Danlos s., OI, PXE AKA composite fibrils, cauliflower fibrils
collagen phagocytosis	multicentric reticulohistiocytosis
collarette	metastatic melanoma, pyogenic granuloma
colloid bodies	eosinophilic degenerated keratinocyte clusters; benign lichenoid keratosis, colloid milium, GVH d., KA, lichen nitidus, lichen planus, lichen striatus, lupus erythematosus, normal skin AKA Civatte bodies, hyaline bodies, cytoid bodies, apoptotic bodies
comma bodies	EM: cytoplasmic curved lipid vacuoles in histiocytes, fibroblasts, & Langerhan's cells; benign cephalic histiocytosis, generalized eruptive histiocytoma, histiocytosis X, infantile self healing reticulohistiocytosis, juvenile xanthogranuloma, multicentric reticulohistiocytosis, sinus histiocytosis with massive lymphadenopathy
composite fibrils	*see collagen flowers*
corneocyte	**retention**: ichthyosis vulgaris, x-linked ichthyosis **proliferation**: epidermolytic hyperkeratosis, lamellar ichthyosis

Dermatopathology Signs & Their Diseases, Definitions, Associations

coronoid lamella	wedge shaped parakeratotic column; actinic keratosis, BCC, eccrine ostial & dermal duct nevus, milium, porokeratosis, punctate kerato-derma, seborrheic keratosis, scar, SCC, wart
corps grains	*see grains*
corps ronds	dyskeratotic acantholytic basophilic keratinocytes with pyknotic nucleus & perinuclear halo; AK, Bowen's d., Darier's d., focal acantholytic dyskeratosis, Grover's d., Hailey-Hailey d., keratoacanthoma, lichen striatus, proliferating trichilemmal cyst, SCC, warty dyskeratoma
Cowdry Type A intra-nuclear inclusions	Herpesvirus infections
curvilinear bodies	*see comma bodies*
cutaneous horn	conical hyperkeratotic papule; AK, BCC, SCC, SK, trichilemmoma, trichilemmal keratosis, verrucae
cytoid bodies	*see colloid bodies*
cytoplasmic inclusions, pleomorphic	multicentric reticulohistiocytosis
dell	depression of epidermal surface; desmoplastic trichoepithelioma, LE, lichen sclerosis
dermal fibrosis	acquired digital fibrokeratoma, acroangiodermatitis, angiofibroma, atrophoderma of Pasini & Perini, BCC, bleomycin administration, blue nevus, collagenoma, cutaneous endometriosis, ductal adenocarcinoma, eccrine spiradenoma, familial & nonfamilial cutaneous fibroma of tuberous sclerosis, fibrous papule of the nose, glomus tumor, hypertrophic scar, intraepithelial epithelioma, keloid, lobomycosis, LSA, lues, Merkel cell carcinoma, metastases, morphea, nevus sebaceous, pearly penile papules, pinta, prurigo nodularis, PSS, radiodermatitis, radiotherapy, spider bites, Talwin injection, morpheaform BCC, desmoplastic trichoepithelioma, SCC, shagreen patch, spindle & epithelial cell nevus, Spitz nevus, syringoma
dermal thickening	scleredema
dermolytic pemphigoid	epidermolysis bullosa acquisita (immunopathologic type)
desmoplasia	dense collagenous hypocellular stroma; desmoplastic spindle cell tumor, desmoplastic trichoepithelioma, epithelioid cell tumor
desmosome absence	BCC, indeterminate cells, Langerhan's cells, sclerodermoid GVHD
desmosome proliferation	benign mucosal pemphigoid
dilapidated brick wall	appearance from acantholysis throughout epidermis; Hailey-Hailey d.
Donovan bodies	oval bipolar staining intracytoplasmic inclusions with surrounding capsule; *Calymmatobacterium granulomatis* (granuloma inguinale)
doubly refractile	cholesterol esters (but not free cholesterol, phospholipids, or neutral fat), gout (urate crystals), silica, splinters, suture, talcum powder

Dermatopathology Signs & Their Diseases, Definitions, Associations

dumbbell shape	cellular blue nevus
dyskeratosis, focal acantholytic	**acantholytic acanthoma,** BCC, CNCH, comedone, condylomata acuminata, **Darier's d.,** dermatofibroma, fibrous papule of the nose, **Grover's d.,** keratosis punctata palmaris et plantaris, **linear epidermal nevi,** melanoma, nevi, oral leukoplakia, papillomas, **papular acantholytic dyskeratosis,** PR, PRP, psoriasiform dermatitis, SCC, seborrheic keratosis, **warty dyskeratoma**
dyskeratotic cells	eosinophilic, shrunken keratinocytes with pynknotic nuclei from abnormal keratinization; acrodermatitis enteropathica, acute GVH, candidiasis, dermatitis herpetiformis, DLE, EM, fixed drug eruption, IP, insect bites, intraepidermal epithelioma, keratoacanthoma, lichen planus, lichen sclerosis, lichen striatus, lichenoid photodermatitis, LE, lymphomatoid papulosis, lymphogranuloma venereum, measles, necrolytic migratory erythema, neutrophilic eccrine hidradenitis, parapsoriasis, pemphigus erythematosus, phototoxic contact dermatitis, PLEVA, proliferating trichilemmal cyst, pseudolymphoma, radiotherapy, SCC, secondary syphilis, solar chelitis, toxic shock s., verrucous incontinentia pigmenti, viral infection, warty dyskeratoma
elastic fiber (gain)	actinic elastosis, dermatofibrosis lenticularis disseminata, Ehlers-Danlos s., elastofibroma, juvenile elastoma, lichen sclerosis, mixed tumor (chondroid syringoma)
elastic fiber (loss)	acrodermatitis chronica atrophicans, actinic elastosis, acrokeratoe-lastosis, adenoma sebaceum, angiofibroma, annular elastolytic granuloma, anetoderma, acquired digital fibroma, atrophoderma, collagenoma, cutis laxa, digital fibrokeratoma, elastosis perforans serpiginosa, hypertrophic scar, keloid, leprechaunism, dermal elastolysis with wrinkling, NLD, necrobiotic xanthogranuloma, nevus sebaceous, progressive nodular histiocytoma, radiodermatitis, restrictive dermopathy, striae, Talwin dermatitis, xanthoma disseminatum (phagocytosis of elastic fibers)
elastic fibers (intraepidermal)	elastosis perforans serpiginosa, keratoacanthoma, SCC
elastin accumulation	Buschke-Ollendorff s., elastoderma, elastofibroma, pseudoxanthoma elasticum, solar elastosis
eosinophils, intraepithelial	halogenodermas, incontinentia pigmenti, keratoacanthoma
epidermal atrophy	acrodermatitis chronica atrophicans, actinic keratosis, atrophoderma, dermatomyositis, GVH d., lentigo maligna, lichen planus, lichen sclerosis et atrophicus, lupus erythematosus, poikiloderma, radiodermatitis, scleroderma, steroid atrophy
epidermal giant cells	pityriasis rosca
epidermal necrosis	erythema multiforme, glucagonoma s., GVH d., hydroa vacciniforme, ischemia, TEN
epidermolytic hyperkeratosis	thickened granular layer with perinuclear halos & swollen keratohyalin granules; actinic keratosis, BCC, benign solid hidradenoma, **bullous congenital ichthyosiform erythroderma,** dermatofibroma, **epidermal nevi, epidermolytic keratosis palmaris et plantaris,**

Dermatopathology Signs & Their Diseases, Definitions, Associations

	GA, hypertrophic scar, intradermal nevus, interferon alpha-2b administration, lichenoid amyloidosis, nevus comedonicus, nummular eczema, sebaceous hyperplasia, **solitary acanthoma**, trichilemmal cyst AKA granular cell degeneration
epidermotropism	lymphoid cell influx to epidermis; large plaque parapsoriasis, metastatic malignant melanoma, mycosis fungoides
epithelial membrane Ag+	Merkel cell carcinoma
epithelial microabscesses	CTCL, histiocytosis X, migratory stomatitis (geographic tongue)
erythrocytes in epidermis	allergic contact dermatitis, drug eruptions, eczematous dermatitis, graft rejection, insect bite, leukocytoclastic vasculitis, lymphomatoid papulosis, PLEVA, pityriasis rosea, polymorphous light eruption
erythrocytes, extravasated	acroangiodermatitis, angiolymphoid hyperplasia with eosinophils, apocrine cystadenoma, cat scratch d., cellulitis, cutaneous cartilage tumor, cutaneous endometriosis, dermatofibroma, erythema annulare centrifugum, erythema multiforme, erythema nodosum, erythropoietic protoporphyria, granuloma faciale, Henoch-Schönlein purpura, Histiocytosis X, Kaposi's sarcoma, lupus erythematosus, lymphomatoid papulosis, meningococcemia, metastatic tumors, migratory panniculitis, parapsoriais variegata, pellagra, peripheral giant cell granuloma, pityriasis rosea, polymorphous light eruption, psoriasis, PLEVA, PMLE, RMSF, ruptured follicular cyst, Schamberg's d., secondary lues, subacute nodular chancroid, Sweet's s., toxic shock s., tuberculosis verrucosa cutis, tularemia, vasculitis
erythrophagocytosis	amebiasis, brucellosis, cytophagic histiocytic panniculitis, familial lymphohistiocytic reticulosis, histiocytosis X, malignant histiocytosis, regional histiocytosis, pancreatic fat necrosis, peripheral giant cell granuloma, pyoderma gangrenosum, regressing atypical histiocytosis
exocytosis	actinic reticuloid, eczema, MF, parapsoriasis en plaque, PLEVA, pityriasis rosea, secondary lues
extracellular cholesterosis	(cholesterol clefts); apocrine cystadenoma (hidrocystoma), EED, necrobiotic xanthogranuloma
extramedullary hematopoiesis	giant cell nevus, neurocristic hamartoma
Farber bodies	*see comma bodies*
festooning	round, irregular papillary dermal projections into subepidermal blister; PCT
fibrinoid deposits	vessel wall fibrin deposition; dermatomyositis, leukocytoclastic vasculitis, rheumatoid nodules, subcutaneous granuloma annulare, SLE
fibrous long-spacing collagen	EM finding; angiofibroma (tuberous sclerosis), BCC (stroma), blue nevus, juvenile hyaline fibromatosis, lepromatous leprosy, melanoma (stroma), SCC (stroma), Schwannoma, scleroderma
fingerprint bodies	eccrine gland cells; ceroid-lipofuscinosis
flame figures	eosinophils, histiocytes & debris surrounding collagen fibers; arthropod bites, dermatophytosis, eczematous dermatitis, eosinophilic cellulitis, hypereosinophilic s., parasites, pemphigoid, prurigo nodularis

Dermatopathology Signs & Their Diseases, Definitions, Associations

florets	conidia that form daisy-like clusters at hyphal branch ends; *S. schenkii*
foam cells	lipid laden macrophage; juvenile xanthogranuloma, leishmaniasis, lepromatous leprosy, reticulohistiocytic granuloma, Weber-Christian d.(idiopathic lobular panniculitis), xanthoma
follicular plugging	Darier's d., lichen sclerosis, LE, pemphigus erythematosus, PRP, seborrheic dermatitis
formalin fixation stable	CEA, EMZ, kappa and lambda chains, keratin epitopes, leukocyte common antigen, myelin basic protein, S-100, salivary mucin, von Willebrand's related antigen
germinal centers	angiolymphoid hyperplasia with eosinophilia, angiomatoid malignant fibrous histiocytoma, lupus panniculitis, malignant fibrous histiocytoma, necrobiotic xanthogranuloma, pseudolymphoma, reactive lymphoid hyperplasia, tick bite granuloma
ghost cells	pale eosinophilic cell with central clearing & absent nucleus; fat necrosis, pilomatricoma AKA shadow cell
giant cells	actinic keratosis, angiofibroma, annular elastolytic granuloma, atypical fibroxanthoma, blastomycosis, Candida granuloma, cat scratch d., chromomycosis, coccidioidomycosis, cryptococcosis, Darier's d. of the nail, desmoid tumor (with muscle involvement), epithelial sarcoma, erythema nodosum, fibrous papule of the nose, giant cell tumor of the tendon sheath, granuloma annulare, Herpesvirus infection, histiocytoma variant of dermatofibroma, histiocytosis X, histoplasmosis, histoplasmosis (African), infarcted lipoma, kala-azar, lichen nitidus, leiomyosarcoma, malignant fibrous histiocytoma, metastatic Crohn's d., multicentric reticulohistiocytosis, mycetoma, NLD, neurofibroma, neurothekioma, palisaded encapsulated neuroma, paracoccidiodomycosis, peripheral ossifying fibroma, phaeohypomycosis, pseudoepitheliomatous hyperplasia, schwannoma, sclerosing lipogranuloma, soft tissue melanoma, sporotrichosis, synovial sarcoma, Talwin injection, tertiary lues, tuberculosis
giant cells, floret type	giant cell fibroblastoma, lepromatous leprosy, pleomorphic lipoma
giant cells, foreign body	actinomycetoma, chronic folliculitis, deep folliculitis eosinophilic cellulitis, juvenile xanthogranuloma, keratoacanthoma, lipodystrophy, lymphogranuloma venereum, necrobiotic xanthogranuloma, nevus sebaceous, nodular vasculitis, ochronosis, peripheral giant cell granuloma, pilomatrixoma, pityrosporon folliculitis, post-steroid fat necrosis, proliferating trichilemmal tumors, subcutaneous fat necrosis
giant cells, Langerhan's	leprosy, leishmaniasis, lymphogranuloma venereum, sarcoidosis, tuberculoid leprosy
giant cells, osteoclast	giant cell malignant fibrous histiocytoma, nodular fasciitis
giant cells, Touton type	dermatofibroma, DFSP, diffuse normolipemic plane xanthoma, histiocytoma, histiocytoma variant of dermatofibroma, histiocytosis X, juvenile xanthogranuloma, necrobiotic xanthogranuloma with paraproteinemia, papular xanthoma, progressive nodular histiocytosis, xanthoma disseminatum, xanthomatous Hand-Schüler-Christian d.

Dermatopathology Signs & Their Diseases, Definitions, Associations

giant melanosome	Albright's s., Becker's melanosis, café-au-lait spots, Chediak-Higashi s., lentigo simplex, lentiginosis profusa, LEOPARD s., melanocytic nevi, nevus spilus, normal skin
grains	cells in stratum corneum with small pyknotic nuclei surrounded by shrunken eosinophilic cytoplasm; Darier's d., Hailey-Hailey d., mycetoma, transient acantholytic dermatosis, warty dyskeratoma
granular cell degeneration	*see epidermolytic hyperkeratosis*
granular cell layer, decreased	AK, Bowen's d., clear cell acanthoma, confluent & reticulated papillomatosis of Gougerot & Cartedeau, harlequin fetus, ichthyosis vulgaris, pilar cyst, proliferating trichellemmal cyst, psoriasis
granular cell layer, increased	angiofibroma, epidermolytic hyperkeratosis, intraepidermal epithelioma, keratosis palmaris et plantaris, lamellar ichthyosis, lichen planus (focal), nevus sebaceous, perforating disorder of renal disease, pseudoepitheliomatous hyperplasia, Refsum's d., seboacanthoma, Spitz nevus, wart, X-linked recessive ichthyosis
granular degeneration	*see epidermolytic hyperkeratosis*
granules	*see sulfur granules*
granuloma, foreign body	asbestos, calcium, carbon, metal, mineral oil, paraffin, quartz, ruptured follicular cyst, silica, spines, splinter, suture, talcum, tattoo, urate, wood
granuloma, necrotizing	allergic granulomatosis, Wegener's granulomatosis
granuloma, palisading	central necrobiosis & peripheral histiocytes, epithelioid cells, lymphocytes & giant cells; gout, GA, NLD, necrobiotic xanthogranuloma, pseudo-rheumatoid nodule, rheumatic fever nodule, rheumatoid nodule
granuloma, sarcoidal	epithelioid & giant cell granuloma; cheilitis granulomatosis, foreign body reactions, MCD, granulomatous rosacea, sarcoidosis, silica, zirconium
granuloma, tuberculoid	epithelioid & giant cell granuloma with cuff of lymphocytes; deep fungal, foreign body, leishmaniasis, leprosy, lupus miliaris disseminatous facei, protothecosis, rosacea, tertiary syphilis, tuberculoid leprosy, tuberculosis
grenz zone	uninvolved margin of dermis; acrodermatitis chronica atrophicans, actinic elastosis, B cell lymphoma, bullous mastocytosis, dermatofibroma, DFSP, granuloma faciale, lepromatous leprosy, leukemia cutis, lymphocytoma cutis, lymphoma cutis, metastatic lesions, Merkel cell carcinoma, neurothekioma, palisaded encapsulated neuroma, parapsoriasis en plaque, pseudolymphoma, sarcoidosis
ground glass cytoplasm	eosinophilic refractile-appearing cytoplasm of histiocytic cells; infantile self healing reticulohistiocytosis, multicentric reticulohistiocytosis, reticulohistiocytoma
Guarnieri bodies	keratinocyte eosinophilic intracytoplasmic inclusions; smallpox, vaccinia
hair germs	congenital vellus hamartoma, trichoepithelioma, trichoblastic fibroma, trichoblastoma

Dermatopathology Signs & Their Diseases, Definitions, Associations

hair matrix	pilomatrixoma
hair pilar canal	trichoadenoma
hair shafts, longitudinal cleft	anhidrotic ectodermal dysplasia
Hassal's corpuscles	epithelial cells aggregated into concentric layers of keratinized cells; thymic cysts
Heinz bodies	denaturation of hemoglobin with formation of precipitates; treatment with dapsone, oxidative stress
hemosiderophage	macrophage or histiocyte containing phagocytized hemosiderin; chronic pigmented purpura, KS, stasis dermatitis
Henderson-Patterson bodies	globules of viral protein; molluscum contagiosum AKA molluscum bodies
herringbone pattern	DFSP, fibrosarcoma
HMB-45 vs. S-100	**HMB-45 negative**; dermal nevus cells, desmoplastic melanoma, neurotropic melanoma **S-100 negative**; blue nevi
hob nailing	endothelial cell projection into lumina; angiolymphoid hyperplasia with e. sinophils, angiosarcoma
Homer-Wright rosettes	concentrically arranged tumor cells; Merkel cell carcinoma, neuroblastoma (metastatic)
horn cyst	seborrheic keratosis, SCC, trichoepithelioma
horn pearls	*see squamous pearls*
hot spots	aggregates of transformed cells in UV-induced neoplasia
Huygens' effect	condenser of microscope defocused to obtain a partial phase effect
hyalin bodies	*see colloid bodies*
hydropic degeneration	basal cell degeneration with vacuole formation; dermatomyositis, discoid lupus, erythema dyschromicum perstans, EM, fixed drug eruption, lichen planus, lichen sclerosis et atrophicus, poikiloderma atrophicans vasculare, poikiloderma congenitale, SCLE, SLE AKA liquefaction degeneration, vacuolar degeneration
hypergranulosis	epidermal nevus, epidermolytic hyperkeratosis, LP, LSC, verruca vulgaris, x-linked ichthyosis
hypogranulosis	ichthyosis vulgaris, normal mucous membrane, psoriasis
immune complexes (perivascular)	bowel bypass s., cryoglobulinemia, drug reaction, EED, erythema nodosum leprosum, erythropoietic protoporphyria, EM, granuloma faciale, leukocytoclastic vasculitis, Lucio phenomenon, lupus profundus, meningococcemia, NLD, nodular vasculitis, polyarteritis nodosa, PCT, Schamberg's d., serum sickness, urticarial vasculitis, Wegener's granulomatosis
immunofluorescence, indirect	pemphigus foliacous 70%, bullous pemphigoid >70%, HG factor 25%, linear IgA disease <25%

Dermatopathology Signs & Their Diseases, Definitions, Associations

immunofluorescence, indirect (intercellular)	blood group A & B antibodies, bullous pemphigoid, burn, cicatricial pemphigoid, lichen planus, myasthenia gravis, pemphigus vulgaris, penicillin reaction, SLE, TEN
inclusions, intracytoplasmic	molluscum contagiosum, orf, paravaccinia (milker's nodules), small pox, vaccinia
inclusions, intranuclear	coxsackie virus, enterovirus, herpesvirus, human papillomavirus, orf, paravaccinia, rubeola
Indian filing	linear infiltration of cells; adenocarcinoma, breast cancer metastasis, granuloma annulare, lymphoma, lymphocytic lymphoma, lymphocytoma cutis, pseudolymphoma
infiltrate, eosinophilic	allergic granulomatosis, angioedema, angiolymphoid hyperplasia with eosinophilia, autoimmune progesterone dermatitis, BP, eosinophilic cellulitis, eosinophilic spongiosis, eosinophilic tongue ulcers, eosinophilic pustulosis of the scalp in children, erythema toxicum neonatorum, granuloma faciale, halogenodermas, herpes gestationis, hypereosinophilic s., infestations, insect bite, Ofuji's d., papular dermatitis of pregnancy, PUPPP
intracellular hyaline globules	Kaposi's sarcoma
intraepidermal spread	Bowen's d., epidermotropic metastatic melanoma, epidermotropic metastatic disease, hidroacanthoma simplex, Paget's d., seborrheic keratosis, superficial spreading malignant melanoma
iron deposits	hemochromatosis, nevus sebaceous, progressive nodular histiocytoma, xanthoma disseminatum
jigsaw puzzle-like	cylindroma
Kamino bodies	eosinophilic aggregations of type IV collagen; epithelioid cell nevus, melanoma, spindle cell nevus
karyorrhexis	nuclear fragmentation with formation of basophilic nuclear dust; leukocytoclastic vasculitis
keratin pearls	*see squamous pearls*
keratinosome body	*see Odland body*
knife marks	seen on a slide; silica granulomas
Kogoj, spongiform pustule of	intraepidermal neutrophil aggregate within sponge-like area; acrodermatitis continua of Hallopeau, candidiasis, dermatophytosis, **geographic tongue**, halogenodermas, impetigo, psoriasis, **Reiter's d.**, subcorneal pustular dermatosis
koilocyte	squamous cell with hyperchromic nuclei surrounded by perinuclear halo; HPV
Kulchitsky cells	endocrine cells with granular or pale pink cytoplasm; argentaffin gut cells; carcinoid
lacunae	splits in basal cell layer; Darier's d. AKA intraepidermal blisters
lacunar cells	immunoglobulin cell with single hyperlobated nucleus with small nucleoli, cytoplasm retracts in formalin fixed tissue with resultant clear space around cell; Hodgkin's lymphoma (nodular sclerosis variant)

Dermatopathology Signs & Their Diseases, Definitions, Associations

lamellar body	*see Odland body*
Langerhan's cells, decreased	HIV, old age, PUVA therapy
Langerhan's cells, increased	early lichen planus, mycosis fungoides
Langerhan's giant cells	multinucleate histiocytic giant cell with peripheral nuclei; foreign body reactions, hypersensitivity reactions
Leishman bodies	epidermal inclusions in leishmaniasis
leukocytoclasis	karyorrhexis and neutrophil degeneration with nuclear dust; leukocytoclastic vasculitis
lichenoid infiltrate	GVH, lichenoid drug eruption, lichenoid keratosis, lichen planopilaris, LP, LE, poikiloderma vasculare atrophicans
lipid vacuoles	Refsum's d., Chanarin-Dorfman s.
Lipshutz bodies/granules	inclusion bodies in cytoplasm of infected ballooned epithelial cells; HSV, molluscum contagiosum (pox virus)
liquefaction degeneration	*see hydropic degeneration*
Luse bodies	long collagen fibers; Hodgkin's lymphoma, lymphoproliferative disease, multicentric reticulohistiocytosis, neural tumors
lymphocytes, satellite	lymphocytes in close apposition to dyskeratotic keratinocytes; GVH d.
lymphoid follicles	angiolymphoid hyperplasia with eosinophilia, dermatofibroma, desmoplastic malignant melanoma, epulis fissuratum, lupus profundus, morphea, lupus panniculitis, necrobiotic xanthogranuloma
lymphoid follicles with germinal centers	ALHE, BCC, Castleman's d., cutaneous lymphoid hyperplasia, inflammatory pseudotumor of the skin, Kimura's d., marginal zone lymphoma, morphea
lymphophagocytosis	cytophagic histiocytic panniculitis, malignant histiocytosis, sinus histiocytosis with massive lymphadenopathy
macromelanosomes	*see melanosomes, giant*
mast cells	androgenic alopecia, atopic dermatitis, keloid, lichen planus, lichen simplex chronicus, lupus erythematosus, mastocytoma, neurofibroma, spindle cell lipoma, synovial sarcoma, trichogerminoma
Max Joseph cleft/space	hydropic degeneration of basal layer leading to epidermal separation; lichen planus
Medlar bodies	intermediate vegetative form of fungi; chromoblastomycosis (pathognomonic) AKA muriform cells
Meischer's microgranuloma	small histiocytes radially arranged around a central cleft; erythema nodosum AKA Meischer's radial granuloma
melanin granules	café-au-lait spots, eruptive nevi, generalized lentigines, metastatic malignant melanoma, xeroderma pigmentosum
melanin granules, giant	Albright's s., melanocytic nevi, multiple lentiginosis s., neurofibromatosis (café-au-lait macules), nevus spilus

Dermatopathology Signs & Their Diseases, Definitions, Associations

melanin macroglobules	Becker's nevus, café-au-lait spots (neurofibromatosis), Chediak-Higashi s., generalized melanosis Hermansky-Pudlak s., LEOPARD s., lentigo simplex, lentigo maligna, leukoderma, nevi, nevus spilus, post PUVA lentigines, tinea versicolor, X-linked ocular albinism, XP
melanin, decreased	albinism, hypopituitarism, monobenzylether of hydroquinone, piebaldism, Tietze's s., Vogt-Koyanagi-Harada s.
melanin, increased	Addison's d., Albright's d., Becker's melanosis, bleomycin administration, busulfan, café-au-lait macules, carbon baby s., chlorpromazine administration, Cronkhite-Canada s., Dowling Degos d., doxorubicin, dyskeratosis congenita, ephelides (or decreased), Fanconi's s., fixed drug eruption, gold administration, hemochromatosis, labial melanotic macule, lamprene administration, lentigo simplex, mechlorethamine, melanosis diffusa congenita, melasma, minocycline administration, neurofibromatosis, nevus spilus, POEMS s., Peutz-Jeghers s., post-inflammatory hyperpigmentation, reticulate acropigmentation of Kitamura, senile lentigo, silver exposure, solar lentigo, tanning, topical psoralens, topical nitrogen mustard, topical 5-FU
melanocytes, absent	chemical depigmentation, halo nevi, piebaldism, pinta, traumatized area, vitiligo, Vogt-Koyanagi-Harada s., Waardenburg's s., Wolf's s., XP
melanocytes, increased	Addison's d., Becker's melanosis, café-au-lait macules in neurofibromatosis, centrofacial neurodysraphic lentiginosis, lentigo maligna, lentigo simplex, LEOPARD s., mechlorethamine, melasma, Moynahan's s., nevus spilus, Peutz-Jeghers s., reticulate acropigmentation of Kitamura, segmental lentiginosis, senile lentigo, Soto's s., tanning
melanocytes, normal	Addison's d., albinism, ash leaf macule of tuberous sclerosis, Chediak-Higashi s., ephelides, labial melanotic macule, melanotic macules of Albright's s., nevus depigmentosus, PKU, Peutz-Jeghers s., sarcoidosis, senile lentigo, Ziprokowski-Margolis s.
melanocytes, reduced	alopecia areata, ash leaf macule of tuberous sclerosis, ephelides, halo nevus, idiopathic guttate hypomelanosis, incontinentia pigmenti achromians, leprosy, lichen planus, Menkes s., pityriasis alba, post-inflammatory hypopigmentation, Vagabond's d., Ziprokowski-Margolis s.
melanophage	phagocytized melanin in histiocyte or macrophage; blue nevus, fixed drug eruption, lichen planus, melanoma, post-inflammatory hyper-pigmentation, seborrheic keratosis
melanosome macrocomplexes	melanosomes sequestered in lysosomes; seborrheic keratoses
melanosomes, giant (macromelanosomes)	unusually large melanin granule aggregations; Albright's s. (rare), alcoholic liver d., Becker's melanosis, café-au-lait macules, Chediak-Higashi s., Hermansky-Pudlak s., lentigines, LEOPARD s., neurofibromatosis, nevus spilus, normal skin, piebaldism, primary biliary cirrhosis, vitiligous achromia with malignant melanoma, XP, XLR ocular albinism

Dermatopathology Signs & Their Diseases, Definitions, Associations

membrane coating granules	*see Odland bodies*
meridional array	quadrennial structure of B-pleated sheet; amyloidosis
Michaelis-Gutman bodies	intracytoplasmic calcified basophilic bodies in phagolysosomes of von Hansemann cells; malakoplakia
Mickulicz cells	large pale foamy histiocytes containing clumps of encapsulated Klebsiella bacteria; rhinoscleroma
microabscess (papillary)	bullous LE, dermatitis herpetiformis
molluscum bodies	globules of viral protein; molluscum contagiosum AKA Henderson-Paterson bodies
mucinoses	**primary**: acquired digital fibrokeratoma, acral persistent papular mucinosis, connective tissue disease, cutaneous mucinosis of infancy, focal mucinosis, granuloma annulare, lichen myxedematosus, melanoma (myxoid melanoma), myxedema (generalized & localized) papular mucinosis, myxoid cyst, plaque-like cutaneous mucinosis, self-healing juvenile cutaneous mucinosis **secondary**: BCC, Degos' d., etretinate therapy, LE, palisading granulomas, PUVA therapy, reticular erythematous mucinosis, skin cancers, toxic oil s.
mucous secretory granules	adenoid cystic carcinoma, apocrine carcinoma, apocrine cystadenoma, apocrine hidrocystoma, chondroid syringoma, clear cell hidradenoma, hidradenoma papilliferum, metastatic tumor of glandular differentiation, mucinous carcinoid, mucinous carcinoma, Paget's d., syringocystadenoma papilliferum
multifocal tumors	Bowen's d., Paget's d., recurrent tumors, sebaceous carcinoma
multinucleated giant cells	multinucleated keratinocytes; HSV infection
Munro microabscess	subcorneal abscess formed by neutrophils; impetigo, psoriasis, Reiter's s., seborrheic dermatitis
muriform cells	intermediate vegetative form of fungi; chromoblastomycosis (pathognomonic) AKA Medlar bodies
myofibroblasts	cranial fasciitis of infancy, dermatofibroma, desmoid, Dupuytren's contracture, fibroma of the tendon sheath, fibrous hamartoma of infancy, infantile myofibromatosis (congenital generalized fibromatosis), infantile digital myofibroblastoma (infantile digital fibromatosis), keloids, malignant fibrous histiocytoma, nodular fasciitis (pseudosarcomatous)
myxoid diseases	see *mucinoses*
n-alkanes	epidermolytic hyperkeratosis, lamellar ichthyosis
necrobiosis	necrosis leading to homogenization of dermal collagen; GA, NLD, NXG, rheumatoid nodule
necrotic nidus	insect bites
needle shaped clefts in subcutaneous fat	post-steroid panniculitis, sclerema neonatorum, subcutaneous fat necrosis of the newborn

Dermatopathology Signs & Their Diseases, Definitions, Associations

neuron specific enolase	BCC, epithelioid sarcoma, Merkel cell carcinoma
neurosecretory granules	Merkel cell carcinoma
neurotropism	congenital nevi, desmoplastic malignant melanoma, microcystic adnexal carcinoma, neurotropic malignant melanoma
neutrophilic micro abscesses, intraepidermal	candidiasis, deep fungal, granuloma inguinale, halogenoderma, impetigo, psoriasis, tuberculosis verrucosa cutis
neutrophilic lysosomes, enlarged	Chediak-Higashi s.
neutrophils, dermal	Behçet's s., cellulitis, familial Mediterranean fever, bowel associated dermatitis-arthritis s., neutrophilic eccrine hidradenitis, pyoderma gangrenosum, rheumatoid nodule, Sweet's s.
neutrophils, epidermal	candidiasis, infantile acropustulosis, impetigo herpetiformis, neutrophilic spongiosis, pustular psoriasis, Reiter's s., subcorneal pustular dermatosis (Sneddon-Wilkinson), transient neonatal pustular melanosis
neutrophils, intraepithelial	acropustulosis of infancy, *Candida* infection, dermatophytes, gonococcemia, halogenodermas, impetigo, keratoacanthoma, miliaria, Reiter's s., pinta, psoriasis, Sneddon-Wilkinson s., sporotrichoid leishmaniasis, secondary syphilis, toxic shock s., yaws
neutrophils, perivascular	cellulitis, erysipelas, neutrophilic urticaria, Still's d., Sweet's s.
nuclear dust	debris from neutrophils; leukocytoclastic vasculitis, Sweet's s.
nuclei, blunt ended	leiomyoma
nuclei, cerebriform	atypical T lymphocyte nuclei; CTCL, Sezary s.
Odland bodies	EM; oval bodies in spinous layer
orthokeratosis	non-nucleated stratum corneum; ichthyosis vulgaris, lichen planus, verruca plana
osseous metaplasia	chondroid syringoma, epithelioid sarcoma, nevi, penile fibromatosis, pilomatrixoma
ossification	BCC, calcifying epithelioma of Malherbe, peripheral ossifying fibroma, Peyronie's d.
osteoblasts	fibro-osseous pseudotumor of the digits (osteoblasts)
osteoclasts	fibro-osseous pseudotumor of the digits, giant cell tumor of tendon sheath, giant cell epulis, giant cell variant of malignant fibrous histiocytoma
osteoid formation	aponeurotic fibromatosis, epithelial sarcoma, fibrosarcoma, giant cell malignant fibrous histiocytoma, malignant mixed tumor, malignant schwannoma, MFH-giant cell type, ossifying fibroma, peripheral giant cell granuloma, peripheral ossifying fibroma, peripheral proliferative myositis (myositis ossificans)
osteoma cutis (secondary)	acne vulgaris, AK, AFX, BCC, bronchogenic carcinoma (metastatic), chondroid syringoma, chondroma, chronic venous insufficiency, dermatofibrom, dermatomyositis, desmoid tumor, desmoplastic

	melanoma, epidermal nevus, folliculitis, Gardner's s., hemangioma, infundibular cyst, lipoma, LE, morphea, myositis ossificans, neurilemmoma, pilar cyst, pilomatrixoma, pyogenic granuloma, scleroderma, syphilis, trauma, trichoepithelioma
Paget cells	large round cells with large nuclei & abundant pink cytoplasm; Paget's d.
panniculitis	**cellular infiltrates** (atypical): leukemia, lymphoma **cellular infiltrates** (lymphoplasma): connective tissue panniculitis, dermatomyositis, lipoatrophy, necrobiosis lipoidica **crystal formation**: subcutaneous fat necrosis, sclerema neonatorum, poststeroid panniculitis, oxalosis, gout **cytophagocytosis**: cytophagic histiocytic panniculitis **ghost cells/saponification**: pancreatic panniculitis **hyalinization/lymphoplasma cellular infiltrates**: lupus panniculitis **palisading granulomas**: granuloma annulare, rheumatoid nodule, necrobiosis lipoidica **septal sclerosis**: morphea profunda, scleroderma, eosinophilic fasciitis **sclerosing lipogranuloma**: implanted lipids **vasculiti**: small vessel vasculitis, polyarteritis, thrombophlebitis **vessel calcification**: calciphylaxis **vessel thrombosis**: coagulopathy, cryoprecipitate
panniculitis	cutaneous periarteritis nodosa, cytophagic histiocytic panniculitis, Rothmann-Makai s., sarcoidosis, scleroderma, sclerosing lipogranuloma
panniculitis, lobular	α-1 antitrypsin deficiency, blunt trauma, cold, connective tissue panniculitis, erythema induratum, infection, leukemia, lipodystrophy, lupus profundus, pancreatic disease, sclerema neonatorum, steroid injection, subcutaneous fat necrosis of the newborn, Weber-Christian
panniculitis, septal	**infections**: blastomycosis, campylobacter colitis, cat-scratch d., chlamydial, coccidioidomycosis, gonorrhea, histoplasmosis, infectious mononucleosis, leprosy, lymphogranuloma inguinale, ornithosis, salmonellosis, shigellosis, streptococcal, syphilis, trichophytosis (deep), tuberculosis, yersiniosis **malignancies**: carcinoma, Hodgkin's d., leukemia, sarcoma **medications**: bromine, iodine, OCPs, penicillin, phenacetin, pyritinol, sulphathiazole **miscellaneous**: Behçet's d., Crohn's d., PAN, pregnancy, Sweet's s., ulcerative colitis
papillary endothelial hyperplasia	cavernous hemangioma, pyogenic granuloma, venous lake, capillary aneurysm, multiple superficial phlebectasia, lymphangiomas, angiolymphomatoid hyperplasia with eosinophilia
papillary mesenchymal bodies	epithelial structures resembling hair papillae; trichoepitheliomas
papillomatosis	elongation of epidermis & papillary dermis; acanthosis nigricans, seborrheic keratosis, verruca
parakeratosis, alternating	retained nuclei in stratum corneum; ILVEN, psoriasis, pityriasis rubra pilaris

Dermatopathology Signs & Their Diseases, Definitions, Associations

parakeratosis, mounded	chronic spongiotic dermatitis, guttate psoriasis, ILVEN, PR, seborrheic dermatitis, xerosis
parakeratosis, shoulder	parakeratotic aggregations at follicular infundibula; seborrheic dermatitis
parasitized histiocytes	American trypanosomiasis, granuloma inguinale, histoplasmosis, leishmaniasis, rhinoscleroma, toxoplasmosis (within keratinocytes)
Paschen bodies	*see Guarnieri bodies*
pattern recognition (instant)	accessory nipple, actinomycosis (eosinophilic sulfur granule), angiokeratoma, calciphylaxis, capillary angioma, clear cell acanthoma, CNCH, eruptive xanthoma, fibroepithelioma, granular cell tumor, harlequin fetus, hibernoma (mulberry cells), molluscum contagiosum (Henderson-Paterson bodies), keratoacanthoma, mucinous carcinoma (aggregates of mucin), neurothekioma, onchocerciasis (aggregate of worms), Paget's, porokeratosis (coronoid lamellae), PXE (dermal dilapidation-calcium), venous lake, verrucae, verruca plana, xanthelasma
Pautrier's microabscess	aggregate of atypical lymphocytes in epidermis with clear surrounding space; contact dermatitis, drug eruption, leukemia cutis, **mycosis fungoides**, PLEVA, PR, poikiloderma vasculare atrophicans
perineural invasion	adenoid cystic carcinoma, BCC, blue nevi, congenital nevi, desmoplastic melanoma, keratoacanthoma, metatypical BCC, microcystic adnexal carcinoma, porocarcinoma, Spitz nevi, Spitz variant of the minimal deviation melanoma
pertinax bodies	acidophilic masses; old nails
pigment incontinence	melanin deposition; erythema dyschromicum perstans, EM, fixed drug eruption, IP, lentigo, lichen planus, lichenoid reaction, LE, poikiloderma, post-inflammatory hyperpigmentation
plasma cells	AK, angiomatoid MFH, BCC, connective tissue disease, desmoplastic malignant melanoma, distinctive exudative discoid and lichen eruption, folliculitis, foreign body granuloma, granuloma inguinale, Kaposi's sarcoma, keratosis lichenoides chronica, lichen sclerosis, lues, LE, MF, NLD, nodular amyloid, papillary adenoma of the nipple, papillary syringoadenoma, periorificial inflammatory infiltrates, plasmacytoma, polyarteritis nodosa, rhinoscleroma, secondary syphilis, SCC, scleroderma, syringocystadenoma papilliferum, Zoon's balanitis
pleated sheets	bilayered lipids in lamellar bodies in the cytoplasm of keratinocytes
polaroscopic positive	erythema elevatum diutinum, dermatofibroma, Fabry's d., Hand-Schüller-Christian d., juvenile xanthogranuloma, normolipemic plane xanthoma, plane xanthoma, sclerema neonatorum, subcutaneous fat necrosis of the newborn, Tangier's d., tuberous xanthoma, xanthelasma
popcorn nuclei	irregular multilobed nuclei; lymphocytic or histiocytic cells in Hodgkin's d. (nodular lymphocyte-predominant)
psammoma bodies	laminated hyalin with calcifications; choroid plexus, cutaneous endometriosis, endosalpingosis, juvenile xanthogranuloma, mammary intraductal papilloma, meningioma, ovarian cancer, pineal gland, pituitary gland, thyroid cancer-papillary type

Dermatopathology Signs & Their Diseases, Definitions, Associations

pseudo Pautrier's microabscesses	chronic actinic dermatitis
pseudocarcinomatous hyperplasia	*see pseudoepitheliomatous hyperplasia*
pseudoepitheliomatous hyperplasia	irregular proliferation of epidermis into dermis; atypical mycobacteria, atypical fibroxanthoma, bacillary angiomatosis, blastomycosis, bromoderma, BCC, burns, cat scratch d., chromoblastomycosis, coccidioidomycosis, cutaneous amebiasis, condyloma lata, Darier's d., **deep fungal infections**, ecthyma contagiosum, epidermal inclusion cyst, keratoacanthoma, grease gun granuloma, granuloma inguinale, **granular cell tumor**, gumma, **halogenodermas**, hidradenitis suppurativa, inflammatory papillary hyperplasia, iododerma, keratoacanthoma, leishmaniasis, lichen planus, lupus vulgaris, lymphogranuloma venereum, malignant melanoma, mycobacterial infection, necrotizing sialometaplasia, osteomyelitis, paracoccidiodomycosis, pemphigoid vegetans, pemphigoid vegetans (Neumann type), phaeohyphomycosis, pigmented spindle cell nevus, podophyllin application, proliferating trichilemmal cyst, prurigo nodularis, pseudoepitheliomatous keratotic and micaceous balanitis, pyoderma gangrenosum, pyoderma vegetans, scrofuloderma, Spitz nevus, sporotrichosis, syphilis, tularemia, **ulcers** (chronic)
pseudohorn cysts	seborrheic keratoses
pseudovascular spaces	compound nevi
psoriasiform epidermal hyperplasia	**usual**: acrodermatitis enteropathica ichthyosis linearis circumflexa, ILVEN, lamellar ichthyosis, lichen simplex chronicus, pellagra, pityriasis rubra pilaris, prurigo nodularis, psoriasis, Reiter's s. **frequent**: contact dermatitis, MF, nummular dermatitis, PR, seborrheic dermatitis, syphilis **occasional**: candidiasis, dermatophytosis, geographic tongue, incontinentia pigmenti, necrolytic migratory erythema, scabies
pustule, eosinophilic	eosinophilic folliculitis, eosinophilic pustulosis of the scalp in children, erythema toxicum neonatorum, halogenodermas, incontinentia pigmenti, keratoacanthoma, pemphigus vegetans
pustule, neutrophilic	acral pustulosis of infancy, pustular psoriasis, subcorneal pustular dermatosis of Sneddon-Wilkinson, transient neonatal pustular melanosis
pustule, subcorneal	candidiasis, dermatophytosis, impetigo, miliaria crystallina, pemphigus erythematosus, pemphigus foliaceus, psoriasis, pyoderma gangrenosum, staphylococcal scalded skin s., subcorneal pustular dermatosis, toxic erythema of the newborn
pustulo-ovoid bodies of Milian	round eosinophilic cytoplasmic granules; granular cell tumor
radiation fibroblasts	radiotherapy
railroad track	appearance of arrangement of bacteria (*Haemophilus ducreyi*); chancroid
Reed-Sternberg cells	mirror image binucleated lymphocytes (classic, infrequent finding); B or T-cell Hodgkin's lymphoma, lymphomatoid papulosis, pseudolymphoma

Dermatopathology Signs & Their Diseases, Definitions, Associations

Rocha-Lima bodies	pink-purple cytoplasmic inclusions in endothelial cells; *Bartonella bacilliformis* (Oroya fever)
Russell bodies	copious homogenous eosinophilic immunoglobulin within plasma cells; chancroid, hidradenitis suppurativa, mucocutaneous leishmaniasis, rhinoscleroma, syphilis
satellite cell necrosis	lymphocytes attached to dead keratinocytes; erythema multiforme, GVHD, TEN
satellitosis	acute GVHD, lichen planus
saw tooth epidermis	serrated appearance of epidermis; lichen planus
Schaumann bodies	calcified inclusions from degenerated lysosomes in macrophages & histiocytes; berylliosis, sarcoid, tuberculosis
school of fish	appearance of arrangement of bacteria (*Haemophilus ducreyi*); chancroid
sclerosis	increased collagen, decreased fibroblasts; morphea, necrobiosis lipoidica, radiodermatitis (chronic), scleroderma
sclerotic bodies	Medlar bodies; chromoblastomycosis
sclerotic stroma	chondroid syringoma, ductal adenocarcinoma, sclerosing BCC, syringoma, trichoepithelioma
scutula	hyphal bodies; favus
secretion, decapitation	apocrine cystadenoma
Sezary cells	atypical T-cells in peripheral smear with cerebriform nuclei; actinic reticuloid, atopic dermatitis, B-cell lymphoma, BCC, chronic dermatoses, DLE, LP, lymphomatoid papulosis, MF, normal persons, parapsoriasis en plaques, PLEVA, Sezary s. (must be 5-10% of total WBC), solar keratosis, psoriasis
shadow cells	pale eosinophilic cell with central clearing & absent nucleus; fat necrosis, pilomatricoma AKA ghost cell
ship pilot's wheel	round yeast cells with narrow necked buds; paracoccidiodomycosis
spaghetti & meatballs	hyphal & yeast elements observed in KOH preparation; *Malessezia furfur* (tinea versicolor)
Splendore-Hoeppli phenomenon	PAS positive amorphous eosinophilic material surrounding granules of clumped bacteria; actinomycosis, botryomycosis, entomophthoromycosis
spongiosis	allergic vesicular id eruption, atopic dermatitis, contact dermatitis, eczematous dermatitis, pityriasis rosea, PMLE, pompholyx, vesicular dermatophytosis
spongiosis, eosinophilic	intracellular epidermal edema with eosinophils; allergic contact dermatitis, **arthropod bite, bullous pemphigoid**, cicatricial pemphigoid, dermatitis herpetiformis, **drug eruption, eczematous dermatitis**, eosinophilic cellulitis (Well's s.), epidermolytic epidermolysis bullosa, erythema toxicum neonatorum, erythromelanoderma, herpes gestationis, hypereosinophilic s., **incontinentia pigmenti** (vesicular stage), milker's nodule, pemphigus foliaceus, pemphigus vegetans, pemphigus vulgaris, polycythemia rubra vera, porokeratosis of Mibelli, **scabies**, subcorneal pustular dermatosis

Dermatopathology Signs & Their Diseases, Definitions, Associations

squamatization	hydropic basal cell layer degeneration; GVH d., lichen planus, lupus erythematosus
squamous eddies	round onion-like aggregate of eosinophilic keratinocytes; AK, keratoacanthoma, **seborrheic keratosis** (irritated), SCC, warty dyskeratoma
squamous pearls	round garlic clove-like aggregate of eosinophilic keratinocytes; SCC, SK
stag horn appearance	hemangiopericytoma
starry sky pattern	Burkitt's lymphoma
stellate abscesses	cat-scratch disease, fungal infections, lymphogranuloma venereum, melioidosis, sporotrichosis, tularemia
storiform pattern	whirling cellular pattern around acellular zones (occasionally around small blood vessels); DFSP
substance P amyloid	normal substance of serum & elastic fibers
sulfur granules	matted colonies of filamentous organisms exuded from skin sinuses; actinomycosis, botryomycosis, mycetoma
sunburn cells	dyskeratotic keratinocytes; actinic skin, AK, SCC
swarm of bees	peribulbar lymphocytic infiltrate; alopecia areata
sweat gland necrosis	barbiturates, gas gangrene (clostridia), hypoxia, pressure
T cell clonality	follicular mucinosis, pagetoid reticulosis, parapsoriasis, MF
T cells	**TH cells**: annular elastolytic granuloma, erythema nodosum leprosum, pseudolymphoma, tuberculoid leprosy; **TS cells**: lepromatous leprosy
telangiectasias	Osler-Weber-Rendu s., trichodiscomas
tingible body macrophages	large macrophages containing fragmented basophilic nuclear & cytoplasm fragments of degenerated lymphoid cells; pseudolymphoma
tombstoning	basal cells of blister floor protrude into blister; pemphigus vulgaris
Touton giant cells	histiocytic multinucleated giant cell with ring of nuclei; xanthogranuloma
transepidermal elimination	calcinosis cutis, CNCH, chromomycosis, elastosis perforans serpiginosa (elastic fibers), granuloma annulare (collagen fibers), hidradenitis suppurativa (elastic fibers), Kyrle's d., lichen nitidus, melanoma, NLD (collagen fibers), nevi, osteoma cutis, perforating disorder of renal disease (collagen fibers), perforating folliculitis (collagen & elastic fibers), pigmented spindle cell nevus, porokeratosis of Mibelli, PXE (altered elastic fibers), reactive perforating collagenosis-collagen, rheumatoid nodules, sarcoidal granuloma, Spitz nevus, vellus hair cysts
triglyceride crystals	sclerema neonatorum, subcutaneous fat necrosis
tuberculosis	bacilli count; primary inoculation TB (+++), miliary TB (++/+), lupus vulgaris (rare), TB verrucosus cutis (rare), scrofuloderma (+), TB cutis orificialis (+++)

Dermatopathology Signs & Their Diseases, Definitions, Associations

ulceration	atypical fibroxanthoma, BCC, DFSP, epithelioid sarcoma (superficial type), malignant melanoma, papillary adenoma of the nipple, SCC
vacuolar degeneration	*see hydropic degeneration*
vasculitis, lymphocytic	angiocentric lymphoma, drug eruptions, lupus, lymphomatoid papulosis, pernio (chilblains), PLEVA, pyoderma gangrenosum
vase-like shape, mononuclear cells	aggregation of mononuclear cells resembling Pautrier's microabscesses; spongiotic dermatitis (not MF)
Verocay bodies	parallel rows of nuclei surrounding homogenous eosinophilic material; neurilemmoma (Antoni type A area), schwannoma
villus	prominent dermal papilla within a blister cavity; Darier's d., pemphigus, warty dyskeratoma
vimentin	chondroblasts, endothelium, fibroblasts, mesothelium, sarcoma, smooth muscle cells, spindle cell SCC
Virchow cells	foamy histiocytes; lepromatous leprosy
wedge shape	arthropod bite, PLEVA, PLC
Weibel-Pelade bodies	EM; electron dense rod-shaped organelles of parallel tubules found in endothelial cells, vascular tumors
Willemze Type A	LP with histiocytes
Willemze Type B	LP with lymphocytes
zebra bodies	EM; lipid vacuoles with transverse membranes; Farber's d., mucopolysaccharidosis

Diagnostic Algorithm

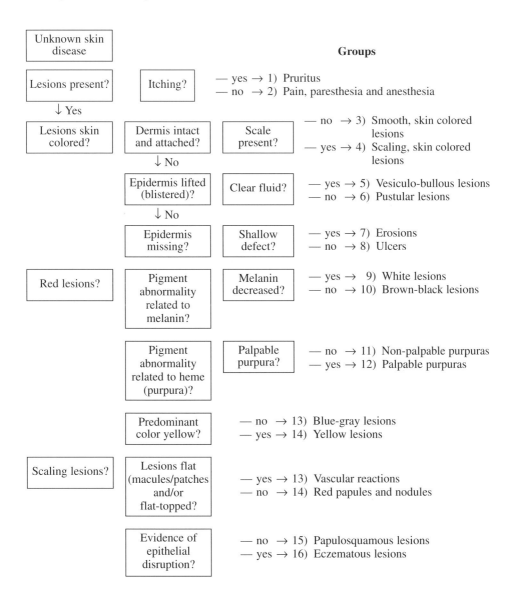

Groups

Unknown skin disease		
Lesions present?	Itching?	— yes → 1) Pruritus — no → 2) Pain, paresthesia and anesthesia
↓ Yes		
Lesions skin colored?	Dermis intact and attached? ↓ No	Scale present? — no → 3) Smooth, skin colored lesions — yes → 4) Scaling, skin colored lesions
	Epidermis lifted (blistered)? ↓ No	Clear fluid? — yes → 5) Vesiculo-bullous lesions — no → 6) Pustular lesions
	Epidermis missing?	Shallow defect? — yes → 7) Erosions — no → 8) Ulcers
Red lesions?	Pigment abnormality related to melanin?	Melanin decreased? — yes → 9) White lesions — no → 10) Brown-black lesions
	Pigment abnormality related to heme (purpura)?	Palpable purpura? — no → 11) Non-palpable purpuras — yes → 12) Palpable purpuras
	Predominant color yellow?	— no → 13) Blue-gray lesions — yes → 14) Yellow lesions
Scaling lesions?	Lesions flat (macules/patches and/or flat-topped)?	— yes → 13) Vascular reactions — no → 14) Red papules and nodules
	Evidence of epithelial disruption?	— no → 15) Papulosquamous lesions — yes → 16) Eczematous lesions

Adapted from Sams WM, Lynch PJ: Principles and Practice of Dermatology, 2nd ed. Philadelphia, Churchill-Livingstone, 1996.

75

Diagnostic Algorithm

I.	No apparent lesions (symptoms only)		
	Pruritus	1.	Pruritus
	Pain	2.	Pain, paresthesia, anesthesia
II.	Skin-colored lesions		
	A. Epidermis intact and attached		
	Scale absent	3.	Smooth skin-colored lesions
	Scale present	4.	Scaling skin-colored lesions
	B. Epidermis lifted (blisters)		
	Blister fluid clear	5.	Vesiculobullous lesions
	Blister fluid white or yellow-white	6.	Pustular lesions
	C. Epidermis missing		
	Defect shallow (epidermis)	7.	Erosions
	Defect deep (dermis)	8.	Ulcers
III.	Non-blanchable, abnormally-colored lesions		
	A. Melanin pigment		
	Hypopigmentation	9.	White lesions
	Hyperpigmentation	10.	Brown or black lesions
	B. Heme pigment		
	Non-palpable	11.	Non-palpable purpuras
	Palpable	12.	Palpable purpuras
	C. Other pigments		
	Blue-gray	13.	Blue-gray lesions
	Yellow	14.	Yellow lesions
IV.	Blanchable, red (Inflammatory) lesions		
	A. Non-scaling red lesions		
	Flat and flat-topped lesions	15.	Vascular reactions
	Rounded and slope-shouldered lesions	16.	Red papules and nodules
	B. Scaling, red lesions		
	Epithelium intact	17.	Papulosquamous lesions
	Epithelium disrupted	18.	Eczematous lesions

Diagnostic Algorithm

Group 1. Pruritus

functional origin	anxiety (especially OCD), depression (esp. elderly)
systemic disorders	hepatic d. (biliary cirrhosis, obstructive d.), iron deficiency, lymphoma (**Hodgkin's**), polycythemia vera, pregnancy, renal d., **thyroid d.**
unapparent skin conditions	AIDS, fiberglass dermatitis, mastocytosis, pediculosis (pubic, head, body), scabies, sweat retention (esp. atopics), **xerosis** (atopy, ichthyosis, excessive bathing)

Group 2. Pain

absent lesions	localized chronic pain s. (glossodynia, vulvodynia, anodynia), neuralgia, post-herpetic neuralgia, reflex sympathetic dystrophy, trigeminal neuralgia
absent pain	congenital absence, leprosy, peripheral neuropathy (esp. diabetes), syringomyelia
lesion-associated	angioleiomyoma, angiolipoma, eccrine spiradenoma, glomus tumor, leiomyoma, neurilemmoma, neuroma
paresthesia	formication ("crawling" sensation in skin) in true infestation & delusions

Group 3. Smooth, Skin-colored Lesions

cysts	epidermoid, mucinous, pilar, synovial
edema & pseudo-edema	angioedema, chronic genital edema, eosinophilic fasciitis, lymphedema, Melkersson-Rosenthal s., scleredema, scleromyxedema
flat & atrophic lesions	lipoatrophy, lipodystrophy, pitted keratolysis, striae
papules, nodules	BCC, chondrodermatitis nodularis, closed comedones, lipomas, molluscum contagiosum, neurofibroma, nevi (intradermal, neural), pearly penile papules, rhinophyma, scars (hypertrophic, keloid), SCC, sebaceous hyperplasia, skin tags (achrocordons), warts
rare lesions	accessory tragus, acrodermatitis chronica atrophicans, anetoderma, arsenical keratoses, basal cell nevus s., calcinosis cutis, connective tissue nevus, Cowden's s., cylindroma, dermoid cyst, Dupuytren's contracture, erythropoietic protoporphyria, fibroma, follicular mucinosis, knuckle pads, lipoidproteinosis, neuroma, nevus sebaceus, osteoma cutis, palmar crease keratoses, palmar/plantar keratoderma, sarcoma, syringoma, thyroglossal cyst, tophi, trichoepithelioma

Diagnostic Algorithm

Group 4. Scaling Skin-colored Lesions

papules & nodules	actinic keratosis, callous, corn, keratoacanthoma, SCC, seborrheic keratosis, verruca
plaques & disseminated disease	epidermal nevus, ichthyosis, nevus sebaceus, porokeratosis of Mibelli, post-inflammatory desquamation & exfoliation, tinea manum, tinea pedis, xerosis
uncommon, rare	acrokeratoelastoidosis, acrokeratosis verruciformis, Cowden's s., disseminated actinic porokeratosis, elastosis perforans serpiginosum, elephantiasis nostra verrucosa, epidermodysplasia verruciformis, hyperkeratosis lenticularis perstans, knuckle pads, Kyrle's d., perforating folliculitis, stucco keratoses, surfer's nodule

Group 5. Vesiculobullous Lesions

vesicular, common	dyshidrosis (pompholyx), herpes simplex, herpes zoster, id reaction, molluscum contagiosum, scabies, tinea pedis (vesicular), vesicular insect bites
vesicular, uncommon & rare	chronic bullous disease of childhood, dermatitis herpetiformis, eczema herpeticum & vaccinatum, Grover's d., hand foot & mouth d., herpes gestationis, hidrocystoma, incontinentia pigmenti, intraepidermal IgA disease, linear IgA d., lymphangioma circumscriptum, pityriasis lichenoides
bullous, common	burns, bullous impetigo, contact dermatitis, friction blisters
bullous, uncommon	bullous disease of dialysis, bullous hemorrhagic pyoderma gangrenosum, chronic bullous disease of children, coma blisters, diabetic bullous d., epidermolysis bullosa, epidermolysis bullosa acquisita, erysipeloid, erythema multiforme, fixed drug eruption, linear IgA disease, milker's nodule, necrotizing fasciitis, orf, pemphigoid, pemphigus, porphyria

Group 6. Pustular Lesions

common	acne vulgaris, acne conglobata, candidiasis, erythema toxicum neonatorum, folliculitis, keratosis pilaris, perioral dermatitis, pyoderma faciale, rosacea, stye
uncommon	acne keloidalis, acne necrotica miliaris, acrodermatitis continua, Behçet's d., bowel bypass s., chloracne, chronic gonococcemia, Crohn's d., dissecting cellulitis, eosinophilic folliculitis, folliculitis decalvans, hidradenitis suppurativa, impetigo herpetiformis, infantile acral pustulosis, intraepidermal neutrophilic IgA dermatosis, myeloma, pityrosporum folliculitis, psoriasis, pustular dyshidrosis, pustular psoriasis, pustulosis palmaris et plantaris, steroid acne, subcorneal pustular dermatosis, transient neonatal pustular melanosis, ulcerative colitis

Diagnostic Algorithm

Group 7. Erosions

common	candidiasis, excoriation, impetigo, unroofed vesiculobullous & pustular lesions
uncommon	acrodermatitis enteropathica, glucagonoma s., SSSS, TEN

Group 8. Ulcers

common	aphthous ulcers, arteriosclerotic, BCC, chondrodermatitis nodularis, decubitus, gangrenous ulcers, neuropathic, SCC, stasis, traumatic
uncommon	actinomycosis, amebiasis, anthrax, aplasia cutis congenita, Bart's s., chancroid, Churg-Strauss d., Crohn's d. of skin, dental sinus, ecthyma, factitial, focal dermal hypoplasia, fungal infection, hemoglobinopathies, herpes infection, chronic (immunosuppressed), congenital sinus, granuloma inguinale, keratoacanthoma, leishmaniasis, lymphoma, lymphomatoid papulosis, mycobacterial infection, nocardiosis, panniculitis, polyarteritis nodosum, pyoderma (blastomycosis-like), pyoderma (malignant), pyoderma gangrenosum, septicemic ulcers, spider bite, syphilis (primary), temporal arteritis, tularemia, Wegener's d.

Group 9. White Lesions

mucous membrane	biting trauma, candidiasis, leukoplakia, lichen planus, lupus erythematosus, secondary syphilis, white hairy leukoplakia
papules	acne vulgaris, calcinosis cutis, hair casts, keratosis pilaris, lichen nitidus, milia, molluscum contagiosum, nits, scars, sebaceous gland hyperplasia, tophus, white piedra
patches, plaques	albinism, atrophie blanche, chemically induced hypomelanosis, Degos' d., halo nevus, hypomelanosis of Ito, hypopigmentation, idiopathic guttate hypomelanosis, leprosy, lichen sclerosis et atrophicus, morphea, piebaldism, pinta, pityriasis alba, poliosis, postinflammatory sarcoid, scleroderma, tinea versicolor, tuberous sclerosis, vitiligo, yaws

Group 10. Brown-black Lesions

generalized	Addison's disease, cancer chemotherapeutic agents, dyskeratosis congenita, exfoliative erythrodermatitis, heavy metals, hemochromatosis, ichthyosis, MSH-related pigmentation in endocrine & malignant d., phenothiazines, porphyria, progeria, Rothmund-Thomson s., scleroderma, Whipple's d., Wilson's d.

Diagnostic Algorithm

Group 10. Brown-black Lesions

macules, papules, nodules	acanthosis nigricans, acrochordon (skin tag), angiokeratoma, black piedra, Bowenoid papulosis, dermatofibroma, dermatosis papulosis nigra, freckles, lentigo, lentigo maligna, lentigo maligna melanoma, nevus (compound, junctional, intradermal), nevus (dysplastic), open comedone, pigmented BCC, seborrheic keratosis, urticaria pigmentosa
patches & plaques	acanthosis nigricans, acral lentiginous melanoma, Albright's s., alkaptonuria, atrophoderma of Pasini & Pierini, Becker's nevus, Berloque (furocoumarin) dermatitis, café-au-lait macules, café-au-lait like birthmarks, chloasma (melasma), confluent & reticulated papillomatosis, congenital pigmented nevus, Dowling-Degos' disease, erythema ab igne, erythrasma, fixed drug eruption, incontinentia pigmenti (late), lentigo maligna, lentigo maligna melanoma, linear nevoid hypermelanosis, morphea, pigmentary demarcation lines (Futcher's line), poikilodermatous pigmentation, postinflammatory hyperpigmentation, tinea nigra palmaris, tinea versicolor

Group 11. Non-palpable Purpura

ecchymotic	actinic purpura, amyloidosis, angioimmunoblastic lymphadenopathy, anticoagulant therapy, calciphylaxis, DIC, Gardner-Diamond s., intravascular coagulation defects (platelets, erythrocytes, coagulation proteins), necrotizing fasciitis, scurvy, steroid purpura, superficial hemorrhagic pyoderma gangrenosum, trauma, vasculitis (polyarteritis nodosa, lymphomatoid granulomatosis)
petechial (primarily)	bacteremia (staphylococcal, meningococcal, bacteria endocarditis), benign pigmented purpuras, black-dot toes & heels, dysproteinemia (cryoglobulinemia), histiocytosis X, hydrostatic petechiae (stasis), intravascular coagulation defects, medication (thiazides)

Group 12. Palpable Purpura

bacteremia	bacteria endocarditis, meningococcal, staphylococcal
non-vasculitic	angiokeratoma, cherry angioma, Kaposi's sarcoma, pyogenic granuloma
rickettsia	RMSF, typhus
venulitis, arteritis	dysproteinemia, Henoch-Schönlein purpura, leukocytoclastic vasculitis, (hypersensitivity vasculitis, rheumatoid vasculitis)

Diagnostic Algorithm

Group 13. Blue-gray Lesions

macules, patches	atrophoderma of Pasini & Pierini, erythema dyschromicum perstans, fixed drug eruption, heliotrope eyelids (dermatomyositis), hemochromatosis, medication (antimalarials, gold, metals, minocycline, phenothiazines, silver), Mongolian spot, Nevus of Ito & Ota, osteoma cutis, tattoo (asphalt, foreign body, graphite, lead), venous lake
papules, nodules	acroangiodermatitis (arteriovenous fistula, pseudo-Kaposi's disease), angiosarcoma, angiolymphoid hyperplasia, blue nevus, collagen vascular d., Glomus tumor, granuloma annulare, hemangioma (esp. cavernous & verrucous), hidrocystoma, Kaposi's sarcoma (esp. classic), leukemia cutis, lichen planus, lymphoma cutis (esp. B-cell), pyogenic granuloma

Group 14. Yellow Lesions

macules, patches	amyloidosis, carotenemia, Fordyce condition (mucous membranes), jaundice, keratoderma of palms & soles, necrobiosis lipoidica diabeticorum, pseudoxanthoma elasticum, solar elastosis, xanthomas (palmar, plantar)
papules, plaques, nodules	amyloidosis, colloid milium, cyst, histiocytic lesion, juvenile xanthogranuloma, mastocytoma, nevus sebaceus, sebaceous hyperplasia, solar elastosis, tophus, xanthelasma, xanthoma (tendinous, tuberous)

Group 15. Vascular Reactions

diffuse, morbilliform	GVH, Kawasaki d., scarlet fever, SSSS, TEN (early erythema chronic migrans), toxic shock s., viral exanthem (erythema infectiosum, roseola, rubella, rubeola)
gyrate, serpiginous, annular	creeping eruption, elastosis perforans serpiginosum, erythema annulare centrifugum, erythema gyratum repens, erythema multiforme, granuloma annulare, sarcoid, SCLE
livedo pattern	antiphospholipid s. (lupus anticoagulant, Sneddon's s.), cholesterol emboli, cutis marmorata telangiectatica, erythema ab igne, erythema infectiosum, large vessel vasculitis, poikiloderma (Civatte, collagen vascular disease, cutaneous lymphoma), polyarteritis
macular localized	acrocyanosis, BCC, Bowen's d., **face** (lupus erythematosus, dermatomyositis, seborrheic dermatitis, photosensitivity reaction), fixed drug eruption, **groin** (intertrigo, erythrasma, tinea cruris, seborrheic dermatitis), **hand** (erythromelalgia, liver d., hereditary redness of the palm, chemotherapy), pernio, tinea versicolor

Diagnostic Algorithm

Group 15. Vascular Reactions

plaques	arthropod assault, cellulitis, erysipelas, erysipeloid, erythema elevatum diutinum, erythema multiforme, erythema nodosum, fixed drug eruption, granuloma faciale, hypocomplementemic vasculitis, juvenile rheumatoid arthritis, nodular vasculitis, panniculitis, PUPPP, relapsing polychondritis, Sweet's s., Well's cellulitis
telangiectatic	angioma serpiginosum, ataxia telangiectasia, erythema ab igne, essential telangiectasia, poikilodermatous conditions, radiodermatitis, telangiectasia of collagen vascular disease (CREST s.), TMEP, unilateral nevoid telangiectasia
transient erythema	anaphylactic reaction, contact urticaria, cutis marmorata, dermographism, erythema marginatum urticaria, flushing (carcinoid, emotional, mastocytosis, medications, pheochromocytoma), physical urticaria

Group 16. Red Papules and Nodules

papules	arthropod assault, cherry angioma, CNCH, coral & marine animal contact, diaper granuloma, elastosis perforans serpiginosum, eosinophilic folliculitis, eruptive xanthoma, foreign body granuloma, Gianotti-Crosti s., Gottron's papules, granuloma annulare, Grover's d., Kaposi's sarcoma, lymphomatoid papulosis, mites, multicentric reticulohistiocytosis, papular urticaria, pityriasis lichenoides, pityriasis rosea, pityrosporum folliculitis, pyogenic granuloma, sarcoid, scabies, secondary stye & hordeolum, syphilis
nodules, plaques	acne conglobata, acne cyst, angiolymphoid hyperplasia with eosinophilia, angiosarcoma, arthropod assault, carbuncle, cylindroma, dissecting cellulitis, erythema elevatum diutinum, erythema nodosum, furuncle, granuloma annulare, hemangioma, hidradenitis suppurativa, inflamed cyst, Kaposi's sarcoma, lupus erythematosus, lymphocytic infiltrate of Jessner, lymphoma & leukemia cutis, milker's nodule, mycobacterial infection, myiasis, nodular vasculitis (erythema induratum), orf, panniculitis, polymorphous light eruption, pseudolymphoma, pyoderma faciale, rheumatoid nodules, sarcoma, sporotrichosis, Sweet's s., vasculitis (esp. polyarteritis nodosum)

Diagnostic Algorithm

Group 17. Papulosquamous Lesions

papules	lichen planus, pityriasis lichenoides, pityriasis rosea, psoriasis, secondary syphilis, viral exanthem
plaques	actinic reticuloid, Basex s., Bowen's d., Darier's d., ichthyosis, ILVEN, keratosis lichenoides chronica, lichen striatus, lupus erythematosus, mycosis fungoides, Pagetoid reticulosis, parapsoriasis, pellagra, photosensitivity eruptions, pityriasis rubra pilaris, psoriasis, Reiter's s., superficial BCC, tinea (capitis, corporis, cruris, pedis)

Group 18. Eczematous Lesions

minimal excoriation	acrodermatitis enteropathica, actinic reticuloid, allergic contact dermatitis, asteatotic eczema, autoeczematization, Darier's d., external otitis, glucagonoma s., Hailey-Hailey d., histiocytosis X, ILVEN, impetigo, infectious eczematoid dermatitis, irritant contact dermatitis, juvenile palmar plantar dermatitis, Leiner's d., lichen striatus, nummular eczema, Paget's d., perioral dermatitis, photosensitivity s., seborrheic dermatitis, winter itch, xerotic eczema
prominent excoriation	atopic dermatitis, dermatitis herpetiformis, dyshidrotic eczema, exfoliative erythrodermatitis, lichen simplex chronicus, neurodermatitis, scabies, stasis dermatitis

Dietary and Foods:
Association, Avoidance, Treatments

actinic keratoses	low fat diet
atopic dermatitis	**avoid**: cow's milk, eggs, fish, peanuts, soy products, wheat
5-hydroxy-indoleacetic acid (5HIAA) excretion, urinary	avocado, bananas, eggplant, red plum, tomatoes, walnut
biotin deficiency	alopecia, intertriginous dermatitis, periorificial dermatitis, xerosis
cobalamin (B12) deficiency	angular cheilitis, beefy red tongue, hyperpigmentation (generalized), hyperpigmented macules, poliosis
carcinoid s., precipitated by	avocados, cheese, chocolate, eating, eggplant, EtOH, hot beverages/foods, red plums, tomatoes, walnuts
cobalt, diet low in	**Avoid**: apricots, beans, beer, beets, cabbage, chocolate, cloves, cocoa, coffee, flour (whole grain), liver, nuts, scallops, tea
copper deficiency	facial abnormalities, light hair, Menkes' s., pili torti
elementary diet	essential and nonessential amino acids and simple sugars, electrolytes, trace elements & vitamins; dermatitis herpetiformis (gluten sensitive enteropathy)
elimination diet (add back one food item per day)	**Avoid**: dairy products, wheat, egg chocolate, cola drinks, nuts, seeds, shellfish, corn, tomato, strawberries, citrus fruits, packaged & prepared meats, dried fruits, sugar substitutes, herbs, spices **Eat**: fresh & frozen vegetables & fruits, fresh meat, poultry, fish baked or broiled (not breaded), water, tea, salt, sugar, fresh lemon
essential fatty acid deficiency	alopecia, increased transepidermal water loss, intertriginous erosions, xerotic dermatitis
flushing	capsaicin (in red pepper), cheese, chocolate, Coprinus mushrooms, dumping s., hot beverages, lemon, monosodium glutamate, nitrites, sodium nitrite (cured meats), sulfites, spiced foods, spoiled fish, spoiled cheese
histamine elimination diet	**Avoid**: beefsteak, cheese, chicken liver, eggplant, red wine, spinach, tomatoes
iron deficiency	alopecia, light hair, koilonychia
Kwashiorkor	crazy paving dermatosis, enamel paint spits, flag sign, flaky paint, hypopigmentation, peripheral edema, xerosis
marasmus	brittle hair, monkey facies, wrinkled skin, xerosis
niacin (P-P) deficiency	angular stomatitis, cheilosis, Casal's necklace, sores (oral, perirectal), symmetric hyperpigmented plaques (sun-exposed)
nickel reduction diet	**Avoid**: shellfish, chocolate milk, beans, kale, leeks, lettuce, lentils, peas, soy protein powder (in prepared meats, soups, bouillon), spinach, sprouts, bran, buckwheat, millet, muesli, multi-grain breads, oat meal, rice (unpolished), rye bran, sesame seeds, wheat bran, cereals, bran biscuits, dates, figs, pineapple, prunes, raspberries, chocolate and cocoa, bottled tea, almonds, baking powder, nuts, licorice, marzipan

Dietary and Foods: Association, Avoidance, Treatments

	Eat: alcohol, asparagus, bananas, beets, berries (except raspberries), broccoli, Brussels sprouts, butter, carbonated beverages, cabbage, cauliflower, cheese, Chinese cabbage, coffee & tea (weak), corn, corn flakes, cornmeal, cornstarch, cucumber, dill, eggplant, eggs, fish, garlic, macaroni, margarine, meat (fresh), mushrooms, onions, parsley, peaches, pears, peppers, popcorn, potatoes, poultry, raisins, rhubarb, rice (polished), spaghetti, wheat flour, whole grain rye & wheat bread, yeast, yogurt
pyridoxine (B6) deficiency	angular stomatitis, cheilosis, glossitis, oral erosions, pellagra-like dermatitis, seborrhea-like dermatitis
riboflavin (B2) deficiency	angular stomatitis, cheilosis, magenta glossitis, scrotal dermatitis, seborrhea-like dermatitis
selenium deficiency	hypopigmentation (generalized), white nails
thiamin (B1) deficiency	edema
urticaria, contact	apricot pit, apple, bean, beer, buckwheat flour, caraway seed, carrot, egg, endive, fish, flour, garlic, kiwi, lettuce, litchi, maize, mango, meat (chicken, lamb, turkey, beef, liver, pork), milk, mustard, peach, peanut, pickle (cucumber), potato, rice, salami casing (mold), shellfish, soybean, spices, strawberry, tomato, watermelon
vitamin A (retinol) deficiency	phrynoderma, xerosis
vitamin C (ascorbic acid) deficiency	corkscrew hairs, follicular hyperkeratosis, friable gums, hemorrhage, poor wound healing, splinter hemorrhages (fingernail) AKA scurvy
vitamin E (tocopherol) deficiency	jaundice, phrynoderma
vitamin K deficiency	intracutaneous hemorrhage, purpura
zinc deficiency	acral & periorificial pustulo-bullous dermatitis, alopecia, angular stomatitis, glossitis, pustular paronychia

Diseases

Albinism, Oculocutaneous

	Hair	Skin	Pigment (nevi, freckles)	Eyes, RR, iris trans-illumination	Melanosomes	Gene mutation	Other
Type Ia, ty-neg	white	pink to red	non-pigmented nevi	gray to blue RR: present poor vision, cartwheel in adults	stage I & II	tyrosinase gene (t-/t-)	scalp biopsy; prenatal diagnosis
Type IB, Ym	white birth, yellow-red by 6 mos.	white at birth, slight tan	present	blue infancy, darkens, RR present	stage III pheomelanosomes	tyrosine gene decreased activity	
Type I, Ts	white birth, yellow scalp, legs brown	creamy white, slight tan	present	blue; no iris pigment, RR present	stages I, II scalp, stages II, III leg hair	tyrosinase gene	T° sensitive loss of activity of tyrosinase above 35-37° C
Type I min. pig.	white birth, white to yellow adults	pink-white, no tan	absent	gray to blue, pupil pigment RR present, clumps at limbus	sate stage II, some with melanin	tyrosinase gene	heterozygotes have zero-normal tyrosinase activity
Type II, ty-pos	white, yellow tan with age	pink-white to cream	present, may be numerous	blue, yellow-brown RR may be absent, limbus/cartwheel	to stage III, eumelanosomes	P gene; 15q	tyrosinase assay suggests heterogeneity
Type IV, Brown	beige to light brown in Africans	cream to light tan exposed skin	uncommon	hazel to lt. tan RR children, may be absent in adults, cartwheel	stage I to II some lightly pigmented stage IV	unknown	tyrosinase normal
Type V, rufous	mahogany red to deep red	reddish brown	may be present	reddish brown to brown, RR unknown	unknown	unknown	New Guineans and Africans
Type VIA, HPS	white, red, brown	cream gray to normal	present	blue-gray to brown, RR in light skinned, not dark, cartwheel	to stage III pheomelanosomes and eumelanosomes	? pallid gene	lysosomal d., heterozygotes; low thioredoxin reductase, Puerto Ricans and Dutch

Diseases

Albinism, Oculocutaneous

	Hair	Skin	Pigment (nevi, freckles)	Eyes, RR, iris trans-illumination	Melanosomes	Gene mutation	Other
Type VIB, CHS	blond to dark brown, steel-gray tint	pink to pink-white	present	blue to dark brown, RR present	macromelano-somes and normal to stage IV	unknown	lysosomal d... susceptible to infection, giant lysosomal granules, lympho-reticular malignancy
Type VII, AD	white to cream, red tint	white to cream	may be present	gray to blue, trans-lucent to cartwheel, RR children	stage I to early stage III, no structural abnormality	unknown	
XL, Nettleship	normal to slightly light	normal to mildly light	present	normal, cartwheel C	macromelano-somes in normal skin of hemi-diaphanous, X RR present X		hypomelanotic macules and patches in some individuals and heterozygotes
XL with deafness	normal to mildly light	normal to mildly light	present	normal, cartwheel C diaphanous, X RR present X	macromelano-somes in normal skin of hemi and heterozygotes		high frequency hearing loss onset puberty to 40 years
AR	normal to slightly light	normal to mildly light	present	normal, cartwheel to diaphanous RR present X	normal		males and females equally affected
OA-lentigines-deafness	normal	normal	lentigines	normal, cartwheel to diaphanous, RR present	macromelano-in lentigines		AD congenital sensorineural deafness

Adapted from Witkop CJ, Quevedo WC, Fitzpatrick TB, et al. Albinism. In: Scriver CR, Beaudet AL, Sly WS, et al. eds. The Metabolic Basis of Inherited Disease, 6th ed. New York: McGraw-Hill 1989:2905-2947.

Diseases

Disorders of Cornification

	Name	Synonyms	Abnormality	
DOC 1	vulgaris	ichthyosis vulgaris	keratohyalin granule; absent profilaggrin	AD
DOC 2	steroid deficient	recessive X-linked ichthyosis	epidermal enzyme; absent cholesterol sulfatase	XR
DOC 3	bullous	epidermolytic hyperkeratosis; bullous congenital ichthyosiform erythroderma	keratin filaments; genetic defect in K1 or K10	AD
DOC 4	lamellar-recessive	lamellar ichthyosis	cornified envelope; defective transglutaminase cross-linking	AR
DOC 5	congenital erythrodermic	lamellar ichthyosis; congenital ichthyosiform erythroderma	lamellar bodies; malformed lipid bilayer; decreased enzyme function	AR
DOC 6	harlequin	harlequin fetus	lamellar bodies & keratohyalin granules; absent lipid bilayer, absent filaggrin	AR
DOC 7	lamellar dominant	autosomal dominant lamellar ichthyosis		AD
DOC 8	Curth-Macklin	ichthyosis hystrix type		AD
DOC 9	Netherton's	Netherton's s., ichthyosis linearis circumflexa		AR
DOC 10	Sjögren-Larsson	Sjögren-Larsson s.		AR
DOC 11	phytanic acid storage	Refsum's d.; heredopathia atactica polyneuritiformis		AR
DOC 12	neutral lipid storage	neutral lipid storage d. Chanarin-Dorfman s.		AR
DOC 13	multiple sulfatase deficiency	multiple sulfatase deficiency s.		AR
DOC 14	trichothio-dystrophy	Tay's s. IBIDS s.		AR
DOC 15	keratitis-deafness	KID s.; atypical ichthyosiform erythroderma with deafness		AD, AR
DOC 16	unilateral hemidysplasia	CHILD s		XD?
DOC 17	chondro-dysplasia punctata	Conradi-Hunermann s.		AR, XD
DOC 18	erythrokerato-derma viriabilis			AD

Diseases

Disorders of Cornification

	Name	Synonyms	Abnormality
DOC 19	erythrokerato-lysis heimalis		AD
DOC 20	erythrokerato-derma progres-siva symmetrica		AD
DOC 21	peeling skin	peeling skin s.; familial continuous skin peeling	AR
DOC 22	Darier's	Darier's d.; keratosis follicularis	AD
DOC 23	Giroux-Barbeau	Giroux-Barbeau s.	AD
DOC 24	keratosis follicularis spinulosa decalvans		XD?

Williams ML, Elias PM. Genetically transmitted, generalized disorders of cornification. The ichthyoses. Dermatol Clin 1987; 5: 155-78.

Diseases

Ehlers-Danlos Syndrome

Type	Inheritance	Defect	Skin Bruising	Skin Elasticity	Skin Fragility	Joint Laxity	Complications
I (gravis)	AD	?	++	+++	+++	+++	aorta, bowel rupture, poor healing
II (mitis)	AD	?	+	++	++	++	minimal; mild form of I
III (hyper-mobile)	AD	?	+	+	+	+++	arthritis, muscle pain
IV (ecchymotic)	AD/AR	type III collagen	+++	-	+++	+	ruptured aneurysm, obstetric hemorrhage, pneumothorax
V	XLR	lysyl oxidase deficiency	+	+++	+	++	mitral/tricuspid valve prolapse, bowel rupture, arthritis, muscle pain
VI	AR	lysyl hydoxylase deficiency	++	+++	++	+++	hypotonia, kyphoscoliosis, osteoporosis; ocular fragility
VII	AD	Missing N-telo-peptide of α_1/α_2 chains type I collagen	+	++	+	++++	severe ligament and joint laxity, hip arthritis and dislocations
VIII (peri-odontal)	AD	?	+	+	+++	+	severe periodontitis
IX (X-linked cutis laxa)	XLR	lysyl oxidase deficiency, abnormal Cu^{2+} metabolism	+	+	++	+	hernia
X	AR	abnormal fibronectin	++	++	+	++	
XI	AD	?	+	+	+	+++	joint dislocations

Diseases

Epidermolysis Bullosa

epidermolysis bullosa simplex	AD, basal cell mutation K5 (12q) K14 (17q) **Weber-Cockayne**: palmoplantar bullae, callous, hyperhidrosis, superinfections **Generalized** (Koebner): generalized bullae **Dowling-Meara**: widespread herpetiform lesions, milia, nail dystrophy, mucous membranes erosions, high morbidity & mortality.
epidermolysis bullosa, junctional	AR, mutation in laminin 5 protein gene, intra-lamina lucida bullae **Herlitz**: bullae without scarring, milia, absent nails, dysplastic teeth, pyloric atresia, anemia, growth retardation, mortality **Non-Herlitz**: bullae of extremities, heal with atrophic scarring, scarring alopecia
epidermolysis bullosa, dystrophic	AD **Cockayne-Touraine**: bullae on extremities, milia, scarring, dystrophic nails **Albopapuloid Pasini** variant: widespread bullae, healing with atrophy, no milia, hypopigmented scars on trunk, dystrophic nails **AR**: generalized bullae with atrophic scarring, hyper/hypopigmentation, dystrophic nails, mitten deformities, flexural contractions, malnutrition, mucous membrane erosions, dysplastic teeth, anemia, SCC

Epidermolysis Bullosa

Type	Inheritance	Onset	Clinical Features	Cleavage	Notes
EB simplex	AD				
1) localized (Weber-Cockayne)		infancy, early childhood	palmoplantar blisters	intraepidermal (basilar)	hyperhidrosis
2) generalized (Koebner)		birth, early infancy	bullae on dorsal hands and feet	intraepidermal, vacuolated basal layer	negative Nikolsky sign
3) herpetiformis (Dowling-Meara)		birth	bullae generalized circinate grouping	intraepidermal, clumped tonofilaments	palmoplantar keratoderma, mucosal erosions
4) superficialis		birth/infancy	peeling skin generalized or extremities	subcorneal, granular	
Junctional EB					
1) generalized lethal (Herlitz, gravis)	AR	Birth	severe generalized blistering and denuded skin, milia, scarring, atrophy, dystrophic or absent nails, pitted tooth enamel	intralamina lucida; hemidesmosome defect	oral erosions, growth retardation, severe anemia, granulation tissue
2) generalized non-lethal (mitis)			as above with no milia and no mucous membrane lesions		
Dystrophic EB					
1) generalized-recessive (Hallopeau-Siemans, gravis)	AR	Birth	hemorrhagic bullae and scarring with milia, mitten deformity, scarring alopecia, mucosal erosions	sublamina densa; anchoring fibril defect, decreased or absent type VII collagen	severe anemia, growth retardation, caries, SCC, high mortality
2) generalized dominant a) Pasini	AD		severe expression; claw-like hands, albopapuloid lesions, white atrophy, scarring with milia	sublamina densa defect; anchoring fibrils	normal growth, ichthyosis, keratosis pilaris, hyperhidrosis
b) Cockayne-Touraine			hemorrhagic bullae, atrophic scars, milia, rare oral cavity lesion, normal teeth		

Diseases

Epidermolysis Bullosa

Type	Inheritance	Level of split	Scarring	Associated features
EB simplex-generalized Koebner	AD	basal cells	none	hyperhidrosis of feet, UVL
EBS localized (Weber-Cockayne)	AD	basal cells	none	hyperhidrosis of feet, hyperkeratotic lesions of palms
EBS-mottled hyperpigmentation	AD	basal cells	none	punctate hyperkeratoses; nails
EBS-herpetiformis (Dowling-Meara)	AD	basal cells	rare	hyperkeratoses of palms/soles
EBS-mottled pigmentation, punctate keratoderma	AD	basal cells	none	nail loss, carous teeth
EBS-localized, anodontia (Kallin s.)	AR	intraepidermal level	none	anodontia, deafness
EBS-Ogna	AD	basal cells	?	onychogrophysis of great toe
EBS-Bart	AD	basal cells	fine	dystrophic nails
EBS-Letalis	AR	basal cells	probably	anemia, frequent fatal
EBS-Mendes de Costa	XLR	basal cells	?	alopecia, microcephaly

Lamina Lucidiolytic Epidermolysis Bullosa (Junctional)

Type	Inheritance	Level of split	Scarring	Associated features
LEB-Gravis (Herlitz, EB hereditaria letalis, generalized atrophic EB gravis)	AR	lamina lucida	atrophy and scarring	nail loss, vegetating lesions, dystrophic teeth (cobblestoning), niciene absent, kalinin decreased
LEB-mitis (generalized atrophic EB mitis)	AR	lamina lucida	atrophic lesions	hair/nail loss, decreased life span, dystrophic teeth
LEB-localized, minimus	AR	lamina lucida	?	nail loss, dystrophic teeth, normal growth and development
LEB-cicatricial	AR	lamina lucida	scarring	syndactyly, hair, esophageal
LEB-inversa	AR	lamina lucida	atrophy	inverse involvement, nail loss
LEB-progressiva (neurotropica)	AR	lamina lucida	atrophy	onset 5-8 years, palmo-plantar involvement

Source: Ryan P. O'Quinn, MD

Diseases

Dermolytic Epidermolysis Bullosa (Dystrophic EB)

Type	Inheritance	Level of split	Scarring	Associated features
DEB-Cockayne-Touraine	AD	below basal lamina, anchoring fibrils decreased	scarring	nail/teeth involvement, SCC, esophageal stenosis, nail involvement
DEB-minimus	AD	sub-basal lamina	?	nails involved, minimal disability
DEB-pretibial	AD	separation in sublamina	scarring, atrophy	normal teeth
DEB-albopouloidea (Pasini)	AD	subbasal lamina lamina blistering	mild scarring	teeth near normal, nails involved, chondroitin sulfate
DEB-Hallopeau-Siemens	AR	sub basal lamina blistering	profound	mitten deformity,syndactyly, dystrophy, SCC, teeth dystrophy, nails normal esophagealinvolvement
DEB-inversa	AR	sub basal lamina	?	nails normal, esophageal involvement severe

Mucopolysaccharidoses

	Eponym	Inheritance	Enzyme defect	Urine MPS
I-H	Hurler	AR	α-L-iduronidase	DS, HS
I-S	Scheie	AR	α-L-iduronidase	DS, HS
I-H-S	Hurler-Scheie	AR	α-L-iduronidase	DS, HS
II-A	Hunter (severe)	XR	iduronate sulfatase	DS, HS
II-B	Hunter (mild)	XR	iduronate sulfatase	DS, HS
III-A	Sanfilippo A	AR	heparan N-sulfatase	HS
III-B	Sanfilippo B	AR	N-acetylglucosaminidase	HS
III-C	Sanfilippo C	AR	acetyl coenzyme A; α-glucosamine-N-acetyltransferase	HS
III-D	Sanfilippo D	AR	N-acetyl-α-glucosamine-6-sulfatase	HS
IV-A	Morquio A (classic)	AR	N-acetyl-α-glucosamine-6-sulfatase	KS
IV-B	Morquio B (mild)	AR	β-galactosidase	KS
VI	Maroteaux-Lamy (severe)	AR	N-acetylgalactosamine sulfatase (arylsulfatase B)	DS
VI	Maroteaux-Lamy (intermediate, mild)	AR	arylsulfatase B	DS
VII	Sly	AR	β-glucuronidase	DS, HS

DS= dermatan sulfate   HS= heparan sulfate   KS= keratan sulfate

Diseases

Osteogenesis Imperfecta

		Biochemical Defect
O. I.	defective biosynthesis of type I, collagen; brittle, osteoporotic bones, blue sclerae, lax joints	
Type I	AD; classic, mild, AKA OI with blue sclerae; normal stature, hearing loss (50%), dentinogenesis imperfecta (rare)	decreased type I procollagen production; substitution other than glycine in $\alpha 1(I)$
Type II	AD, AR, AD new mutation; perinatal lethal, beaded ribs, compressed femurs, platyspondylisis AKA OI congenita	rearranged COL1A1 & COL1A2 genes; substitution for glycyl residues in $\alpha 1(I)$ or $\alpha 2(I)$ chain
Type III	AD, AR (rare), new mutation; progressive deforming type, very short stature, variable sclerae hue, dentinogenesis common, hearing loss common	frame shift mutation prevents incorporation of $pro\alpha 2(I)$ into molecules (non-collagenous defect)
Type IV	AD; normal sclerae, mild bone deformity, short stature, dentinogenesis common, hearing loss (some)	point mutation in $\alpha 2(I)$ chain, rare point mutation in (1(I) chain, small deletions in $\alpha 2(I)$ chain

Diseases

Palmoplantar Ectodermal Dysplasias

	inheritance	inhuman	bone	cardiac	cysts	deafness	eye	hair	infection	malignancy	nail	neural	oral	pigment	teeth
I	AD	-	-	-	-	-	-	-	-	-	+	-	+	-	-
II	AD	-	-	-	+	-	-	+	-	-	+	-	-	-	+
III	AD	-	-	-	-	-	-	-	-	+	-	-	-	-	-
IV	AR	-	+/-	-	-	-	-	+/-	+	-	+	-	+	-	+
V	AR	-	-	-	-	-	+	-	-	-	-	+/-	-	-	-
VI	AR/AD	+	-	-	-	+	+	+	-	-	+	-	+	-	+
VII	AD	+	-	-	-	+	-	+	-	-	+	+	-	-	-
VIII	AR	+	+/-	-	-	-	-	-	-	+	+	+/-	+	-	-
IX	AD	-	+/-	-	-	-	-	-	-	+	+/-	-	-	-	-
X	AD	-	+/-	-	-	+/-	+	+	-	+	+	+/-	+	-	-
XI	AD	-	-	-	-	-	-	-	-	-	+/-	-	-	+	+/-
XII	AD	-	-	-	-	-	-	-	-	-	-	-	-	+	-
XIII	AD	+/-	-	-	-	-	+	+	-	-	+	-	+/-	+	+/-
XIV	AR/AD	-	-	+	-	-	-	+	-	-	-	-	-	-	-
XV	AD	+	-	-	-	+	-	-	-	-	+/-	-	-	-	-
XVI	AR	-	+	-	-	+	+	+/-	+	+	+/-	+	+	-	-
XVII	AD	-	+	-	-	-	+	-	-	-	+	+	-	-	+
XVIII	AD	-	+/-	-	-	-	-	-	-	-	+/-	+	-	-	-
XIX	AR	-	-	-	+	-	-	+	-	+	+	-	-	-	+
XX	AR	-	-	+	-	-	-	+	-	-	+	-	-	-	+

Modified from: Fitzpatrick, p. 607

Diseases

Palmoplantar Ectodermal Dysplasia: Eponyms & Synonyms

I. Jadassohn-Lewandowsky s.; **II.** Jackson-Sertoli s., Jackson-Lawler ; **III.** PPK associated with esophageal cancer, tylosis; **IV.** Papillon-Lefèvre s.; **V.** tyrosinemia type II, Richer-Hanhart s.; **VI.** Olmsted s., mutilating palmoplantar keratoderma with periorificial keratotic plaques, polykeratosis of Touraine; **VII.** Vohwinkel's s., keratoma hereditaria mutilans; **VIII.** mal de Meleda, mutilating PPK of the Gamborg-Nielsen type, acral keratoderma; **IX.** Huriez s., PPK with sclerodactyly, scleroatrophic & keratotic dermatosis of limbs, sclerotylosis; **X.** hidrotic ectodermal dysplasia, Fischer-Jacobsen-Clouston s., alopecia congenita with keratosis palmoplantaris, keratosis palmaris with drumstick fingers, PPK & clubbing; **XI.** congenital poikiloderma with traumatic bulla formation, anhidrosis, & keratoderma, Naegeli-Franceschetti-Jadassohn s.; **XII.** acrokeratotic poikiloderma, hyperkeratosis-hyper-pigmentation s.; **XIII.** dermatopathia pigmentosa reticularis, dermatopathia pigmentosa reticularis et atrophica, dermatopathia pigmentosa reticularis hyperkeratotica et mutilans; **XIV.** Woolly hair & endomyocardial fibrodysplasia; **XV.** palmoplantar keratoderma with sensorineural deafness, Bart-Pumphrey s.; **XVI.** keratosis-ichthyosis-deafness s., KID s., ichthyosiform erythroderma corneal involvement & deafness, Desmon's s.; **XVII.** corneodermatosseous s., CDO s.; **XVIII.** palmoplantar keratoderma & spastic paraplegia, Charcot-Marie Tooth d. with PPK & nail dystrophy; **XIX.** eyelid cysts palmoplantar keratosis hypodontia & hypotrichosis, Schöpf-Schulz-Passarge s.; **XX.** cardiofaciocutaneous s.

Pemphigus Diseases

	Pemphigus Vulgaris	Pemphigus Foliaceus	IgA Pemphigus	Pemphigus Foliaceus	Paraneoplastic Pemphigus
Epidemiology	Most common type, Ashkenazi jews	idiopathic, drug-induced, endemic	rare		neoplasms
Antigen	desmoglein 3, 130-kd cadherin	desmoglein 1, 160-kd cadherin	unknown, some desmocollins I and II		250-kd desmoplakin I 230-kd BP1 antigen 210-kd desmoplakin II
HLA	DR4, DR6	DR1, DQ1 and DR4			
Clinical Features	flaccid bullae, denuded areas, Nikolsky sign, painful oral erosions	superficial crusts, erosions, hypertrophic lesions	superficial crusts		mucosal erosions progress to intractable stomatitis, poly-morphous skin eruption, lichenoid eruptions

Diseases

Pemphigus Diseases

	Pemphigus Vulgaris	Pemphigus Foliaceus	IgA Pemphigus	Foliaceus Paraneoplastic Pemphigus
Sites of predilection	mouth, spread to head, neck, upper trunk, intertriginous areas, esophagus, cervix	central face, then head, neck, upper trunk, extremities. Rare oral lesions		stomatitis orally, head and neck, trunk, extremities, palms and soles
Histology	suprabasilar cleft, basal "row of tombstones" acantholytic cells in blister. Eos and spongiosis in lower epidermis. Scant infiltrate; eos, PMN, lymphs	vacuolization, acantholytic clefting in granular or sub-granular layer. Denuded roof, epidermal spongiosis with eos, perivascular infiltrate with eos, lymphs	1) subcorneal pustule with acantholytic cells 2) intraepidermal pustule with eos and rare acantholytic cells	variable, most suprabasilar acantholysis and inflammation. Lichenoid infiltrate, keratino-cyte necrosis
Immunofluorescence	linear IgG and C3 on epidermal cell surfaces	linear/granular IgA on epidermal cell surfaces	linear/granular IgA	IgG and complement in epidermal intercellular spaces, granular/linear complement along basement membrane zone
Notes	p. vegetans is variant: persistent hypertrophic lesions of flexures and umbilicus. Ab titers and d. activity correlate well. Loss of attachment of cell membrane between desmosomes.			Poor prognosis, stomatitis is refractory
Treatment	prednisone, azathioprine, chlorambucil, methotrexate, cyclophosphamide, gold, cyclosporine, plasmapheresis	prednisone, topical steroids, antimalarials, methotrexate, cyclophosphamide, azathioprine	dapsone, prednisone ?etretinate	treat the tumor, prednisone or immunosuppressive medications

Diseases

Porphyria

Porphyria	Inheritance	Enzyme deficiency	Erythrocyte	Feces	Plasma	Urine
acute intermittent porphyria	AD	porphobilinogen deaminase	—	—	—	ALA, PBG
ALA dehydratase deficiency porphyria	AR	ALA dehydratase	ZnPROTO	COPRO, PROTO	ALA	ALA
congenital erythropoietic porphyria	AR	uroporphyrinogen III cosynthase	URO I > COPRO I	COPRO I > URO I	URO I > COPRO I	URO I > COPRO I
erythropoietic protoporphyria	AD, variable	ferrochelatase	PROTO	PROTO	PROTO	—
hepatoerythropoietic porphyria	AR	uroporphyrinogen decarboxylase	ZnPROTO	COPRO, ISOCOPRO	URO, COPRO	URO, ISOCOPRO
hereditary coproporphyria	AD	coproporphyrinogen oxidase	—	PROTO > COPRO	COPRO	COPRO: acutely, ALA, PBG
porphyria cutanea tarda	AD, acquired	uroporphyrinogen decarboxylase	—	ISOCOPRO	URO, COPRO	URO I> III; 7-COOH-P III > I
variegate porphyria	AD	protoporphyrinogen oxidase	—	PROTO > COPRO	COPRO, PROTO	COPRO > URO acutely, ALA, PBG

Eponyms and Syndromes

Achard-Thiers s.	postmenopausal women, excess adrenocortical androgens; diabetes, hirsutism & masculinization
acquired circumscribed dermal melanocytosis of the face	Hori's nevus
acquired partial face-sparing lipodystrophy	Dunnigan s.
acrodermatitis enteropathica	AR; disorder of zinc uptake, vesiculopustulous dermatitis of head, body orifices, hands & feet with alopecia, diarrhea & steatorrhea
acrodermatitis papulosa infantum	Gianotti-Crosti s.
actinic prurigo	Hutchinson's prurigo
acute disseminated histiocytosis X	Letterer-Siwe d./s.
acute hemorrhagic edema of infancy	Finkelstein's d., Seidlmeyer's s.
Adams-Oliver s.	AD/AR; aplasia cutis congenita of scalp with terminal transverse limb defects
Adamson's fringe	bottom one-third of hair follicle
Addison's d.	adrenal insufficiency; hyperpigmentation, longitudinal nail bands, hypotension, altered serum electrolytes, vitiligo, weakness
adenosine deaminase deficiency	erythrocyte enzyme; thymic involution, decreased T cell survival, abnormal B cell function: mucocutaneous candidiasis, bacterial, protozoal & viral infections
adiposis dolorosa	Dercum's d.
Albright's s.	McCune-Albright s.
Alezzandrini's s.	unilateral tapetoretinal degeneration followed by alopecia areata, facial vitiligo, poliosis, sometimes deafness
alkaptonuria	AR, homogentisic acid accumulation due to deficient homogentisate 1,2-dioxygenase; elevated urine homogentisic acid, ochronosis, arthritis
Ambras s.	AD; hypertrichosis of face, ears, shoulders with facial dysmorphism & dental abnormalities
Ancell-Spiegler s.	multiple cylindromas
angiokeratoma corporis diffusum	Fabry's d.
angry back s.	excited skin s.
anhidrotic ectodermal dysplasia	Christ-Siemens-Touraine s.
anticardiolipin Ab s.	arterial & venous thromboses, elevated anticardiolipin antibody, livedo reticularis, SLE
antiphospholipid Ab s.	lupus anticoagulent s.

Eponyms and Syndromes

Apert's s.	acrocephalosyndactyly, associated with cutis verticis gyrata
Argyll-Robertson pupil	irregular, small, unequal pupils that react weakly to light; syphilis
Ascher s.	blepharochalasis, double lip & nontoxic thyroid enlargement
ataxia-telangiectasia	Louis-Bar s.
Auspitz sign	punctate bleeding at the sites of scale removal; psoriasis (except inverse or pustular psoriasis)
Böök's s.	palmar hyperhidrosis
BADS s.	black locks, oculocutaneous albinism & deafness of sensineuronal type
Bannayan s., Bannayan-Zonana s.	Proteus s.
Baraitser's s.	atrichia, MR
Bart's s.	AD; aplasia cutis congenita (esp. of legs); dominant epidermolysis bullosa dystrophica
Bart-Pumphrey s.	AD; palmoplantar keratoderma with sensorineural deafness AKA PED type XV
basal cell nevus s.	Gorlin's s., Gorlin-Goltz s.
Basan's s.	AD; fine dermal ridges, single flexion crease, xerosis, long philtrum, thin upper lip, nail ridges
Bateman, herpes iris of	large lesions of EM with central bulla & marginal vesicle ring
Bateman's purpura	actinic (solar) purpura
Battle's sign	skin discoloration over mastoid area of skull; basilar skull fracture
Bazex's s.	1) AD; follicular atrophoderma of dorsal hands, abnormal hair & sweat glands, multiple BCC 2) acquired eczematous & psoriasiform lesions (ear, nose, dorsal hands, feet, knees), nail dystrophy & paronychial inflammation with SCC (GI, respiratory) (100%) AKA paraneoplastic acrokeratosis
Bean s.	AD, sporadic, rare; rubbery cutaneous venous malformations with GI bleeds & hemangiomas, anemia AKA blue rubber bleb nevus s.
Beane-Stevenson s.	AD, 10q26, FGFR2; cutis gyrata, craniofacial dysostosis
Beau's lines	transverse depression across nail plate; cytotoxic drugs, dysmenorrhea, MI, post fever, psoriasis
Becker's nevus	common, sharply demarcated hyperpigmented patch of shoulder, chest, scapula AKA Becker's melanosis
Beckwith-Wiedemann s.	AD with variable penetrance; sporadic; mid-facial capillary malformation, macroglossia, HSM, omphalocele, gigantism, hemihypertrophy, Wilms' tumor, adrenal cortical carcinoma, hepatoblastoma AKA EMG s. & exomphalos-macroglossia-gigantism s.
Bednar tumor	pigmented dermatofibrosarcoma protuberans
Behçet's d.	aphthosis (oral & genital), arthritis, cutaneous pustular vasculitis, meningoencephalitis, posterior uveitis, thrombophlebitis, intestinal inflammation

Eponyms and Syndromes

benign familial pemphigus	Hailey-Hailey d.
Bezold sign	inflammatory edema below apex of mastoid process; mastoiditis
BIDS s.	*b*rittle hair, *i*ntellectual impairment, *d*ecreased fertility, *s*hort stature
Biederman's sign	dark red color of anterior pillars of throat; syphilitics (some)
Bier spots	light macules on arms & legs of young adults; benign physiologic vascular anomaly
Biette's collarette	thin white ring of scales on papule surface; secondary syphilis
biotin dependent carboxylase deficiency	CNS disease; alopecia, ataxia, *Candida* dermatitis, decreased IgA, defective T cells, keratoconjunctivitis, seizures
biotinidase deficiency	AR; deficiency causes multiple carboxylase deficiency
bird-headed dwarfism	Seckel's s.
Birt-Hogg-Dube s.	fibrofolliculomas (>5) of the ear, forehead, nose, temporal region
Björnstad's s.	AR; pili torti & sensorineural deafness
Blaschko's lines	CHILD s., chondrodysplasia punctata, Delleman-Oorthuys s., focal dermal hypoplasia (Goltz's s.), hypomelanosis of Ito, incontinentia pigmenti, incontinentia pigmenti achromians, lichen striatus, linear & whorled nevoid hypermelanosis, linear epidermal nevus, linear lichen planus, linear nevus sebaceous, linear psoriasis, linear sclero-derma, mosaic EHK, Proteus s., Schimmelpenning-Feverstein-Mims s.
Blaschko's lines, linear	ILVEN, lichen striatus, linear Darier's d., linear LP, linear poroker-atosis, nevus comedonicus
Blaschko's lines, x-linked	CHILD s., Conradi-Hunermann s., focal dermal hypoplasia, hypo-hidrotic ectodermal dysplasia, incontinentia pigmenti, Menkes' kinky hair s., orofacial-digital s, Partington's s.
blastomycosis, N. American	Gilchrist's d.
blind loop s.	bowel bypass s.
Bloch-Sulzberger s.	XLD male lethal, Xp11; cutaneous, ocular, CNS & skeletal abnor-malities AKA incontinentia pigmenti
Bloom's s.	AR, 15q26; photodistributed erythema with telangiectasia, chelitis, café-au-lait, craniofacial abnormalities, growth retardation, hypogo-nadism, leukemia, lymphoma, breast cancer, GI adenocarcinoma AKA congenital telangiectatic erythema
blue rubber bleb nevus s.	Bean s.
Borsieri's sign	fingernail drawn along skin produces white demarcation line which quickly turns red; scarlet fever (early)
Bourneville's s., Bourneville-Pringle s.	AD; adenoma sebaceum, brain hamartomas, café-au-lait spots, MR, seizures, shagreen patches, subungual fibromas, vitiligo AKA tuber-ous sclerosis
bowel bypass s.	(20%) post jejunal bypass; malaise, myalgia, polyarthralgia, rash, sterile skin pustules
Bowen's d.	SCC of genitals

Eponyms and Syndromes

Brachmann-de Lange s.	Cornelia de Lange s.
Brill-Zinsser d.	recurrent epidemic typhus (*Rickettsia prowazeki*)
Brocq, pseudopelade of	end-stage scarring alopecia caused by favus, LE, LP, sarcoidosis, scarring folliculitis, scleroderma
Brooke-Fordyce	hereditary benign cystic epitheliomas
Brooke-Spiegler s.	multiple trichoepitheliomas & cylindromas
Brunauer-Fuhs-Siemens PPK	AD; mild PPK AKA striate PPK, Wachters PPK, keratosis palmoplantaris varians
Brunsting-Perry pemphigoid	similar to cicatricial pemphigoid with predominant head & neck scarring involvement
Buckley's s.	hyperimmunoglobulin E s. with asthma & coarse facial features
Buerger's d.	thromboangiitis obliterans
burning feet s.	Goplans' d.
Burns' s.	KID s.
Buruli ulcer	*Mycobacterium ulcerans* skin ulcer
Buschke-Fischer-Brauer d.	keratosis punctata palmaris et plantaris
Buschke-Lowenstein tumors	dysplastic genital warts
Buschke-Ollendorff s.	AD; dermatofibrosis lenticularis disseminata, elastin nevi, osteopoikilosis
Bywater's lesions	digital pulp papules (leukocytoclastic vasculitis); autoimmune disease, especially RA
Calabar swellings	localized angioedema from adult worm migration through subcutis, usually around joints: loiasis
Campbell-DeMorgan spots	cherry angioma
candidiasis, chronic mucocutaneous	severe combined immunodeficiency s., Nezelof's s., DiGeorge's s. **chronic oral candidiasis**: onset any age, no inheritance pattern; oropharyngeal, sparing skin & nails **chronic candidiasis with endocrinopathy**: AR; onset childhood, one or more: hypoadrenalism, hypoparathyroidism hypothyroidism, hypogonadism, antibodies to endocrine glands, alopecia, vitiligo **chronic localized candidiasis**: (*Candida* granuloma) onset childhood, may be associated with endocrinopathy, mucosal, nail & skin, hyperkeratotic, granulomatous, vegetating *Candida* **chronic diffuse candidiasis**: AD/AR; nails, skin, mucous membranes, no endocrinopathy **chronic candidiasis with thymoma**: adult onset; myasthenia gravis, aplastic anemia, decreased neutrophils & immunoglobulins
Cannon's d.	white sponge nevus
Cantu's s.	AD; brown macules on face, forearms, feet with hyperkeratosis of palms & soles
carbon baby s.	rare; hyperpigmentation progressing from groin & face to entire skin surface birth-2 years AKA universal acquired melanosis

Eponyms and Syndromes

carcinoid s.	pronounced flushing, with wheezing, diarrhea, abdominal pain; carcinoid cancer of bowel, bronchus, pancreas, thyroid, teratomas
cardio-facio-cutaneous s.	abnormal facies, cardiac anomalies, eczema, follicular hyperkeratosis, growth retardation, ichthyotic changes, MR, occasionally palmoplantar hyperkeratosis, splenomegaly
Caripito itch	irritating setae of genus *Hylesia* caterpillar AKA butterfly itch, moth dermatitis
Carney's s.	lentigines, myxomas (cardiac, skin, breast), endocrine abnormalities
Carrion's d.	Oroya fever
Casal's necklace	broad band of dermatosis around neck; pellagra (niacin deficiency)
Castleman's d.	lymphoproliferative disorder presenting as isolated mediastinal mass or solitary cutaneous tumor AKA angiofollicular lymphoid hyperplasia
Chadwick's sign	dark blue or purple color of vaginal mucosa; pregnancy
Chagas' d., Chagas-Cruz d.	American trypanosomiasis, *Trypanosoma cruzi*, reduviid bug (vector) erythematous nodule (chagoma), at bite site, high fever, unilateral facial & eyelid edema (Romaña's sign) regional LAD, HSM & meningoencephalic irritation
Chanarin-Dorfman s.	AR; disordered lipid metabolism, erythroderma, fine white scaling & lichenification over dorsal hands, myopathy, vacuolated leukocytes; increased in Middle Eastern or Mediterranean descent AKA neutral lipid storage d.
chancriform s.	nodule/chancre on distal extremity with chain of nodules extending proximally; sporotrichosis
Chediak-Higashi s.	AR, lethal; oculocutaneous albinism, absent elastase, increased cAMP, decreased cGMP, poor melanosome transport, ecchymoses, pigmented nevi, gray hair, pancytopenia, bleeding diathesis, lymphoma, HSM, giant lysosomal granules, histiocytic infiltration of organs, pulmonary pyogenic infections, leukocyte deficiencies (chemotaxis, adherence, killing, deformability)
CHILD s.	XLD; *c*ongenital *h*emidysplasia with *i*chthyosiform erythroderma & *l*imb *d*efects
CHIME s.	*c*oloboma, *h*eart defects, *i*chthyosiform dermatosis, *m*ental retardation & *e*ar anomalies AKA Zunich-Kaye s.
chondrodysplasia punctata	Conradi's d.
Christ-Siemens-Touraine s.	XLR; anodontia, cataracts, frontal bossing, MR, pseudorhagades, saddle nose, sebaceous gland hyperplasia, sparse dry hair, thickened lips, thin brittle nails AKA anhidrotic ectodermal dysplasia
chronic granulomatous d.	**XLR**, AR, AD; cutaneous/systemic pyogenic infections, defective oxidative metabolism of neutrophils and monocytes; abscesses, acne (severe), diarrhea, FTT, furuncles, hidradenitis suppurativa, infections, paronychia (chronic), perirectal ulcerative stomatitis
Churg-Strauss s.	allergic granulomatous angiitis; rare-vasculitis with asthma, peripheral eosinophilia & recurrent pneumonia

Eponyms and Syndromes

Clark's nevi	dysplastic melanocytic nevi
Clouston's s.	AD; alopecia, cataracts, nail dystrophy & clubbing, MR (some), palmoplantar hyperkeratosis, seizures (some), xerosis, French Canadians AKA hidrotic ectodermal dysplasia
Coat's d.	retinal telangiectasias & occasional skin telangiectasias
Cobb's s.	sporadic; dermatomal capillary malformation over spinal vascular malformation, angiokeratoma circumscriptum
Cockayne's s.	AR; aged appearance, cachexia, cataracts, growth arrest, microcephaly, neurological deterioration, photodistributed erythema, subcutaneous fat loss, early death
Cockayne-Touraine s.	dominant dystrophic epidermolysis bullosa
Coffin-Siris s.	AD; MR, sparse scalp hair, lax joints, bushy eyebrows, low nasal bridge, hypertrichosis
common variable immunodeficiency s.	late onset decreased immunoglobulins IgA, IgG, IgM; autoimmune diseases, alopecia areata, chronic giardiasis, eczema, recurrent otitis media, *Trichophyton rubrum*, URI infections, vitiligo
congenital self-healing reticulohistiocytosis	Hashimoto-Pritzker d.
congenital telangiectatic erythema	Bloom's s.
congenital total lipodystrophy	Lawrence-Seip s.
congenital varicella s.	chorioretinitis, cortical atrophy, cutaneous scars, limb hypoplasia
Conradi-Hünermann s.	X-dominant, male lethal ichthyosiform erythroderma in Blaschko's lines, cataracts & asymmetric limb defects AKA chondrodysplasia punctata
Consular d.	gnathostomiasis
contact urticaria s.	**stage 1**: localized urticaria restricted to the area of contact **stage 2**: generalized urticaria, including angioedema **stage 3**: urticaria associated with bronchial asthma **stage 4**: urticaria associated with anaphylactic reactions
COPS s.	calcinosis cutis, osteoma cutis, poikiloderma & skeletal abnormalities
Cornelia de Lange s.	de Lange s.
Corrigan's sign	purple line at junction of teeth & gum; chronic copper poisoning
Coulomb, pseudoscars of	stellate scars of the hands
Cowden's s., Cowden d.	AD; oral papillomatosis, palmoplantar keratoses, arched palate, fissured tongue, caries, GI hamartomatous polyps, GU cysts, breast cancer AKA multiple hamartoma s.
craniofacial dysostosis	Crouzon's d.
CREST s.	*c*alcinosis cutis, *R*aynaud's phenomenon, *e*sophageal dysfunction, *s*clerodactyly, *t*elangiectasia
cri du chat s.	partial 5p deletion; hypertelorism, microcephaly, MR, high-pitch cry, simian crease

Eponyms and Syndromes

Crocker, dermatitis repens of	acrodermatitis continua (Hallopeau)
Cronkhite-Canada s.	alopecia, diffuse palmar hyperpigmentation, spotty hypopigmentation of dorsal hands, nail dystrophy, GI polyposis & adenocarcinoma (15%), malabsorption with hypoproteinemia, electrolyte disturbance
Cross-McKusick-Breen s.	AR; oculocutaneous albinism, gingival hypertrophy, microphthalmus, small opaque corneas, oligophrenia with spasticity, high arched palate & scoliosis AKA oculocerebral-hypopigmentation s.
Crouzon's d.	AD, 10q26; craniofacial dysostosis
Crowe's sign	café-au-lait macules of axillae (axillary freckling); neurofibromatosis
Crow-Fukase s.	POEMS s.
Cullen's sign	blue periumbilical discoloration; acute pancreatic blood extravasation
Curth & Macklin, ichthyosis hystrix of	AD, very rare; resembles EHK with variable involvement, porcupine-like or verrucous hyperkeratosis
Cushing's s.	excessive glucocorticoids; characteristic habitus, cutis marmorata, easy bruising, ecchymoses, impaired wound healing, petechiae, striae, transparent epidermis, thinned dermis
cutis marmorata telangiectatica congenita	sporadic; atrophic reticulated vascular patch, ipsilateral hemiatrophy/hypertrophy, glaucoma, MR
Dabska's tumor	endovascular papillary angioendothelioma
Danoff s.	AD?; adrenocortical micronodular dysplasia, atrial myxoma, lentigines, spindle cell tumors
Darier's d., Darier-White d.	AD, 12q23-24.1, disrupted keratin tonofilament-desmosome complex; keratotic papules in seborrheic distribution, nail dystrophy, palmar pits, acrokeratoses AKA keratosis follicularis
Darier's sign	firm stroking of pigmented macule leads to mast cell mediator release & edema; urticaria pigmentosa (pathognomonic)
Davis Colley d.	keratosis punctata palmaris et plantaris
de Lange s.	brachycephaly, bushy eyebrows, carp mouth, coarse hair, depressed nose bridge, dwarfism, low set ears, MR, simian crease, webbed neck AKA Cornelia de Lange s.
De Sanctis-Cacchione s.	AR; subset of xeroderma pigmentosum with MR, retarded growth, gonadal hypoplasia, sometimes neurologic degeneration & ocular abnormality AKA xerodermic idiocy
DeBarsy's s.	cataracts, corneal opacities, ear dysplasia, growth retardation, joint hypermobility, microcephaly, MR, progeroid facies, pronounced nasolabial fold, skin wrinkling
Degos' acanthoma	benign epidermal tumor with glycogen containing epidermal cells AKA clear cell acanthoma
Degos' s.	multisystem lymphocytic vasculitis CNS & GI involvement AKA malignant atrophic papulosis

Eponyms and Syndromes

Delleman-Oorthuys s.	sporadic; cutis aplasia, skin tags, ocular defects, CNS defects
delusion of parasitosis	Ekbom's d.
Dennie-Morgan lines	accentuated folds of lower eyelid; atopic patients (non-diagnostic)
Dercum's d.	multiple painful lipomas; AKA adiposis dolorosa
dermatitis exfoliativa neonatorum	Ritter's d., staphylococcal scalded skin s.
dermatomyositis	Wagner-Unverricht d.
Desmons' s.	KID s.
DiGeorge s.	teratogen caused; abnormal development of 3rd & 4th pharyngeal pouches; thymic & parathyroid hypoplasia, deficient cell mediated immunity; abnormal facies, congenital heart defects, decreased T cells, esophageal atresia, severe recurrent candidiasis infections
disseminated pagetoid reticulosis	Ketron-Goodman d.
Donohue's s.	absent subcutaneous fat, elfin face, hirsutism, thickened skin AKA leprechaunism
Dowling-Degos' d./s.	AD; brownish reticulate macules in flexural areas AKA reticulate pigmented anomaly of the flexures
Dowling-Meara EBS	epidermolysis bullosa herpetiformis
Down s.	trisomy 21; epicanthal fold, flat nose, short phalanges, widened spaces between 1st & 2nd digits of hands & feet, MR
Dubois' sign	short 5th digit; congenital syphilis
Dubokowitz's s.	broad nasal tip, eczematous lesions in infancy, epicanthal folds, micrognathia, MR, ptosis, sparse scalp hair, subcutaneous tissue diminished
Dukes' d.	mild febrile childhood illness with erythematous exanthem; Coxsackie ECHO virus group AKA scarlatinella, fourth d.
Duncan's d.	X-linked lymphoproliferative d.; abnormal immune response to EBV infection, early death or acquired dysgammaglobulinemia, chronic infectious mononucleosis, malignant lymphoma, T-lymphocyte depletion
Dunnigan s.	fat loss of limbs associated with DM AKA acquired partial face-sparing lipodystrophy
Dupuytren's d.	palmoplantar fibromatosis; dimpled palmar skin over 4th metacarpal, progressing to contracture
dyskeratosis congenita	Zinsser-Cole-Engman s.
dysplastic nevus s.	dysplastic nevi in patient at risk for familial or nonfamilial malignant melanoma
EEC s.	AD; *e*ctodermal dysplasia with *e*ctrodactyly, *c*left lip/palate, blepharitis, speckled irides, MR
Ehlers-Danlos s.	*see table in Diseases section*
Ekbom's d.	delusion of parasitosis

Eponyms and Syndromes

Elejalde s.	AR; bronze skin after sun exposure, CNS dysfunction, hypotonia, MR, seizures, silver hair
Elliot's sign	induration of edge of syphilitic skin lesion
EMG s.	*e*xomphalos, *m*acroglossia, *g*igantism AKA Beckwith-Wiedemann s.
Enroth's sign	abnormal fullness of eyelids; Graves' disease
eosinophilic cellulitis	Well's s.
eosinophilic fasciitis	Schulman's s.
epidermal nevus s.	sporadic; ILVEN; café-au-lait macules, epidermal nevi, hemangiomas, kyphoscoliosis, limb deformities, lipodermoid tumors, MR, seizures AKA Schimmelpenning s., Solomon s.
Epstein's pearls	milia in oral cavity (palate) usually in infants
erythema multiforme major	Stevens-Johnson s.
erythema multiforme minor	Hebra's d.
erythrokeratoderma viriabilis	Mendes de Costa s.
erythroplasia of Queyrat	SCC of glans penis
erythropoietic porphyria	Günther d.
excited skin s.	patch testing; false + reactions (up to 40%), hypersensitivity caused by strong + reaction to one allergen AKA angry back s.
exomphalos-macroglossia-gigantism s.	Beckwith-Wiedemann s.
Fabry's d.	XLR; storage disease of glycosphingolipid catabolism, deficiency of α-galactosidase A leading to accumulated ceramide trihexoside in CV & renal systems; telangiectases in bathing suit distribution, corneal opacities, burning pain of palms, soles & abdomen; leg edema, osteoporosis, retarded growth, delayed puberty AKA angiokeratoma corporis diffusum
familial atypical multiple mole melanoma s.	dysplastic nevi with GI & pancreatic malignancy AKA FAMMM s.
familial dysautonomia	Riley-Day s.
familial dyskeratotic comedones	AD; widespread comedonal lesions on extremities
familial Mediterranean fever	AR; fever, peritonitis, pleurisy, purpura, renal amyloidosis, synovitis, urticaria, vasculitis nodules
FAMMM s.	familial atypical multiple mole melanoma s.
Fanconi's s.	vitamin D resistant rickets, glucosuria, aminoaciduria, acidosis, hypouricemia, hypokalemia, flexion deformities, generalized ichthyosis & FTT
Farber's d.	lipogranulomatosis

Eponyms and Syndromes

Favre-Racouchot d.	open comedones in background of dermatoheliosis on temples AKA nodular elastosis with cysts & comedones
Felty's s.	anemia, frequent leg ulcers, leukopenia, pigmented lower extremity macules, RA, splenomegaly, thrombocytopenia
Feuerstein & Mims s.	epidermal nevus s. AKA Schimmelpenning s., Solomon s.
fifth d.	erythema infectiosum
Filipovitch's sign	yellow discoloration of palms & soles; typhoid fever AKA palmo-plantar sign
Finkelstein's d.	acute hemorrhagic edema of infancy
Fisch's s.	deafness, partial heterochromia, premature graying hair
Fischer-Jacobsen-Clouston s.	AD; "drumstick fingers," growth retardation, hair abnormalities, MR, palmoplantar scaling, thickened nails AKA hidrotic ectodermal dysplasia, PED type X
Fitzpatrick sign	lateral compression produces dimpling; dermatofibroma
Flegel's d.	keratinous papules of calves AKA hyperkeratosis lenticularis perstans
focal dermal hypoplasia	Goltz s.
folliculitis decalvans	Quinquaud's d.
Fordyce's angiokeratoma	small benign blood vessel tumor on scrotum & labia majora
Fordyce's condition	benign ectopic sebaceous glands on oral mucosa, genital mucosa, esophagus or larynx
Forscheimer spots	pinpoint rose colored macules & petechiae on soft palate; rubella
fourth d.	Dukes' d.
fourth venereal d.	gangrenous & ulcerative balanoposthitis or granuloma inguinale
Fox-Fordyce d.	females (9x); chronic, pruritic follicular eruption of apocrine glands of axillae and pubic area
François s.	AR; nodules of hands, nose, ears, osteochondrodystrophy AKA ocu-lomandibulofacial s.
Franceschetti-Jadassohn s.	AD, onset >2 years old; heat intolerance, hypohidrosis, palmoplan-tar hyperkeratosis, reticular hyperpigmentation, yellow teeth
Frey's s.	auriculotemporal s.; gustatory sweating in malar area following parotid gland damage
Futcher's line	pigmentary demarcation between dorsal & ventral forearm AKA type A lines, Voigt's lines
Gamborg-Nielson PPK	AD; diffuse glove & stocking keratoderma with constricting digital bands, nail abnormalities, angular chelitis, hyperhidrosis, develop-mental retardation AKA mal de Meleda
Gardner's s.	AD; colon polyps progressing to carcinoma, dental anomalies, desmoid tumors, epidermal cysts, fibromas, ocular fundus pigmenta-tion, osteomas, retroperitoneal fibrosis, thyroid cancer
Gardner-Diamond s. (purpura)	autoerythrocyte sensitivity (thought to be psychogenic); painful bruises & ecchymoses (on legs, arms, face), syncope, abdominal pain, vomiting

Eponyms and Syndromes

Gaucher's d.	AR; lysosomal storage disease, deficiency of β-glucocerebrosidase; café-au-lait macules, collodion baby, ichthyosis
Gianotti-Crosti s.	young children; HBV, coxsackie A16, EBV, CMV, parainfluenza virus, RSV, group A streptococcal; fever, malaise, HSM, copper red flat topped firm papules; face, extremities & buttocks-progress to plagues & scales AKA acrodermatitis papulosa infantum, infantile papular acrodermatitis, papular acrodermatitis of childhood
Gilchrist's d.	North American blastomycosis
Giroux-Barbeau s.	AD; erythrokeratoderma with ataxia
glucagonoma s.	glucagon-producing pancreatic tumor; dermatitis, necrolytic migratory erythema, anemia, carbohydrate intolerance, hypoaminoacidemia, stomatitis, weight loss
Goldenhar's s.	triad of accessory tragi, auricular fistulas, epibulbar dermoids or lipodermoids
Goldstein's sign	wide space between first two toes; cretinism, Down s.
Goltz s.	focal dermal hypoplasia
Good's s.	thymoma with acquired hypogammaglobulinemia
Goplans' d.	localized hypohidrosis & painful feet AKA burning feet s.
Gorham's d.	sporadic; venous malformations, lymphatic malformations, replacement of bone with fibrous tissue
Gorlin's s., Gorlin-Goltz s.	AD, 9q21; early BCC's, palmoplantar pits, cysts of mandible & maxilla, bone, intracranial calcification, eye & reproductive tract abnormalities, medulloblastomas, mental retardation, characteristic facies AKA basal cell nevus s.
Gorlin's sign	ability to touch tip of nose with tongue; Ehlers-Danlos s., normal persons
Gottron's papules	inflammatory papules over dorsal hand joints; dermatomyositis
Gottron's sign	violaceous erythema over knuckles, elbows, medial malleoli, patella; dermatomyositis (pathognomonic)
Gougerot-Blum s.	pigmented purpuric lichenoid dermatitis
Graham-Little s., Graham-Little-Feldman s.	cicatricial alopecia with follicular lichen planus of skin & scalp, may be associated with noncicatricial alopecia of axillae & pubic areas AKA Graham-Little-Piccardi-Lassueur s.
granuloma multiforme	Mkar d.
granulomatous cheilitis	Melkersson's s., Melkersson-Rosenthal s.
Greenblatt's sign	linear depression over Poupart's ligament separating draining lymph nodes; lymphogranuloma venereum AKA groove sign of Greenblatt
Greither's s.	palmoplantar keratoderma with transgrediens to dorsal surfaces
Griscelli s.	AR; albinism with hypomelanosis, silver hair, pyogenic infection, HSM, thrombocytopenia, immune deficiency AKA hypopigmentation-immunodeficiency d.
Grisolle's sign	when skin is stretched, a papule is felt; smallpox (historical)

Eponyms and Syndromes

Grover's d.	pruritic erythematous papules typically middle aged or older males on trunk, shoulders, neck, thighs AKA transient acantholytic dermatosis
Gunther's d.	AR, 10q25.2-q26; uroporphyrinogen III cosynthetase; **early**: immediate photosensitivity with burning, edema, erosions **late**: mutilating scarring in sun exposed areas, cicatricial alopecia, hypertrichosis, brown teeth, photophobia, hemolytic anemia, splenomegaly AKA erythropoietic porphyria
Haarscheibe receptor	receptor associated with Merkel cells AKA Pinkus corpuscle, hederiform ending
Hailey-Hailey d.	AD, defect in tonofilament-desmosome complex, adhesion molecule abnormalities(?); recurrent vesicles & bullae in intertriginous areas AKA benign familial pemphigus
Hallermann-Streiff s.	dyscephaly, parrot nose, mandibular hypoplasia, proportionate nanism, hypotrichosis, bilateral congenital cataracts, and microphthalmia AKA oculomandibulofacial s.
Hallopeau, acrodermatitis continua of	sterile pustular eruption of fingers or toes that extends proximally
Hallopeau, pemphigus vegetans of	localized pemphigus vulgaris
Hallopeau-Siemens	generalized recessive dystrophic epidermolysis bullosa
Hand-Schüller-Christian d.	Langerhan's cell histiocytosis
Hansen's d.	leprosy
harlequin s.	unilateral facial flushing & sweating
Hartnup's d.	AR, 2pter-q32.3, defective amino acid transport; photodistributed erythema, scale, ataxia, psychiatric disturbances, aminoaciduria, stomatitis
Hashimoto-Pritzker d.	congenital self-healing reticulohistiocytosis
Hatchcock's sign	tenderness elicited when running finger toward angle of jaw; mumps
Hebra's d.	erythema multiforme (minor)
Heck's s.	focal epithelial hyperplasia; mucosal HPV, primarily in native American children
Heerfordt s.	chronic sarcoid, anterior uveitis, parotid gland enlargement, facial nerve palsy
Heller, median canaliform dystrophy of	split midline nail with fir tree-like appearance, especially of thumbs
hemochromatosis	AR, or acquired; deposition of hemosiderin in parenchymal cells, causing bronze skin pigmentation, dysfunction of liver, pancreas, heart, pituitary, arthropathy, diabetes, cirrhosis, HSM, hypogonadism, loss of body hair
hepatolenticular degeneration	Wilson's d.
hereditary hemorrhagic telangiectasia	Osler-Weber-Rendu s.

Eponyms and Syndromes

hereditary painful callosity s.	PPK with oral mucosa hyperkeratosis
heredopathia atactica polyneuritiformis	Refsum's d.
Herlitz variant	junctional epidermolysis bullosa AKA JEB-gravis, JEB-lethal
Hermansky-Pudlak s.	AR; pigment dilution, nevi, SK, SCC, BCC, ecchymoses, petechiae, cream colored hair & skin, photophobia, strabismus, hemorrhage, granulomatous colitis, cardiomyopathy
Hertogh's sign	lateral thinning of eyebrow hair; atopic dermatitis, hypothyroidism
Heubner's arteritis	endarteritis of medium & large arteries resulting in thrombotic infarction; syphilis
HID s.	sporadic; AKA hystrix-like ichthyosis with deafness
hidrotic ectodermal dysplasia	Clouston's s.
Higoumenakis sign	unilateral irregularly enlarged medial clavicle; late congenital syphilis
Hines & Bannick s.	hyperhidrosis & hypothermia associated with diencephalic epilepsy or hypothalamic storm
Hippocratic nail	onychogryphosis AKA Osler's toe, ram's horn nail
Hoffman-Zurhelle s.	nevus lipomatosis cutaneous superficialis
Hoigne reaction	psychotic symptoms secondary to procaine in procaine penicillin, pseudo-anaphylactic reaction; syphilis
Holmes-Adie s. with anhidrosis	Ross s.
homocystinuria	AR or non-genetic; developmental delay, failure to thrive, neurologic abnormalities, hematologic abnormalities
Hopf, acrokeratosis verruciformis of	AD; small warty papules on extensor surfaces with punctate keratoses of palm
Hori's nevus	acquired circumscribed dermal melanocytosis of the face
Howel-Evans' s.	AD; 17q23, palmoplantar keratoderma (tylosis) ages 5-15, later esophageal cancer
Hunt's s.	Ramsay-Hunt s.
Hunter s.	XLR; mucopolysaccharidosis; deficiency of iduronate-2-sulfatase, similar to Hurler s.
Huriez s.	AD; mild keratoderma with scleroatrophy & sclerodactyly, nail changes; SCCs of dorsal hand
Hurler s.	AR; mucopolysaccharidosis, deficiency of L-iduronidase; thick hyperpigmented inelastic skin, corneal clouding, death by age 10
Hutchinson's freckle	large lentigo with grossly irregular borders; may progress to lentigo maligna melanoma
Hutchinson's prurigo	actinic prurigo
Hutchinson's sign	diffusion of pigment from proximal nail matrix; melanoma

Eponyms and Syndromes

Hutchinson's teeth	widely spaced small notched upper incisors; congenital syphilis (pathognomonic)
Hutchinson-Gilford s.	progeria
Huygens' effect	condenser of microscope defocused to obtain a partial phase effect
hyalinosis cutis et mucosae	Urbach-Wiethe d.
hyper IgE s.	eczema, recurrent cutaneous & systemic infections, decreased neutrophil chemotaxis, reversible ichthyosis, fungal infections, CMC, urticaria, incontinentia pigmenti
hypereosinophilic s.	eosinophilia & eosinophilic infiltrate of organs
hyperkeratosis lenticularis perstans	Flegel's d.
hypervitaminosis A s.	dry lips & skin, hair loss, sticky skin sensation, extraosseous calcifications, embryotoxic & teratogenic effects from systemic retinoids
hypocomplementemic urticarial vasculitis s.	urticarial vasculitis, angioedema, eye inflammation, arthritis/arthralgia, mild renal d., obstructive pulmonary d., serum complement activation with hypocomplementemia, C1q precipitin
hypohidrotic ectodermal dysplasia	AR, similar to Christ-Siemens-Touraine s.
hypomelanosis of Ito	AD; guttate & whorled hypopigmentation, conductive hearing loss, ocular abnormalities, MR, seizures, skeletal deformities, female predominant AKA incontinentia pigmenti achromians
IBIDS s.	*i*chthyosis plus BIDS (*b*rittle hair, *i*ntellectual impairment, *d*ecreased fertility, *s*hort stature) AKA Tay's d.
IFAP s.	*i*chthyosis *f*ollicularis with *a*lopecia & *p*hotophobia
IgA deficiency s.	AR; 1:600, atopy, asthma, autoantibodies, chronic gastroenteritis, DM, milk allergy, non-tropical sprue, PA, SLE, thyroiditis, URI
IgM deficiency s.	1:1000, infections; pneumococci, meningococci, verrucae, eczema, autoimmune features
incontinentia pigmenti	Bloch-Sulzberger s.
incontinentia pigmenti achromians	hypomelanosis of ITO
infantile papular acrodermatitis	Gianotti-Crosti s.
intestinal lipodystrophy	Whipple's d.
Jackson-Sertoli s.	AD, disruption of K17 expression; limited focal plantar keratoderma, woolly scalp hair, straight eyebrow hair, natal teeth AKA pachyonychia congenita type II, PED type II
Jadassohn-Lewandowsky s.	AKA pachyonychia congenita AD; **Type I**: thickened dystrophic nails, blisters around callosities, palmoplantar hyperhidrosis, leukokeratosis oris, follicular keratosis, laryngeal keratosis with hoarseness **Type II**: natal teeth and premature anodontia, steatocystoma multiples, follicular & palmoplantar keratosis without oral leukokeratosis **Type III**: corneal dystrophy, mucocutaneous keratosis

Eponyms and Syndromes

Jadassohn-Pellizari anetoderma	postinflammatory anetoderma
Janeway lesion	non-tender erythematous macule on proximal palms & soles; endocarditis (5%), gonococcemia, hemolytic anemia, SLE, typhoid fever
Jarisch-Herxheimer reaction	febrile reaction in patients treated with penicillin from unknown cause; syphilis
Jellinek's sign	brownish pigmentation on lid margins; hyperparathyroidism AKA Rasin's sign
Job s.	hyper IgE s. with red hair, atrophic nails, hyperextensible joints, cold abscesses
Johanson-Blizzard s.	AR; microcephaly, MR, congenital absent skin posterior of midline scalp, sparse hair, ala nasi hypoplasia, café-au-lait macules, hypoplasia of nipples & areola
Johnston's s.	XLR/monogenic autosomal; hyperkeratotic collodion baby-type skin with arthrogryposis & posterior column hypoplasia
Jones-Mote reaction	cutaneous basophil hypersensitivity; may occur with allergic contact dermatitis
Kallmann's s.	anosmia & hypogonadotrophic hypogonadism, associated with X-linked ichthyosis
Kanagawa phenomenon	hemolysin produced by *Vibrio parahaemolyticus* associated with diarrhea
Kaposi-Irgang d.	lupus panniculitis, lupus profundus
Kasabach-Merritt s.	sporadic; infancy-platelet trapping in large hemangioma leading to anemia, consumption coagulopathy, CHF, DIC, GI bleed, thrombocytopenia
Kast's s.	Maffucci's s.
Kawasaki s.	infants/children; fever, edematous reddened palms & soles, polymorphous truncal exanthem, bilateral conjunctivitis, mucosal erythema & strawberry tongue, cervical LAD, ulcerative gingivitis, enlarged cervical lymph nodes, cardiac complications (25%) AKA mucocutaneous lymph node syndrome
keratoma hereditaris mutilans	Vohwinkel's s.
keratosis follicularis	Darier's d., Darier-White d.
keratosis punctata palmaris et plantaris	Buschke-Fischer-Brauer d.
Kerr's sign	alteration of the texture of skin below the somatic level of spinal cord lesion
Ketron-Goodman d.	generalized (disseminated) pagetoid reticulosis (mycosis fungoides)
KID s., keratitis-ichthyosis-deafness s.	sporadic, AR, AD; keratitis, ichthyosiform erythroderma, & profound neurosensory deafness, alopecia, decreased sweating, malformed teeth, nail dystrophy, sometimes inflammatory corneal vascularization, SCC may develop in childhood AKA Senter s., Desmons' s., PED type XVI

Eponyms and Syndromes

Kimura's d.	angiolymphoid hyperplasia with eosinophilia with different nature of proliferating vascular cells
Kindler-Weary s., Kindler s.	acral blistering, poikiloderma, reticulate hyperpigmentation, sclerodactyly, scleroatrophy
kinky-hair s.	Menkes s.
kissing d.	popular name; infectious mononucleosis
Kitamura, reticulate acropigmentation of	AD; reticulate, slightly depressed pitting brown hyperpigmentation initially on dorsal hand, & then generalizing
Klippel-Trenaunay-Weber s., Klippel-Trenaunay s.	sporadic, usually unilateral lower extremity lesions; angiokeratomas, AV fistulas, hemangiomas, hypertrophy of bone & soft tissue, lymphatic malformation, nevus flammeus, skin varices AKA Parkes-Weber s.
Koebner phenomenon	physical trauma leading to lesion spread; acquired perforating dermatosis, bullous pemphigoid, contact dermatitis, Darier's d., erythema multiforme, Grover's d., Hailey-Hailey d., lichen nitidus, lichen planus, porokeratosis of Mibelli, psoriasis (20%), pyoderma gangrenosum, sarcoid, verrucae, vitiligo (30%) AKA isomorphic phenomenon
Koebner, EBS of	generalized epidermolysis bullosa simplex
Koenen tumors	fibromas developing around fingers & toes; tuberous sclerosis
Koplik spots	white spots on buccal mucosa; coxsackievirus A16, echovirus 9, measles
Krisovski's sign	cicatricial lines radiating from the mouth; congenital syphilis
Kwashi shakes	Parkinsonian-like tremors in recovery phase; kwashiorkor
Kyrle's d.	AR(?); rare perforating disorder; papules with hyperkeratotic plugs coalescing to plaques
LAMB s.	*l*entigines, *a*trial myxoma, *m*ucocutaneous myxomas, & *b*lue nevi
Langer-Giedion s.	AAD, 8q24.11; redundant skin, sparse hair, bulbous nose, MR, hyperextensible joints
Langerhan's cell histiocytosis	malignant lymphoma, lung carcinoma, post-chemotherapy leukemia (esp. etoposide) AKA Hand-Schüller-Christian d.
Laugier-Hunziger s.	lentigines of lips, mouth, genitalia, perineal, nail changes (pigmented bands, hyperpigmentation)
Lawrence-Seip s.	AR; near total fat loss with somatic hypertrophy, acanthosis nigricans, diabetes mellitus AKA congenital total lipodystrophy
Leiner's d.	C5 dysfunction leading to decreased serum phagocytosis (opsonic activity); eczema, seborrhea, erythroderma, diarrhea, recurrent gram negative infections, muscle wasting, & FTT in infants
LEOPARD s.	AD; *l*entigines, *e*lectrocardiographic abnormalities, *o*cular hypertelorism, *p*ulmonary stenosis, *a*bnormal genitalia, *r*etarded growth & development, *d*eafness
leprechaunism	Donohue's s.
leprosy	Hansen's d.

116

Eponyms and Syndromes

Leroy's s.	rare lipomucopolysaccharide disorder with skin thickening & bone changes
Leser-Trelat sign	multiple eruptive SK's with pruritus; acanthosis nigricans, cancer (breast, colon, lung, prostate, stomach), lymphoma, malignant melanoma, mycosis fungoides, primary lymphoma (brain)
Letterer-Siwe d./s.	AR; reticuloendotheliosis of childhood, eczema, hemorrhage, hepatosplenomegaly, progressive anemia AKA acute disseminated histiocytosis X
leukocyte alkaline phosphatase deficiency	AR; defective antibacterial & antifungal protection, increased IgE & eosinophils, normal chemotaxis; eczema, pulmonary infections
leukocyte myeloper-oxidase deficiency	AR; defective antibacterial, antifungal protection
Lewis hunting response	alternating vasodilatation & vasoconstriction during cold exposure (especially of hands)
linear sebaceous nevus s.	nevus sebaceous of Jadassohn
lipoid proteinosis	Urbach-Wiethe d.
Lisch nodules	melanocytic iris hamartomas; neurofibromatosis
Loffler's s.	pulmonary infiltration & eosinophilia; rarely occurring with cutaneous larva migrans
Lofgren's s.	arthralgia, bilateral hilar adenopathy, cough, erythema nodosum, fever
Louis-Bar s.	AR, 11q22; ataxia, cutaneous & bulbar telangiectasias, café-au-lait macule, decreased IgA, IgE & lymphocytes, granuloma, lymphoma, nystagmus, respiratory infections, sclerodermoid changes, solar lentigines AKA ataxia-telangiectasia
Lovibond's angle	cuticle angle greater than 180° indicates clubbing
low sulphur hair s.	trichothiodystrophy
Lucio phenomenon/ reaction	hemorrhagic infarcts; Latapi's lepromatosis
Lyell's s.	toxic epidermal necrolysis
Madelung's d.	benign symmetric lipomatosis
Maffucci's s.	sporadic; enchondromatosis, limb deformities, multiple cutaneous/visceral hemangiomas, venous malformations, short stature, sarcomas AKA Kast's s.
MAGIC s.	*m*outh *a*nd *g*enital ulcerations with *i*nflamed *c*artilage
Majocchi's d.	purpura annularis telangiectoides
Majocchi's granuloma	deep fungal infection producing granulomatous response AKA trichophytic granuloma
Mal de Meleda	AR; palmoplantar keratoderma with transgrediens
malignant atrophic papulosis	Degos' s.
Marfan s.	AD, sporadic 5 & 15 elastic degeneration; striae distensae, elastosis perforans serpiginosa, arachnodactyly, ocular defects, skeletal defects

Eponyms and Syndromes

Marinesco-Sjögren s.	AR; cerebellar ataxia, mental & growth retardation, cataracts, brittle fingernails, sparse incompletely keratinized hair
Marjolin's ulcer	carcinoma appearing in any type of skin scar
Maroteaux-Lamy s.	mucopolysaccharidosis; deficiency of *N*-acetylgalactosamine-4-sulfatase, dermatan sulfate in urine & metachromatic granules in leukocytes
Masson's pseudoangiosarcoma	intravascular papillary endothelial hyperplasia
mastocytosis s.	episodic s. in some patients with systemic mastocytosis; bone lesions, HSM, skin lesions
Mauserung phenomenon	stratum corneum shed in full-thickness sheets, leaving red tender base; bullous ichthyosis
McCune-Albright s.	sporadic; hyperthyroidism, precocious puberty, café-au-lait macule, polyostotic fibrous dysplasia, AKA Albright's s.
McDonald's acne	acne exacerbation from work near a deep fat fryer
Mee's lines	paired narrow white transverse nail lines; arsenic poisoning
Meischer's granuloma	actinic GA; annular elastolytic granuloma, erythema nodosum, Sweet's s. AKA actinic granuloma
Meischer's nevi	dome shaped nevi on face
Meissner's receptor	upper dermal papillae receptors; unknown function
Meleney's gangrene	progressive bacterial synergistic gangrene
Meleney's ulcer	Meleney's gangrene with burrowing necrotic fistulas through tissue planes
Melkersson's s., Melkersson-Rosenthal s.	AD; triad of recurrent noninflammatory orofacial swelling, relapsing facial paralysis & fissured tongue (lingua plicata) AKA granulomatous chelitis
Mendes de Costa s.	AD; ichthyosis with transient migratory macular erythroderma & fixed hyperkeratotic plaques AKA erythrokeratoderma viriabilis
Menkes' s., Menkes' kinky hair s.	XLR, copper transport abnormality, tyrosinase deficiency; characteristic facies, trichorrhexis nodosa, pili torti, monilethrix, severe cerebral degeneration & arterial change, death in infancy
Mibelli, porokeratosis of	AD, rare; plaques with coronoid lamellae usually on acral surfaces AKA classic porokeratosis
Michelin tire baby	appearance of rolls of fatty tissue; generalized congenital smooth muscle hamartoma, generalized nevus lipomatosus
MIDAS s.	*mi*crophthalmia, *d*ermal *a*plasia, *s*clerocornea
Miescher-Melkersson-Rosenthal s.	Melkersson's s.
Milroy's d.	primary (essential) lymphedema
Mkar d.	granuloma multiforme
Mondor's d.	thrombophlebitis of large subcutaneous veins of lateral chest & breast

Eponyms and Syndromes

Mongolian spots	blue-brown pigmented patch on lower back & buttocks of infants; Asians, blacks, inborn error of metabolism; GMI type 1 gangliosidosis
monilethrix	AD; beaded hair that breaks less than an inch long
Montgomery's s.	xanthoma disseminatum
Moon's molars	abnormal teeth; congenital syphilis AKA mulberry molars
Morquio's s.	AR; mucopolysaccharidosis, excretion of keratan sulfate in urine, genu valgum, pectus carinatum, deafness, corneal clouding, platyspondyly, short neck & trunk
Morton's neuroma	3rd or 4th inter-metatarsal foot space fibrosis & vascular proliferation with nerve entrapment
Moynahan's s.	multiple symmetric lentigines, congenital mitral valve stenosis, dwarfism, genital hypoplasia, MR AKA progressive cardiomyopathic lentiginosis
Mucha-Habermann d.	PLEVA
Muckle-Wells s.	AD; chronic relapsing urticaria, fever, arthralgias, deafness, renal amyloidosis
mucocutaneous lymph node s.	Kawasaki d.
mucopolysaccharidoses	*see table in Diseases section*
Muehrcke's lines	paired white parallel transverse nail bands; hypoalbuminemia
Muir-Torre s.	AD, 2p; multiple sebaceous tumors; adenoma, multiple GI carcinomas, hyperplasia, BCC, KA, GU & GI carcinoma. AKA Torre s.
multiple carboxylase deficiency	deficiency of holocarboxylase synthetase or biotinidase, causing deficiency of carboxylase; alopecia, ataxia, developmental delay, hyperammonemia, hypotonia, metabolic ketoacidosis, organic aciduria, seizures, rash
multiple hamartoma s.	Cowden's s.
multiple lentigines s.	LEOPARD s., Moynahan s.
multiple mucosal neuroma s.	Sipple's s., multiple endocrine neoplasia type 2b
mutilating keratoderma	Vohwinkel's s.
Naegeli-Franceschetti-Jadassohn s.	AD; reticulate hyperpigmentation hypohidrosis, severe enamel defects with loss of dentition
nail-patella s.	hereditary osteo-onychodysplasia; absent patella, clinodactyly, micronychia, triangular lunulae
NAME s.	AD; *n*evi, *a*trial myxoma, *m*yxoid neurofibromas, *e*phelides, plus testicular tumors, adrenocortical d., pituitary adenomas
Nekam d.	keratosis lichenoides chronica
NERD s.	*n*odules, *e*osinophilia, *r*heumatism, *d*ermatitis; articular nodules, dermographism, episodic hand & foot edema, eosinophilia, generalized pruritic dermatitis, urticaria

Eponyms and Syndromes

Netherton's s.	AR; ichthyosis linearis circumflexa (pathognomonic), trichorrhexis invaginata (hair shaft defect), atopic diathesis, sometimes MR & aminoaciduria
Neu-Laxova s.	AR, fatal; abnormal face, eclabion, ectropion, IUGR, limb deformities, microcephaly, severe hyperkeratosis
Neumann, pemphigus vegetans of	more extensive than pemphigus vegetans of Hallopeau
neutral lipid storage d.	Chanarin-Dorfman s.
nevus elasticus	pseudoxanthoma elasticum
nevus fuscocaeruleus opththalmomaxillaris	unilateral, usually facial, slate-gray macules AKA nevus of Ota
nevus lipomatosus cutaneous superficialis	Hoffman-Zurhelle s.
nevus sebaceous of Jadassohn	linear sebaceous nevus s.
Nezelof's s.	AR, XL, spontaneous; thymic dysplasia with normal immunoglobulins, absent T cell function, chronic infections, chronic mucocutaneous *Candida*, purine nucleoside phosphorylase deficiency (some)
Nicolaides-Baraitser s.	brachydactyly, MR, prominent lower lip, sparse hair, short metacarpals
Niemann-Pick d., Niemann's d.	Five types; lysosomal storage disease deficiency of sphingomyelin phosphodiesterase with sphingomyelin accumulation in reticuloendothelial system
Nikolsky's sign	separation of dermal/epidermal layer with stroking; bullous impetigo, bullous pemphigoid, epidermolysis bullosa, GVH d., intracutaneous bulla formation, pemphigus erythematosus, pemphigus foliaceus, pemphigus vulgaris, SSSS, Stevens-Johnson s., toxic epidermal necrolysis
Nissl arteritis	endarteritis of small arteries & arterioles resulting in thrombotic infarction; syphilis
Noonan's s.	congenital heart disease, hypogonadism, ptosis, short stature, webbed neck
occipital horn s.	XLR form of cutis laxa
oculocerebral-hypopigmentation s.	Cross-McKusick-Breen s.
oculomandibulofacial s.	François s., Hallermann-Streiff s., mandibulo-oculofacial dyscephaly
Ofuji's d.	eosinophilic pustular folliculitis; sterile annular pustules-face, trunk, extremities
Ogna, EBS of	Norwegian cases of EBS
Olmsted's s.	massive, mutilating keratoderma with hyperkeratotic plaques & severe nail dystrophy with alopecia, follicular hyperkeratosis, oral leukokeratoses, psychomotor delay, short stature
Omenn's s.	AR; combined T & B cell immunodeficiency with alopecia, diffuse erythema, FTT, hyperkeratosis & recurrent infections

Eponyms and Syndromes

Osler's nodes	painful erythematous or hemorrhagic macules, papules or nodules on distal fingers; gonococcemia, hemolytic anemia, SLE, typhoid fever (*see also Janeway lesion*)
Osler's sign	small painful erythematous swellings (Osler's nodes) in skin of hands & feet; subacute bacterial endocarditis (10%), SLE
Osler's toe	onychogryphosis AKA Hippocratic nail, ram's horn nail
Osler-Weber-Rendu s.	AD, 9q33; punctate telangiectasias of ears, feet, hands, lips, tongue; epistaxis, GI & GU telangiectasias GI hemorrhage, recurrent epistaxis in childhood, pulmonary & hepatic AV fistulas, CNS aneurysms, AV malformations AKA hereditary hemorrhagic telangiectasia
osteogenesis imperfecta	*see table in Diseases section*
Ostertag s.	AD; hereditary systemic amyloid, hepatomegaly, hypertension, nephropathy
Ota, nevus of	unilateral, usually facial, slate-gray macules AKA nevus fusco-caeruleus opththalmomaxillaris
pachydermoperiostosis	Touraine-Solente-Golés.
pachyonychia congenita	Jadassohn-Lewandowsky s.
Pacinian corpuscles	receptors in deep dermis or subcutis especially in digits, associated with blood vessels, serving as rapidly adapting mechanoreceptors to vibrational stimuli
PACK s.	primary biliary cirrhosis, anti-centromere antibody, CREST (calcinosis cutis, Raynaud's phenomenon, esophageal dysfunction, sclerodactyly, telangiectasia) and keratoconjunctivitis sicca
pagetoid reticulosis	Woringer-Kolopp d.
painful bruising s.	women; purpuric painful ecchymoses with emotional stress, without preceding trauma
Pallister-Killian s.	circumscribed hypopigmentation on cranium, sparse eyebrows & eyelashes, sparse scalp hair, severe MR, hearing loss, seizures, ptosis, high forehead, hypertelorism, facial defects
Papillon-Lefèvre s.	AR; palmoplantar keratoderma with transgrediens, keratotic plaques of elbows, knees, periodontitis, tooth loss, falx calcification
papular purpuric gloves and socks s.	Parvovirus B-19 in adults
paraneoplastic acrokeratosis	Bazex's s.
parasitic melanoderma	vagabond's d.
Parkes-Weber s.	Klippel-Trenaunay-Weber s.
Parrot's lines	depressed linear scars radiating from anus, mouth, & nose like wheel spokes; congenital syphilis AKA rhagades
Parry-Romberg s.	facial hemiatrophy, hyperpigmentation & atrophy of dermis, subcutaneous fat, muscle & bone
Partingtons s.	FTT, hemiplegia, recurrent pneumonia, hyperpigmentation (generalized reticulate), seizures

Eponyms and Syndromes

Pasini	dominant dystrophic epidermolysis bullosa albopapuloid
Pastia's lines	linear petechiae; Kawasaki d., scarlet fever
Paterson's s., Paterson-Brown Kelly s., Paterson-Kelly s.	Plummer-Vinson s.
peeling skin s.	AR; cycles of spontaneous desquamation of full thickness stratum corneum sheets, generalized hyperkeratosis, palmoplantar hyperkeratosis with pruritus, underlying erythroderma
PEP s.	POEMS s.
Peruvian wart	vascular papules & nodules developing in crops; Carrion's d. AKA verruga peruana
Peutz-Jeghers s.	AD; lentigines (around mouth, eyes, lips, oral mucosa, hands, feet), GI polyps, GI malignancies (3%), cancer (breast, pancreas, reproductive organs), colic, intussusception, GI bleeding
Peyronie's d.	induration of corpora cavernosa of penis, producing fibrous chordee
phenylketonuria	AR; hyperphenylalaninemia due to phenylalanine 4-monooxygenase deficiency; eczema, hypopigmentation of hair & skin, MR, seizures, tumors, mousy odor
PIBIDS	*p*hotosensitivity plus IBIDS (*i*chthyosis, *b*rittle hair, *i*ntellectual impairment, *d*ecreased fertility, *s*hort stature)
piebaldism	AD, c-kit on 4q12; depigmented patches, white forelock
pigmented purpuric lichenoid dermatitis	Gougerot-Blum s.
Pinkus corpuscle	*see Haarscheibe receptor*
plasma cell balanitis (vulvitis)	Zoon's balanitis (vulvitis)
PLEVA	Mucha-Habermann d.
Plummer-Vinson s.	angular cheilitis, dysphagia, hypochromic anemia, koilonychia & painful tongue AKA Paterson's s., Paterson-Brown Kelly s., Paterson-Kelly s., sideropenic dysphagia, Vinson's s.
POEMS s.	*p*olyneuropathy, *o*rganomegaly, *e*ndocrinopathy, *M* protein & *s*kin changes AKA Crow-Fukase s.
Pohl-Pinkus marks	hair shaft constrictions, acquired trichodystrophy; antimitotic drugs, emotional stress, systemic d.
poikiloderma congenitale	Rothmund-Thompson s.
polycystic ovary s.	Stein-Leventhal s.
popliteal web s.	congenital popliteal webs, cleft palate, pits (lower lip), toenail dysplasia
porphyria cutanea tarda	AD, 1p34, uroporphyrinogen decarboxylase gene, & sporadic/acquired; delayed photosensitivity, facial hypertrichosis, **scarring alopecia, milia, hypermelanosis**
porphyria, acute intermittent	AD 11q24, porphobilinogen deaminase; no skin features, acute attacks with seizures, peripheral neuropathy, weakness, abdominal pain, tachycardia, hyponatremia secondary to ADH secretion

Eponyms and Syndromes

porphyria, erythropoietic	AR, 10q25.2-q26; uroporphyrinogen III cosynthetase; **early**: immediate photosensitivity with burning, edema, erosions **late**: mutilating scarring in sun exposed areas, scarring alopecia, hypertrichosis, brown teeth, photophobia, hemolytic anemia, splenomegaly AKA Günther's d.
porphyria, hepatoerythropoietic	AR, 1p34, uroporphyrinogen decarboxylase gene, homozygous form of familial PCT; onset infancy, very rare, severe photosensitivity, hemolytic anemia, splenomegaly, dark urine, hypertrichosis, hyperpigmentation, sclerodermoid change, mutilating scars
porphyria, variegate	AD 14q32, protoporphyrinogen oxidase; bullae, erosions, scarring, milia, hypertrichosis, acute attacks precipitated by drugs, infection fever, alcohol, pregnancy
porphyria; erythropoietic coproporphyria	extremely rare, little is known; elevated PROTO & COPRO in red blood cells.
porphyria; erythropoietic protoporphyria	AD, 18pter-p11.2, ferrochelatase deficiency; onset 1-4 years old. **early**: burning erythematous plaques in sun distribution. **late**: waxy thickened scarring with cholelithiasis, jaundice, anemia
porphyria; hereditary coproporphyria	AD, 9, coproporphyrinogen oxidase gene; onset young adults, delayed photosensitivity, acute attacks similar to PCT precipitating factors, usually less severe
postphlebitic s.	complications of deep venous thrombosis; chronic venous insufficiency, persistent edema, pain, purpura, increased cutaneous pigmentation, eczematoid dermatitis, pruritus, ulceration, & indurated cellulitis
Pott's d.	scrotal cancer in chimney sweeps from polycyclic aromatic hydrocarbons
Preus s.	arched palate, cataracts, dolichocephaly, generalized hypopigmentation, growth retardation, hypochromic anemia, psychomotor retardation, small teeth
primary (essential) lymphedema	Milroy's d.
progeria	unknown inheritance; thin, atrophic skin, mottled hyperpigmentation, sparse hair, large cranium, micrognathia, osteoporosis, premature atherosclerosis, CHF, MI, short stature, short life span
progressive cardio-myopathic lentiginosis	Moynahan's s.
progressive pigmented purpuric dermatosis	Schamberg's d.
prolidase deficiency	AR; aminoacidopathy, deficiency of X-Pro dipeptidase, urinary excretion of imidodipeptides; chronic skin lesions, impaired motor & cognitive development, frequent infections, bone abnormalities
proteus s.	AD, sporadic; AV malformations, capillary malformation, growth & mental retardation, linear epidermal nevi, intracranial tumors, large at birth, lipomas, lymphatic-venous malformations, macrocephaly, macrodactyly, pigmented penile macules, scoliosis, soft tissue & bony hypertrophy of extremities, subcutaneous masses AKA Bannayan s.

Eponyms and Syndromes

pseudo-Darier's sign	urticarial wheal, induration, piloerection with stroking; congenital smooth muscle hamartoma
pseudo-Hutchinson's sign	discoloration of nail matrix; subungual hematoma
pseudopelade of Brocq	end stage cicatricial alopecia & fibrosis from; favus, folliculitis (scarring), LE, lichen planus, sarcoidosis, scleroderma
pseudoxanthoma elasticum	AR; basophilic degeneration of elastic tissue; flexural yellow macules & papules forming plaques, lax inelastic redundant skin, angioid streaks (retina), arterial insufficiency of lower extremities, calcified arteries, coronary insufficiency, hypertension, mitral valve prolapse, GI hemorrhage AKA nevus elasticus
purpura annularis telangiectoides	Majocchi's d.
Quincke pulsation	flushing of nail beds synchronous with heartbeat; aortic regurgitation
Quinquaud's d.	folliculitis decalvans
Rabson-Mendenhall s.	acanthosis nigricans, dental dysplasia, dystrophic nails, premature puberty
Raeder's s.	Horner's s., plus frontal/temporal headache & lacrimal sweating
Ramsay-Hunt s.	herpes zoster of facial & auditory nerves, external ear with ipsilateral facial paralysis occasional deafness, tinnitus, vertigo AKA geniculate neuralgia, herpes zoster auricularis, neuralgia facialis vera, otic neuralgia, Hunt's s.
Rapp-Hodgkin s.	AD, AR?; absent dermatoglyphics, cleft lip/palate, coarse scalp hair, dry skin, epiphora, ectropion AKA anhidrotic ectodermal dysplasia
Rasin's sign	brownish pigmentation on lid margins; hyperparathyroidism AKA Jellinek's sign
Raynaud's sign	acrocyanosis
Reed's s.	familial leiomyomatosis cutis et uteri
Refsum's d.	AR; phytanic oxidase deficiency; arrhythmias, ataxia, bony anomalies, deafness, hyperkeratosis, lenticular opacity, retinitis pigmentosa AKA heredopathia atactica polyneuritiformis
Reiter's s.	seronegative asymmetric arthropathy with one or more; cervicitis, circinate balanitis, conjunctivitis, dysentery, keratoderma blennorrhagicum, stomatitis, urethritis; males 9:1, HLA-B27 (80%)
REM s. , reticular erythematous mucinosis s.	women; photosensitive reticulated erythematous macules & papules with dermal mucin
Rendu-Osler-Weber s.	hereditary hemorrhagic telangiectasia AKA Osler-Weber-Rendu s.
reticulate pigmented anomaly of the flexures	Dowling-Degos' d.
Reye's s.	acute noninflammatory encephalopathy (lethargy, confusion, vomiting), hepatitis preceded by varicella (20-40%) & usually aspirin AKA infantile digital fibromatosis
Richner-Hanhart s.	AR; 16q22, AKA tyrosinemia type II; tyrosine aminotransferase deficiency, MR, palmoplantar keratoderma, severe keratitis

Eponyms and Syndromes

Richter's s.	development of large cell lymphoma in patient with chronic lymphocytic lymphoma
Riley-Day s.	AR; defective lacrimation, skin blotching, emotional instability, motor incoordination, absence of pain sensation leading to burns & bitten tongue, hyporeflexia, erythema of face & trunk, cyanosis of extremities, corneal anesthesia, hyperhidrosis, hypertension AKA familial dysautonomia
Riley-Smith s.	AD; multiple lymphatic venous malformations & pseudo-papillomas, macrocephaly
Ritter's d.	*S. aureus* infection elaborating exfoliatin, leading to denuded skin AKA staphylococcal scalded skin s.
Riyadh chromosome breakage s.	depigmentation, MR, silver hair
Roberts phocomelia s.	upper limb reduction malformation, flexion contractures of knees, silver hair, IUGR, MR
Romana's sign	unilateral bipalpebral edema; Chagas' d., oculoglandular s.
Rombo s.	AD; atrophoderma vermiculatum, BCC, hypotrichosis, milia, peripheral vasodilation with cyanosis
Rosai-Dorfman s.	sinus histiocytosis with massive LAD
Rosenthal-Kloepfer s.	corneal leukomata, acromegaloid appearance, cutis verticis gyrata
Ross s.	progressive segmental anhidrosis with tonic pupils, absent DTRs
Roth's spots	conjunctival petechiae; subacute bacterial endocarditis
Rothmann-Makai s.	lipogranulomatosis subcutanea; idiopathic lobular panniculitis with fat cell necrosis, lipophagic granuloma, cysts
Rothmund-Thomson s.	AR, 8; mostly females (some have C1q deficiency); atrophic hyperpigmented reticulated telangiectatic cutaneous plaques, alopecia, bone defects, cancer, dental dysplasia, hypogonadism, hypoparathyroidism, nail dystrophy, photosensitivity AKA poikiloderma congenitale
Rothschild's sign	loss of hair from lateral third of eyebrows; hypothyroidism (nonspecific)
Rowell's s.	erythema multiforme-like lesions occurring in patients with SLE & La/SS-B autoantibodies
Rozychi's s.	achalasia, congenital deafness, leukoderma, muscle wasting
rubber man s.	Ehlers-Danlos s.
Rubinstein-Taybi s., Rubinstein's s.	mental & motor retardation, broad thumbs & great toe, keloid formation, short stature, characteristic facies, high palate, beaked nose, large foramen magnum, vertebral abnormalities
Rud's s.	AR (?); associated with recessive X-linked ichthyosis, hypogonadism, MR, obesity, retinitis pigmentosa [may be the same disease as X-linked recessive ichthyosis]
Ruffini's corpuscle	rare, subcutaneous acral skin receptor; unknown function
runting s.	GVH with diarrhea, dermatitis, HSM, hemolytic anemia, pancytopenia

Eponyms and Syndromes

Russell's sign	callous (or calluses) on the dorsum of dominant hand; purging eating disorder
Russell-Silver s., Russell's s.	café-au-lait spots, incurved fifth fingers, lateral asymmetry, low birth weight, precocious puberty, short stature, syndactyly, triangular-shaped face, turned down corners of mouth
Ruvalcaba-Myhre-Smith s.	bony & craniofacial abnormalities, genital macules, intestinal polyposis
Sabinas s.	AR; brittle hair, MR, nail dystrophy, ocular dysplasia, xerosis
Sanfilippo's s.	mucopolysaccharidosis, excretion of heparan sulfate in urine; generalized hirsutism, hepatomegaly, macrocephaly, MR, death before age 20
SAPHO s.	*s*ynovitis, *a*cne, *p*ustulosis, *h*yperostosis, *o*steitis
Satoyoshi's s.	early onset alopecia areata, malabsorption, painful muscle spasms, short stature, skeletal defects
scalded skin s.	AKA dermatitis exfoliativa neonatorum, Ritter's d.
SCARF s.	XLR (?); *s*keletal abnormalities, *c*raniostenosis, cutis laxa, *a*mbiguous genitalia, *r*etardation, *f*acial anomalies
scarlatinella	Dukes' d.
Schäfer's s., Schäfer-Branauer s.	pachyonychia congenita with physical & mental retardation
Schamberg's d.	progressive pigmented purpuric dermatosis; tan macules with minute petechiae on lower extremities
Schimmelpenning s.	sporadic, AD; AKA epidermal nevus s.
Schimmelpenning-Feverstein-Mims s.	systemic nevi in Blaschko's lines, mild MR, skeletal abnormalities
Schinzel-Giedion s.	AR: narrow, deep set triangular nails, telangiectasias of nose & cheeks, dermatoglyphic changes, simian crease, hypertrichosis
Schnitzler's s.	monoclonal IgM, arthralgia, bone pain, fever, lymphadenopathy, hepatomegaly, hyperostosis, nonpruritic urticarial vasculitis
Schnyder's s.	progressive partial symmetrical erythrokeratoderma with deafness
Schönlein-Henoch s.	nonthrombocytopenic purpura due to vasculitis in children; arthropathy, arthritis, erythema, GI symptoms, renal disease, urticaria AKA Henoch-Schönlein purpura
Schopf-Schulz-Passarge s.	AR, diffuse symmetric PPK; fragile nails, sparse hair, eyelid cysts, hypodontia, hypotrichosis, longitudinal & oblique nail furrows AKA PED type XIX
Schultz-Charlton phenomenon	(historic test) intradermal injection of 0.1 mL of antitoxin into area of scarlet fever rash producing blanching at site of injection; scarlet fever
Schwachman's s.	AR; exocrine pancreatic insufficiency, growth retardation, impaired neutrophil chemotaxis, neutropenia, recurrent infections, skeletal defects, with ichthyosiform or eczematous change
Schweninger-Buzzi anetoderma	idiopathic anetoderma without preceding lesions

Eponyms and Syndromes

Seckel's s.	AR; hypodontia, pancytopenia, simian crease, skeletal defects, trident hands AKA bird-headed dwarfism
Secretans s.	traumatic edema of dorsal hand (factitial)
Seeligmuller's sign	mydriasis of side of face affected by neuralgia
Seidlmeyer's s.	acute hemorrhagic edema of infancy
Seip's s.	accelerated osseous maturation, lipodystrophy, muscular hypertrophy
Senear-Usher s.	pemphigus erythematosus
Senter s.	KID s.
serum sickness s.	develops 8-12 days after administration of serum proteins; albuminuria, arthralgia, fever, hypocomplementemia, LAD, leukopenia, nephritis, splenomegaly, urticaria
severe combined immunodeficiency s. (SCIDs)	XLR, sporadic, AR; decreased humoral & cell-mediated immunity, absence of delayed hypersensitivity, lack of immunoglobulins, lymphocytopenia, GVH in utero, eczema, recurrent infections, recurrent Candidiasis, diarrhea, FTT, death by age 2
Sezary s.	CTCL with generalized exfoliative erythroderma, intense pruritus, LAD, Sezary cells (skin, lymph nodes, blood)
Shab-Waardernburg s.	Waardenburg's s.
Shapira's s.	ataxia, developmental delay, hair defects (sparse, brittle, light color), short stature
Shprintzen's s.	marfanoid features with craniosynostosis AKA Shprintzen-Goldberg s.
Shulman's s.	eosinophilic fasciitis
sideropenic dysphagia	Plummer-Vinson s.
Siegert's sign	short, medially curved 5th fingers; Down syndrome
Siemens, ichthyosis bullosa of	AD, keratin 2e mutations; similar to EHK
Siemerling-Creutzfeldt d.	adrenal atrophy, early death, hyperpigmentation, leukodystrophy
Silex's sign	furrows radiating from mouth; congenital syphilis
Silver-Russell s.	Russell-Silver s.
Silvestrini-Corda s.	elevated levels of circulating estrogens from liver failure; atrichia, eunuchoid body, gynecomastia, hypogonadism, sterility
Sipple's s.	AD, sporadic; mucosal neuromas, medullary carcinoma of thyroid, pheochromocytoma, marfanoid body habitus AKA multiple mucosal neuroma s., multiple endocrine neoplasia type IIa
sister chromatid exchanges	Bloom's s., Cockayne s., dyskeratosis congenita, Fanconi's anemia
Sister Marie Joseph sign	umbilical metastasis; colon, **gastric**, ovarian
sixth d.	exanthema subitum (HHV 6)
Sjögren's s.	keratoconjunctivitis sicca, xerostomia with connective tissue disease; polymyositis, RA, scleroderma, SLE
Sjögren-Larsson s.	AR; congenital oligophrenia, ichthyosis, spastic pyramidal symptoms

Eponyms and Syndromes

Sneddon's s.	livedo vasculitis with cerebral infarction; aphasia, hemiplegia, &/or hemianopsia
Sneddon-Wilkinson d.	subcorneal pustular dermatosis
Sobye's massage	BID facial massage; rosacea
Solomon s.	epidermal nevus s.
Soret band	390-410 nm radiation band; absorbed by porphyrins
Sotos' s.	abnormal facies, genital lentigines, macrocephaly, skeletal defects
Spiegler-Fendt sarcoid	pseudolymphoma
Spitz's nevi	dysplastic nevi
Splendore-Hoeppli phenomenon	refractile amorphous eosinophilic matrix; immunoglobulin to *S. aureus, P. aeruginosa*, coagulase-negative staphylococci, streptococcal species, *Escherichia coli, Proteus* species
staphylococcal scalded skin s.	Ritter's d.
steatocystoma multiplex	AD; presents at puberty, numerous cysts over sternum, chest, axillae, proximal arms
Steijlen's s.	atrichia, MR, palmoplantar keratoderma, tooth loss
Stein-Leventhal s.	anovulation, hirsutism, oligomenorrhea, polycystic ovaries AKA polycystic ovary s.
Stevens-Johnson s.	erythema multiforme minor with mucocutaneous & systemic lesions AKA erythema multiforme major
Stewart-Treves s.	lymphangiosarcoma following lymphedema/lymphadenectomy, usually after radical mastectomy
stiff hand s.	fibrosis of hand leading to stiffness; diabetes
Still's d.	juvenile RA
Sturge-Weber s.	sporadic; usually unilateral nevus flammeus over trigeminal nerve, progressive tissue & bone hypertrophy beneath nevus, vascular malformation in leptomeninges, hemiparesis, MR, seizures
subcorneal pustular dermatosis	Sneddon-Wilkinson d.
Sucquet-Hoyer canal	contains glomus cells giving rise to glomus tumors
Sulzberger-Garbe s.	exudative discoid & lichenoid dermatitis
Sutton's nevus	halo nevus
sweat retention s.	occlusion of sweat ducts; pruritus, dermatitis, miliaria
Sweet's s.	acute febrile neutrophilic dermatosis
Takayasu's d.	vasculitis of aortic arch & its major branches
Tangier d.	AR, lipoprotein & lipid metabolism disorder; absence of HDL, deficient apolipoproteins A-I & A-II, low to normal LDL, high triglycerides, accumulation of cholesteryl esters, enlarged orange tonsils, pharyngeal mucosa, rectal mucosa, recurrent peripheral neuropathy, splenomegaly, corneal infiltration

Eponyms and Syndromes

Tay's d.	(P)IBIDS = trichothiodystrophy
Tay's s.	bone defects, café-au-lait spots, hypersplenism, lentigines, MR, physical retardation, vitiligo
Texier's d.	allergic reaction to Vitamin K injection
Tietze's s.	AD; albinism, with normal eye pigment, deaf-mutism, eyebrow hypoplasia
TORCH s.	*t*oxoplasmosis, *o*ther (syphilis, bacterial sepsis), *r*ubella, *C*MV, *h*erpes; chorioretinitis, deafness, HSM, jaundice, microcephaly, purpura, thrombocytopenia
Torre's s.	Muir-Torre s.
Touraine-Solente-Golè s.	AD; cutis verticis gyrata, short stature, thin yellow nails AKA pachydermoperiostosis
toxic epidermal necrolysis	Lyell's s.
toxic shock s.	desquamation 1-2 weeks after onset, disorientation, fever, GI upset, hepatic changes, hypotension, mucous membrane hyperemia, myalgia, rash, renal abnormalities, thrombocytopenia
transient acantholytic dermatosis	Grover's d.
trench mouth	Vincent's infection
trichomegaly	excessive eyelash & eyebrow hair growth associated with dwarfism, MR, retinal pigment degeneration
trichothiodystrophy	Tay's d., (P)IBIDS
triparanol s.	use of triparanol causing alopecia, poliosis, ichthyosis, irreversible cataracts, impotence
Trousseau's s.	hypercoagulable state secondary to malignancy of pancreas, stomach, lung, prostate, colon, ovaries, gallbladder leading to thrombophlebitis
tuberous sclerosis	Bourneville's s., Bourneville-Pringle s.
Turcot's s.	familial adenomatous polyps, CNS tumors
Turner s.	XO or 45X; disorder of gonadal differentiation, short stature, undifferentiated gonads, neck webbing, low posterior hair line, cardiac defects, sterility
Turner's sign	blood causing blue discolored skin at costovertebral angle; acute hemorrhagic pancreatitis
twenty nail s.	trachyonychia
Tyndall effect	blue appearance of melanin in dermal lesions due to selective light absorption
Tyson's glands	sebaceous glands of prepuce
Ullrich-Turner s.	45X, female phenotype; lymphedema, melanocytic nevi, mild MR, short stature, sexual infantilism, webbed neck
uncombable hair s.	AD; pili torti & canaliculi; blond, dry, thick, shiny hair

Eponyms and Syndromes

unilateral nevoid telangiectasia	generalized essential telangiectasia of vascular nevus under influence of estrogen
Unna's nevi	exophytic nevi with silhouette of fibroepithelial polyps
Unna-Thost s.	AD; diffuse palmoplantar keratoderma
Unverricht's d.	Baltic myoclonic epilepsy
Urbach-Wiethe d.	AR; infiltrative hyaline deposits in skin, mucous membranes & internal organs AKA lipoid proteinosis, hyalinosis cutis et mucosae
vagabond's d., vagrant's d.	skin discoloration due to chronic *Pediculus humanus corporis* bites AKA parasitic melanoderma
Van Lohuizen's s.	cutis marmorata telangiectasia congenita
Venus' necklace	hypopigmented macules on liner pigmented reticulae patches; secondary syphilis AKA leukoderma colli syphiliticum
Verbov-Sharland s.	palmoplantar keratoderma with neurosensory deafness
Vincent's infection	acute necrotizing ulcerative gingivitis AKA trench mouth
Vinson's s.	Plummer-Vinson s.
Vogt triad	epilepsy, MR, skin abnormalities (adenoma sebaceum); <1/3 of patients have full triad
Vogt-Koyanagi-Harada s., Vogt-Koyanagi s.	alopecia, bilateral uveitis, choroiditis, deafness, headache, meningism, poliosis, retinal detachment, vision loss, vitiligo, vomiting, sometimes glaucoma or vertigo
Vohwinkel's s.	AD; palmoplantar keratoderma with digital pseudoainhum, scarring alopecia & high frequency hearing loss AKA keratoma hereditaris mutilans, mutilating keratoderma
Voigt's lines	pigment demarcation lines of dorsolateral arms; blacks & Asians AKA Futcher's lines
von Hippel-Lindau d.	AD, 3p25-26; hereditary phakomatosis; angiomatous lesions (kidneys, liver, pancreas), capillary malformation (rare), café-au-lait macules, pheochromocytoma, renal cell cancer, vascular malformations in cerebellum & brain stem, retinal hemangioblastoma
von Recklinghausen's d.	AD 17q11.2; neurofibromatosis type I
Vorner's s.	clinical appearance of Unna-Thost s. with epidermolytic hyperkeratosis on biopsy
Waardenburg's s.	AD, 2q35; white forelock, neurosensory deafness, wide nasal bridge, heterochromia of iris
Wachters PPK	Brunauer-Fuhs-Siemens PPK
Wagner-Unverricht d.	dermatomyositis
Watson's s.	deletion of NF1 gene; variant of neurofibromatosis 1, multiple café-au-lait macules, neurofibromas (few), MR, pulmonary valvular stenosis, short stature
Weber-Christian s.	idiopathic lobular panniculitis; relapsing febrile nodular nonsuppurative panniculitis/arthralgias, fever, malaise
Weber-Cockayne s.	localized epidermolysis bullosa simplex

Eponyms and Syndromes

Wegener's granulomatosis	+ C-ANCA, facial and periauricular lesions; malignant pyoderma
Weil's d.	*Leptospira interrogans serovar icterohemorrhagiae*; hepatorenal failure, jaundice, oliguria, purpura
Well's s.	eosinophilic cellulitis
Werner's s.	AR, 8p12; premature aging with baldness, cataracts, muscular atrophy, osteoarthritis, scleroderma, subcutaneous calcification, telangiectasias, diabetes mellitus tendency, neoplasms, short stature
Westerhof's s.	AD; café-au-lait macules, growth retardation, hyper & hypopigmented macules, MR
Whipple's d.	abdominal pain, anorexia, arthritis, CNS disturbance, diarrhea, fever, LAD, skin pigment changes, steatorrhea AKA intestinal lipodystrophy
Wickham's striae	reticulate white lines on top of papules & buccal mucosa; lichen planus
Williams s.	AD; dysmorphic facies, supravalvular aortic stenosis, velvety skin
Wilson's d.	AR, q13; copper metabolism defect of ceruloplasmin, copper accumulates (in liver, brain, kidney, cornea), azure lunulae, hyperpigmented legs, Kayser-Fleischer ring AKA hepatolenticular degeneration
Wimberger sign	osteochondritis of medial proximal tibial metaphysis; congenital syphilis AKA cat bite sign
Winterbottom's sign	enlarged posterior cervical lymph nodes; trypanosomiasis (Gambian)
Wiskott-Aldrich s.	XLR, immunodeficiency; autoimmune phenomena, cyclic neutropenia, decreased chemotaxis, eczema, increased malignancy, recurrent pyogenic infections, thrombocytopenia, decreased IgA & IgE, normal/increased/decreased IgM, platelet dysfunction
Woolf's s.	piebaldism with deafness
Woringer-Kolopp d.	localized pagetoid reticulosis
Woronoff's ring	white blanching skin ring (leukoderma); psoriasis
Wyburn-Mason's s.	sporadic; facial nevus flammeus, ataxia, AV malformation of optic nerve & retina, enlarged facial veins, MR, nystagmus, seizures
xeroderma pigmentosa	AR; deficient enzyme in excisional repair of UV-damaged DNA; extreme UV photosensitivity; keratoses, malignancies (BCC, SCC), papillomas, telangiectasia
xerodermic idiocy	De Sanctis-Cacchione s.
X-linked hypogammaglobulinemia	decreased IgM, IgG, IgA, C1q, cutaneous & systemic pyogenic infections, chronic echovirus infection with dermatomyositis-like finding, eczema, URI, osteomyelitis, pneumonia, joint infections, large joint arthritis, no B cells
yellow nail s.	lymphedema with smooth, thickened, curved, yellow discolored nails
Zinsser-Cole-Engman s.	XLR/AD; reticular pigmentation progressing to atrophy & telangiectasia, bullous conjunctivitis, esophageal strictures, leukoplakia (mucous membranes), mental deficiency, nail dystrophy, palmoplantar hyperkeratosis & hyperhidrosis, pancytopenia, skeletal disorders,

Eponyms and Syndromes

	thrombocytopenia AKA dyskeratosis congenita
Ziprowski-Margolis s.	XLR, males; Xg26.3-q27.1; deaf-mutism, heterochromic irides, piebald-like hypomelanosis of skin & hair
Zoon's balanitis (vulvitis)	variant of lichen planus (?) of genitalia AKA plasma cell balanitis (vulvitis)
Zunich-Kaye s.	CHIME s.

Classifications of Syndromes

Autosomal dominant	acrokeratosis verruciformis of Hopf, Adams-Oliver s., albinism, albinism and deafness, anonychia ectrodactyly, Bannayan's s., Bart's s., basal cell nevus s., Basan's s., Beckwith-Wiedemann s., blue rubber bleb nevus s., bullous ichthyosiform erythroderma, Buschke-Ollendorff s., Clouston's s., cold hypersensitivity, congenital scalp defect, Cowden's s., cutis laxa, Darier's d., distichiasis and lymphedema, dyskeratosis congenita, EB-Cockayne, EB-dystrophica, EB-simplex, EEC s., Ehlers-Danlos s., epidermolysis bullosa simplex, epidermolysis bullosa dystrophica, epitheliomas, erythrokeratoderma viriabilis, familial angioedema, familial dyskeratotic comedones, familial localized heat urticaria, familial Mediterranean fever, familial pachydermoperiostosis, Gardner's s., glomus tumors, Hailey-Hailey d., hereditary hemorrhagic telangiectasia, hereditary koilonychia, hereditary sclerosing poikiloderma, hidrotic ectodermal dysplasia, Howel-Evans' s., Huriez s., hypertrichosis universalis, hypomelanosis of Ito, ichthyosis hystrix gravior, ichthyosis vulgaris, incontinentia pigmenti achromians, Jadassohn-Lewandowsky s., keratoderma palmaris et plantaris, keratoderma with esophageal cancer, LEOPARD s., leukonychia totalis, lipoatrophic diabetes, lymphedema and distichiasis, lymphedema-hereditary, Maffucci's s., Marfan's s., Marie-Unna hair dystrophy, melanoma, Melkersson's s., milia and decreased hair density, monilethrix, Muir-Torre s., multiple benign ring-shaped skin creases, multiple cylindromas, multiple leiomyomata, multiple lipomatosis, Naegeli-Franceschetti-Jadassohn s., Naegeli's s., nail-patella s., NAME s., neurofibromatosis, Osler-Weber-Rendu s., pachydermoperiostosis, pachyonychia congenita, Peutz-Jeghers s., piebaldism, pili annulati, porphyria cutanea tarda, porphyria-acute intermittent, porphyria-variegate, porphyria- erythropoietic protoporphyria, porphyria-hereditary coproporphyria, Rapp-Hodgkin s., Riley-Smith s., sclerotylosis, uncombable hair s., steatocystoma multiplex, trichorhinophalangeal s., tuberous sclerosis, urticaria-deafness-amyloidosis, Vohwinkel's s., von Hippel-Lindau d., von Recklinghausen's d., Waardenburg's s., Westerhof's s., woolly hair
autosomal recessive	acrodermatitis enteropathica, albinism, alkaptonuria, arginosuccinic aciduria, aspartylglycoaminuria, ataxia-telangiectasia, biotinidase deficiency, Björnstad's s., Bloom's s., cartilage-hair hypoplasia, cerebrotendinous xanthomatosis, Chanarin-Dorfman s., Chediak-Higashi s., circumscribed keratoderma, Cockayne's s., Conradi's d., Cornelia de Lange s., Cross-McKusick-Breen s., cutis laxa, De Sanctis-Cacchione s., Desmons-Britten s., EB-dystrophica, EB-

Eponyms and Syndromes

Classifications of Syndromes

letalis, EB-junctional, Ehlers-Danlos s., epidermodysplasia verruci-
formis, erythropoietic porphyria, familial dysautonomia, Fanconi's
s., Farber's lipogranulomatosis, fucosidosis type II, Gaucher's d.,
Hallermann-Streiff s., harlequin fetus, Hartnup's d., hemochromato-
sis, Hermansky-Pudlak s., homocystinuria, Hunter's s., Hurler s.,
hypohidrotic ectodermal dysplasia, ichthyosiform erythroderma
(non-bullous), ichthyosis-lamellar, IgA deficiency s., juvenile fibro-
matosis, KID s., keratitis-ichthyosis-deafness s., keratoderma palmaris et plantaris, lamellar ichthyosis, Lawrence-Seip s., Letterer-
Siwe d., leukocyte alkaline phosphatase deficiency, leukocyte
myeloperoxidase deficiency, lipoid proteinosis, Mal de Meleda,
Marinesco-Sjögren s., Morquio's s., mucopolysaccharidoses, multiple sulfatase deficiency, Netherton's s., Neu-Laxova s., Nezelof s.,
Niemann-Pick d., Omenn's s., Papillon-Lefèvre s., peeling skin s.,
phenylketonuria, porphyria-erythropoietic, porphyria-hepatoerythro-
poietic, progeria, prolidase deficiency, pseudoxanthoma elasticum,
Refsum's d., Richner-Hanhart s., Rothmund-Thomson s., Rud's s.,
Sabinas s., Schwachman's s., Seip-Lawrence s., sialidosis-juvenile
type II, Sjögren-Larson s., Swiss type aggamaglobulinemia, Tangier
d., trichorrhexis invaginata, trichothiodystrophy, tyrosinemia II,
Urbach-Wiethe d., vitamin D-resistant rickets (type II0 with alopecia, Werner's s., Wilson's d., Wilson's d., xeroderma pigmentosum

chemotactic abnormalities	**neutrophils**: lazy leukocyte s., Chediak-Higashi s., hyperim-munoglobulin E s., Shwachman s. **leukocytes**: Wiskott-Aldrich s.
chromosomal fragility	ataxia-telangiectasia, Bloom's s., Cockayne s., Fanconi's anemia
Lyonization (functional mosaicism)	Conradi s., incontinentia pigmenti
non-Mendelian	Delleman-Oorthuys s., Klippel-Trenaunay-Weber s., McCune-Albright s., Neurocutaneous melanosis, proteus s., Schimmelpenning s., Sturge-Weber s.
X-linked dominant	Albright's d., atrichia with keratin cysts, Bloch-Sulzberger s., chondrodystrophia congenita punctata (Conradi-Hünermann type), congenital hemidysplasia with ichthyosis and limb defects (CHILD s.), Conradi-Hünermann s., craniofrontal dysplasia, focal dermal hypoplasia (Goltz s.), incontinentia pigmenti, keratosis follicularis spinulosa de Calvans, orofacialdigital s.,type II vitamin D resistance
X-linked recessive	anhidrotic ectodermal dysplasia (Christ-Siemens-Touraine s.), Bruton's X-linked aggamaglobulinemia, chronic granulomatous d., Crandall's s., cutis verticis gyrata with thyroid aplasia, dyskeratosis congenita (Zinsser-Cole-Engman s.), Ehlers-Danlos s. type V and IX, Fabry's d., keloids, keratosis pilaris decalvans, Mendes de Costa s., Menkes Kinky hair s., Hunter's s., ichthyosis follicularis, keratosis follicularis spinulosa decalvans, Lesch-Nyhan s., occipital horn s., properdin dysfunction, renal dysplasia, severe combined immunodeficiency s., rhabdomyomatous mesenchymal hamartoma, SCIDS, torticollis, Wiskott-Aldrich s., X-linked ichthyosis, Ziprowski-Margolis s.

Exanthems

Exanthems: Viral

Disease	Age	Season	Incubation/Prodrome	Morphology	Distribution/Features	Findings	Diagnosis	Management
measles, 1st d. (rubeola) paramixovirus-RNA	infants to young adults	Winter & Spring	1 week, high fever, URI symptoms, conjunctivitis	erythematous macules & coalescing papules	face first, then covers whole body; non-pruritic	Koplik spots, cough, fever, photophobia, SM, LAD	acute & convalescent hemagglutinin serology	report to public health, oral vitamin A
rubella, 3rd disease (rubella virus)	> 15 YO usually non-vaccinated	Spring	15-21 days, fever; absent or low grade, malaise, cough	rose-pink nonconfluent papules	face first, then moves to body	LAD; post-auricular & occipital, H/A malaise	rubella IgM or acute & convalescent hemagglutinin	reportable, avoid exposure to pregnant women
erythema infectiosum; 5th disease (parvovirus B19-ssRNA)	5-15 years	Winter & Spring	rare (fever, malaise, H/A)	'slapped cheeks' reticulate or maculopapular erythema	arms & legs, but may be generalized	waxing & waning rash, occasional arthritis, H/A malaise	clinical, acute & convalescent serology	
roseola 6th disease, exanthem subitum (HSV 6 & 7)	6 months-3 year	Spring & Fall	5-15 days. High fever for 3-5 days	maculopapular rash appears after fever declines	trunk, neck, generalized; lasts hours to days	cervical & postauricular adenopathy	usually clinical	
HIV (human immunodeficiency virus)	adults > children	—	fever, malaise, sore throat, diarrhea	roseola-like hemorrhagic hacules	upper body, palms, soles	LAD	acute & convalescent HIV serology	
chickenpox (varicella-zoster virus)	1-14 years	late fall to spring	none	macules, papules rapidly become vesicles, erythematous base, crusts	scalp & face more profuse on trunk than extremities	pruritus, fever, oral lesions	clinical, Tzanck prep, DIF or viral culture	aspirin contra-indicated (risk of Reye's s.)

Exanthems

Exanthems: Viral

Disease	Age	Season	Incubation/ Prodrome	Morphology	Distribution/ Features	Findings	Diagnosis	Management
Enterovirus (coxsackie, echo, polioviruses)	children	leading cause of summer & fall exantems	3-5 days. Occasional fever	pleomorphic; macular, papular, petechial, purpura, vesicles	generalized, may be acral	low-grade fever, occasional myocarditis, aseptic meningitis, pleurodynia, malaise	clinical, viral culture from throat, rectal swab	petechiae or purpura may indicate meningococcemia
Epstein-Barr virus	young children to adolescents	any	fever, LAD, sore throat	macular, papular, morbilliform	trunk, extremities	cervical LAD, HSM	Monospot; EBV nuclear antigen acute/convalescent IgG-viral capsule antigen	
Gianotti-Crosti s. (HBV, coxsackie virus, EBV)	1-6 years	any	none	papules, papulo-vesicles, may coalesce	face, arms, legs, buttocks, spares torso	occasional LAD, hepatosplenomegaly	clinical; hepatitis B & EBV serology	
asymmetric flexural exanthem of childhood (virus unknown)	children				extensor surface joint involvement, generalizes in 3-4 days	low grade fever, diarrhea, abdominal pain, LAD; cervical, axillary, inguinal		

Exanthems

Exanthems: Bacterial and Rickettsial

Disease	Age	Season	Prodrome	Morphology	Distribution	Findings	Diagnosis	Management
SSSS (S aureus epidermolytic toxin)	neonates, infants	any	none	abrupt onset, tender erythroderma	diffuse with perioral & perinasal scaling	fever, conjunctivitis, rhinitis	clinical; culture of S aureus from systemic site	neonate: if blistering present, hospitalize, IV nafcillin
toxic shock s. (Staphylococcal toxin)	adolescent/ young adult	any	none	macular erythroderma	generalized	hypotension, fever, myalgia, diarrhea, vomiting	clinical definition criteria, isolation of S aureus cervix	treat hypotension
scarlet fever (2nd disease) β-streptococcus	children	fall to spring	acute onset with fever, sore throat	diffuse erythema with sandpaper texture	facial flushing with circumoral pallor, linear erythema in skin folds	exudative pharyngitis, palatal petechiae, abdominal pain	throat culture	penicillin
meningococcemia	< 2 years	winter to spring	malaise, fever, URI symptoms	papules, petechiae, purpura	trunk, extremities, palms, soles	temp > 40° C, meningismus, circulatory collapse	blood culture, lumbar puncture	STAT IV penicillin, treat for shock
RMSF (Rickettsia rickettsii)	any	summer	fever, malaise	macular papular, petechial rash	wrists, ankles, palms, soles, later trunk	CNS, pulmonary, cardiac lesions	serology	treat presumptively
Kawasaki d. (etiology unknown)	6 months to 6 years	winter to spring	irritability	polymorphous-papular morbilliform, erythema with desquamation	generalized, often with perineal accentuation	conjunctivitis, cheilitis, glossitis, peripheral edema, LAD	clinical	IV Ig, salicylates

Adapted from; Williams ML, Frieden IJ. Dermatologic disorders. In Grossman M, Dieckman RA (eds). Pediatric Emergency Medicine: A Clinician's Reference. Philadelphia: JB Lippincott, 1991.

Hair

alopecia areata	acrodermatitis enteropathica, Addison's d., adrenal d., Alezzandrini's s., asthma, atopic dermatitis, connective tissue d., diabetes mellitus, *Candida* endocrinopathy s., Down s., Hashimoto's thyroiditis, LP, LE, myasthenia gravis, pernicious anemia, polymyalgia rheumatica, RA, stress, **thyroid d.** (8-12%), ulcerative colitis, vitiligo, Vogt-Koyanagi s.
alopecia universalis	loss of all body hair; alopecia areata, exfoliative erythroderma
alopecia, cicatricial	acne keloidalis, CTCL, dissecting cellulitis of the scalp, DLE, dystrophic epidermolysis bullosa (Hallopeau-Siemens), folliculitis decalvans, Graham-Little s., Gunther's d., hemochromatosis, ichthyosis (congenital erythrodermic), lichen planopilaris, lupus pernio, metastatic disease, mixed inflammatory scarring alopecia, Parry-Romberg s., PCAS, PCT, pseudopelade, PSS, pustular psoriasis, scleroderma, traction alopecia, ulcerative lichen planus, Vohwinkel's s.
alopecia, moth eaten	secondary syphilis
alopecia, noncicatricial	acrodermatitis enteropathica, AIDS, alopecia areata, biotin deficiency, Clouston's s., Cronkhite-Canada s., dermatomyositis, erythroderma, follicular eczema, follicular mucinosis, Hodgkin's d., IFAP s., KID s., lipoid proteinosis, lupus erythematosus, multiple carboxylase deficiency, Olmsted's s., PRP, psoriasis, Rothmund-Thomson s., Satoyoshi's s., Sezary's s., sprue, Vogt-Koyanagi-Harada s., zinc deficiency
alopecia, patchy	lipoid proteinosis
alopecia, primary scarring; lymphocyte associated	alopecia mucinosa, discoid lupus, lichen planopilaris, pseudopelade of Brocq
alopecia, primary scarring; pustulofollicular	acne keloidalis nuchae, dissecting cellulitis of scalp, erosive pustular dermatosis of the scalp, favus, folliculitis decalvans, kerion, tinea capitis
alopecia, primary scarring; vesiculobullous	cicatricial pemphigoid, epidermolysis bullosa
anagen effluvium	boric acid intoxication, colchicine, mercury intoxication, protein malnutrition, radiation therapy, systemic chemotherapy, thallium poisoning
anagen/telogen ratio, decreased	alopecia areata
atrichia	AD, alopecia areata, alopecia-onychodysplasia-hypotrichosis s., AR, atrichia with papular lesions, Baraitser's s., CL, demotrichic s., ectodermal dysplasia with severe MR, Hayden's s., Jeanselme and Rime hypotrichosis, Marie-Unna hypotrichosis, Mendes da Costa s., Moynahan's s., odonto-onychodysplais with alopecia, Perniola's s., Shokeir's s., Silvestrini-Corda s., Steijlen's s., Tricho-onychodysplaia with xeroderma, Wilson's s.
balance beam alopecia	pressure alopecia in gymnasts
bamboo hair	ball & socket deformity-trichorrhexis invaginata; Netherton's s.

Hair

bayonet hair	acquired pigmented nodal swelling of hair shaft
beaded hair	monilethrix
black dot hair	appearance with fungal infection; *Trichophyton tonsurans, Trichophyton violaceum*
brittle hair	BIDS s., IBIDS s., Sabinas s., Shapira's s.
broomstick eyelashes	unruly fine eyelashes; kwashiorkor
bubble hair	acquired open areas of hair shaft; hair dryer induced
coarse hair	de Lange s., Rapp-Hodgkin s.,
corkscrew hairs	wound hairs of lower extremities; scurvy, vitamin C deficiency
doll's hair	follicular convergence; lichen planopilaris
ectothrix	fungal arthrospores surrounding hair shaft; *Microsporum andouinii, M. canis, M. ferrugineum, M. gypsum, M. phanum, M. fulvum, Trichophyton verrucosum, T. mentagrophytes, T. rubrum*
endothrix	fungal spores growing within hair shaft; *Trichophyton tonsurans, T. violaceum, T. schoenleinii, T. gourvilli, T. soudanense, T. youandei*
exclamation point hairs	shortened hair from fracture at weak points, distal broader than proximal; alopecia areata
exclamatory hair	tapering proximal hair shaft; anagen effluvium
eyebrow aplasia	anhidrotic ectodermal dysplasia, atrichia congenita, isolated familial characteristic, keratosis pilaris atrophicans, KID s., monilethrix, oculomandibular dysostosis, oculovertebral dysplasia, pili torti, polydysplastic epidermolysis bullosa, progeria, Rothmund-Thomson s., Tietze's s.
eyebrow confluence	Cornelia de Lange s., hypertrichosis lanuginosa, isolated familial characteristic, kwashiorkor, Waardenburg's s.
eyebrow hair loss	alopecia areata, atopic dermatitis, follicular mucinosis, Graham-Little-Feldman s., hypothyroidism, leprosy, myxedema, Netherton's s., progeria, Rapp-Hodgkin s., retinoids, secondary syphilis, Tietze's s., trichotillomania, ulerythema oophyrogenes
eyebrow hypertrophy	Cornelia de Lange's s., Hurler's s., hypertrichosis lanuginosa, idiopathic gingival fibromatosis and hypertrichosis, isolated familial characteristic, trichomegaly
eyelash hypertrophy	AIDS, trichomegaly
flag sign	bands of light & dark dyspigmented hair; kwashiorkor
forelock, white	piebaldism, poliosis with multiple malformations, Waardenburg's s., Woolf's s.
gray hair, premature	ataxia telangiectasia, B12 deficiency, Book's s., coup de sabre, Chediak-Higashi s., Fisch's s., prolidase deficiency, Rothmund-Thomson s., Seckel's s., vitiligo, Waardenburg's s., Werner's s.
gray patch	discrete, gray, lusterless hair; tinea capitis
Hertogh's sign	lateral thinning of eyebrow hair; atopic dermatitis, hypothyroidism

Hair

hirsutism	anorexia, cancer (ovary, testicular), congenital, Cushing's s., dermatomyositis, Donohue's s., hypothyroidism, malnutrition, medications, Sanfilippo's s., severe head injury, Stein-Leventhal s. (polycystic ovaries)
hyperthyroidism	alopecia areata, hair shedding, thyroid disease
hypertrichosis, generalized	**acquired**: acrodynia, acromegaly, anorexia nervosa, Cushing's s., dermatomyositis (juvenile), diabetes mellitus, drugs, head injury, hyperostosis interna, hypothyroidism, idiopathic gingival fibromatosis and hypertrichosis, malabsorption s., multiple sclerosis, PCT, POEMS s., post encephalitis, schizophrenia **congenital**: Ambras s., Coffin-Siris s., congenital generalized hypertrichosis, congenital hypertrichosis lanuginosa, congenital macrogingiva & giant fibroadenomas, Cornelia de Lange's s., DEB-Cockayne Touraine, erythropoietic protoporphyria, faun tail, fetal alcohol s., generalized smooth muscle hamartoma, Gorlin's s., Gunther's d., hepatoerythropoietic porphyria, hereditary gingival fibromatosis/hypertrichosis, Hurler's s., hyperkinetic circulatory disorder, Lawrence-Seip s., leprechaunism (Donohoe's s.), LSA in female children, melorheostosis, neurofibromatosis, osteochondrodysplasia with hypertrichosis, PCT, POEMS s., PSS, Schinzel-Giedion s., stiff skin s., total lipodystrophy, variegate porphyria
hypertrichosis, localized	**acquired**: Becker's nevus, bites, burns (periphery), chickenpox, chromic osteomyelitis, congenital AV fistula, denervated areas, HIV (eyelashes), immunization sites (smallpox, diphtheria-tetanus), insect bites, irritants, lichen simplex, lymphedema, melorheostotic scleroderma, osteosclerotic myeloma, post morphea, pressure, stasis, sympathetic dystrophy, trauma, under casts **congenital**: congenital smooth muscle hamartoma, diastematomyelia, hairy elbows, hairy pinna, pigmented nevus, spina bifida, spina bifida occulta, trichomegaly, traction, Winchester s.
hypomelanosis	Book s, Down s., Fanconi's s., Hallermann-Streiff s., myotonic dystrophy, Pierre-Robin s., progeria, Rothmund-Thomson s., Seckel's s., Treacher-Collins s., tyrosinuria, Werner's s.
hypopigmentation	phenylketonuria
hypotrichosis (*see also pili torti & trichoschisis*)	argininosuccinicaciduria, cartilage hair hypoplasia, ectodermal dysplasia, Hallermann-Streiff s., Jeanselme & Rime hypotrichosis, Kalin's s., lipoid proteinosis, Marie-Unna hypotrichosis, regional choridal atrophy & alopecia, Rombo s., Schopf-Schulz-Passarge s. **nutritional deficiency**: biotin, calorie malnutrition, essential fatty acid, Hartnup d., homocytinuria, protein, zinc
IBIDS s.	birefringence of hair, pili torti, sparse hair, trichorrhexis nodosa, trichoschisis
loose anagen s.	hair sheding; absent root sheath, normal anagen bulb, ruffled cuticle
lupus hairs	short, fractured hairs from increased hair fragility; LE
Maria-Unna hereditary hypotrichosis	AD; sparse, absent at birth, wiry hair in childhood, variable loss at puberty; twisting, longitudinal ridging, cuticle peeling
melanin casts	amorphous intrafollicular deposits of melanin pigment

Hair

monilethrix	AD, AR; mutation in hair keratin hHb6, type II keratin genes, hHb1, chromosome 12q13 keratin cluster; elliptical nodes on hair shaft
moth-eaten hair	patchy alopecia; syphilis
ophiasis pattern	periphery of scalp with hair loss; alopecia areata
pili annulati	AD, sporadic; alternating bright & dark bands of hair shaft
pili bifurcati	division of hair into two hair shafts; congenital, damaged hair, pseudopelade, pili torti, trichotillomania
pili canaliculi	grooved hair; trichothiodystrophy AKA spun glass hair, uncombable hair, triangle hair
pili multigemini	multiple buds within hair follicle
pili spinulosis	dilated pore containing multiple tufted white hairs; eruptive hair cysts, keratosis pilaris, seborrheic keratosis
pili torti	twisted, tort hair; arginosuccinicaciduria, arthrogryposis & ectodermal dysplasia, Bazex's s., Björnstad's s., citrullinemia, Conradi-Hunermann chondrodysplasia punctata, Crandall's s., ectodermal dysplasia with syndactyly, etretinate, hypohidrotic ectodermal dysplasia, isotretinoin, Menkes' kinky hair s., monilethrix, Netherton's s., PIBIDS s., pili canaliculis, pili torti & enamel hypoplasia, pseudomonilethrix, Salamon's s., Salti-Salem s., striate keratoderma, Tay's s., tricho-odontonychial dysplasia with pili torti, trichorrhexis nodosa, trichothiodystrophy
pili torti; AD	AD; flattened, twisted hair shaft; citrullinemia, dental & ocular abnormalities, ichthyosis, keratosis pilaris, sensorineural deafness, trichothiodystrophy
Pohl-Pinkus marks	hair shaft constrictions, acquired trichodystrophy; antimitotic drugs, emotional stress, systemic d.
premature graying	antimalarial ingestion, ataxia telangiectasia, B12 deficiency, chloroquine ingestion, Cockayne's s., dystropia myotonia, prolidase deficiency, pernicious anemia, pangeria, progeria, poikiloderma congenitale
pseudo pili annulati	non-hereditary, no hair shaft cortex abnormality, alternately flattened hair shaft
pseudomonilethrix	irregular flattened & expanded hair shaft; compressed overlapping hairs, trauma
pull test	gentle traction at base of 25-50 terminal hairs; loss of 2-3 hairs per pull is pathologic
silver color hair	Chediak-Higashi s., Elejalde s., Griscelli s., Hermansky-Pudlak s., infantile sialic acid storage d., Menkes kinky hair s., Riyadh chromosome breakage s., Robert's phocomelia s., selenium deficiency
sparse eyebrow/eyelash	Pallister-Killian s.
sparse hair	Dubokowitz's s., Langer-Giedion s., Marinesco-Sjögren s., Nicolaides-Baraitser s., Pallister-Killian s., progeria, Schopf-Schulz-Passarge s., Shapira's s.
swarm of bees	peribulbar lymphocytic infiltrate; alopecia areata

Hair

telogen effluvium	**endocrine**: hyperthyroidism, hypothyroidism, perimenopause, post-menopause, postpartum **medications**: anticoagulants, ACE inhibitors, antimitotic agents, β-blockers, lithium, OCPs, retinoids, valproic acid, vitamin A toxicity **nutritional**: caloric deprivation, deficiency (biotin, essential fatty acid, iron, zinc), protein deprivation **other**: physical stress, psychological stress
trichoclasis	transverse fractures through cortex; chemical or physical trauma, trichothiodystrophy
trichodystrophy, acquired	structural abnormality of hair shaft; bleaching, drying, frequent combing & brushing, intense sunlight exposure, permanent waving, systemic d.
trichomalacia	alopecia areata, traction alopecia, trichotillomania
trichomegaly	long eyelashes; interferon, cyclosporine A, erythrocytic porphyria, HIV, kala-azar
trichonodosis	AD; knotted hair
trichoptilosis	split ends; congenital hypotrichosis (Marie-Unna), normal, uncombable hair s.
trichorrhexis invaginata	ball & socket intussusception of distal hair into proximal shaft; congenital ichthyosiform erythroderma, ichthyosis linearis circumflexa, lamellar ichthyosis, **Netherton's s.**
trichorrhexis nodosa	intrashaft node (paint brush node); Apert's s., arginosuccinic aciduria, biotin deficiency, citrullinemia, KID s., lamellar ichthyosis, Menkes' kinky hair s., Netherton's s., PIBIDS s., sulfur-deficient hair, trauma
trichoschisis	transverse fractures through hair; chemical trauma, physical trauma, PIBIDS s., trichothiodystrophy
trichothiodystrophy	brittle hair from decreased sulfur content; pili torti, trichoschisis alternating bands under polarization; BIDS s., hyperammonemia, IBIDS s., Marinesco-Sjögren s., PIBIDS s.
woolly hair	axially twisted hair shaft; normal (blacks) 1) AR; striated palmo-plantar keratoderma, cardiac abnormalities 2) AD; palmoplantar keratoderma (Unna-Thost), right ventricular dysfunction Jackson-Sertoli s.

Infectious Diseases and Agents

abscess	*Staphyloccoccus aureus, S. epidermidis,* α-hemolytic & non-hemolytic streptococci, *Bacteroides*
acrodermatitis chronica atrophicans	*Borrelia burgdorferi* (America), *B. garinii, B. afzelii* (Europe); vector is *Ixodes ricinus* (sheep tick)
actinomycosis	***Actinomyces israelii***, *Streptomyces somaliensis, Actinomadura madurae, Actinomadura pelleterii, Nocardia asteroides, N. brasiliensis, N. caviae*
adult T-cell leukemia & lymphoma	human T-lymphocyte virus type 1 (HTLV-1)
ancylostomiasis	*Ancylostoma duodenale, Strongyloides stercoralis*
anthrax	*Bacillus anthracis*
aphthae, minor	*?Streptococcus sanguis* strain 2A
aspergillosis	*Aspergillus flavus* (primary cutaneous aspergillosis) *A. fumigatus* (disseminated aspergillosis), *A. niger*
bacillary angiomatosis	*Bartonella henselae, B. quintana*
bacteremia, gram negative	***Pseudomonas aeruginosa***, *Escherichia coli, Serratia marcescens, Aeromonas hydrophila, Vibrio vulnificus*
bacteremia, gram positive	*Staphylococcus aureus, Nocardia spp.*
Bartonella	bartonellosis, cat scratch d.
bartonellosis	*Bartonella bacilliformis*; vector is *Phlebotemus sandfly*
bedbug bites	*Limex lectularis*
bejel (endemic syphilis)	*Treponema pallidum*
black dot hair	*Trichophyton tonsurans, T. violaceum*
blastomycosis	*Blastomyces dermatitidis*
blastomycosis-like pyoderma	coagulase positive staphylococci, β-hemolytic streptococci
blistering distal dactylitis	group A β-hemolytic streptococci, *Staphylococcus aureus,* ***Streptococcus pyogenes***
Borrelia	Lyme d., morphea (Europe)
Boston exanthem	echovirus 16
Botryomycosis (actinophytosis)	*Staphlyococcus aureus, Escherichia coli, Proteus, Pseudomonas*
bowenoid papulosis	HPV-16
bullous impetigo	staphylococci phage 71 (coagulase positive)
buruli ulcer	*Mycobacterium ulcerans*
candidiasis	***Candida albicans***, *C. tropicalis, C. parapsilosis, C. krusei, C. kefyr, C. glabrata (Torulopsis glabrata)*
candidiasis, disseminated	*Candida albicans, C. tropicalis*
carbuncle	*Staphylococcus aureus*

Infectious Diseases and Agents

Castleman's d. (plasma cell variant)	HHV-8
cat scratch disease	*Bartonella henselae, B. clarridgeiae*
cellulitis	*Staphylococcus aureus, Streptococcus pyogenes* facial cellulitis in children; *Haemophilus influenzae* post dog or cat bite; *Pasteurella multocida*
Chagas disease	*Trypanosoma cruzi* vector; reduviid bug
chancroid	*Haemophilus ducreyi*
Chlamydia	lymphogranuloma venereum
Chlamydia	psittacosis
chromoblastomycosis	*Cladosporium carrionii, Fonsecaea compacta, **Fonsecaea pedrosoi**, Phialophora verrucosa, Rhinocladiella aquaspersa*
CMV	Giannoti-Crosti s.
coccidioidomycosis	*Coccidioides immitis*
condyloma acuminata	HPV 6, 11, 16, 18
cryoglobulinemia	hepatitis B
cryptococcosis	*Cryptococcus neoformans*
cutaneous larva currens	*Strongyloides stercoralis*
cutaneous larva migrans	*Ancylostoma braziliense* (#1 cause in US), *A. cninum, A. duodenale, Bunostomum phlebotomum, Necator americanus, Uncinaria steno-cephala*
cutaneous small vessel vasculitis	group A β-hemolytic Streptococcus, *Staphylococcus aureus, Mycobacterium leprae*, HAV, HBV, HCV, HSV, influenza virus, *Candida albicans, Plasmodium malariae, Schistosoma haemato-bium, Schistosoma mansoni, Onchocerca volvulus*
cysticercosis	*Taenia solium* (pork tapeworm)
Dengue fever	arbovirus, vector is *Aedes aegypti* mosquito
diptheria	*Corynebacterium diphtheriae*
dimorphic fungi	*Blatomyces dermatitidis, Coccidiodes immitis, Parcoccidioides immitis, Histoplasma capsulatum, Sporothrix schenkii*
dirofilariasis	*Dirofilaria tenuis, D. immitis*
donovanosis (granuloma inguinale)	*Calymmatobacterium granulomatis*
dracunculosis (Guinea worm d.)	*Dracuncula medinensis*; vector is *Cyclops* (water flea)
EBV	exanthem, Giannoti-Crosti s., mononucleosis
ecthyma	group A, β-hemolytic streptococci &/or Staphylococcus aureus
ecthyma contagiosum (orf)	parapox virus
ecthyma gangrenosum	*Pseudomonas aeruginosa*
eczema herpeticum	**HSV-1**, HSV-2

Infectious Diseases and Agents

eczema vaccinatum	*vaccinia* (cowpox virus) – military contacts
enterobiasis	*Enterobius vermicularis*
epidermodysplasia verruciformis	HPV 5, 8, 9, 10, 12, 14, 15, 17, 19-29
erysipelas	β-hemolytic group A streptococci, group B, C, G streptococci
erysipeloid	*Erysipelothrix rhusiopathiae*
erythema infectiosum (5th d.)	parvovirus B19
erythrasma	*Corynebacterium minutissimum*
eumycetoma	*Exophiala jeanselmii, Madurella mycetomi, Madurella grisea, Pseudallescheria boydii; also Acremonium flaciforme, Acremonium kiliensis, Acremonium recifei, Aspergillus flavus, Aspergillus nidulans, Corynespora cassicola, Curvularia geniculata, Curvularia lunata, Cylindrocarpon cyanescens, Cylindrocarpon destructans, Fusarium moniliforme, Fusarium oxysporum, Fusarium solani, Hormonema sp., Leptosphaeria senegalensis, Leptosphaeria tompkinsii, Neotestudina rosatii, Phialophora verrucosa, Plenodomus avramii, Polycytella hominis, Pseudochaetosphaeronema larense, Pyrenochaeta mackinnonii, Pyrenochaeta romeroi, Scopulariopsis brumptii*
exanthems, viral	coxsackievirus, EBV, enterovirus, HBV, HIV, HSV-6, parvovirus, rubella, rubeola
fascioliasis	*Fasciola hepatica, F. gigantica*
favus	*T. schoenleinii*
felon	*Staphylococcus aureus, Streptococcus pyogenes*, gram negative bacilli
filariasis	*Brugia malayi, Brugia timori, Wuchereria bancrofti*, vector is *Culex, Aedes, Mansonic, Anopheles* mosquitos
fish tank granuloma	*Mycobacterium marinum*
flea-borne	dog tapeworm, murine typhus, plague
fly-borne	African trypanosomiasis, bartonellosis, leishmaniasis, loiasis, myiasis, onchocerciasis, tularemia, viral sand fly fever
focal epithelial hyperplasia	HPV 13, 32
fogo selvagem	vector is *Simulium privinosum*
folliculitis	**gram negative**: Enterobacter, Klebsiella, Proteus, Pseudomonas aeruginosa (hot tub) **gram positive**: Staphylococcus aureus **other**: Pityrosporum orbiculare, Demodex follicularum, Propionibacterium acnes (?)
Fournier's gangrene	group A β-hemolytic streptococci, mixed aerobic & anaerobic infection
fungi, dimorphic	*Blastomyces dermatitidis, Coccidiodes immitis, Parcoccidioides immitis, Histoplasma capsulatum, Sporothrix schenkii*

Infectious Diseases and Agents

furuncle	*Staphylococcus aureus*
genital warts	HPV 16, 18, 31, 33, 35
Giannoti-Crosti s.	BCG, Coxsackie A16, CMV, EBV, group A streptococcus, HAV, **HBV**, parainfluenza virus, polio virus, rotavirus, RSV, vaccinia virus
glanders	*Pseudomonas mallei*
gnathostomiasis	*Gnathosoma spinigeum, G. hispidum, G. hipponicum;* intermediate host is *Cyclops*
gonorrhea	*Neisseria gonorrhoeae*
grains/granules	**black**: *Curvularia geniculata, Helminthosporium spiciferum, Leprosphaeria senegalensis, Madurella grisea, M. mycetomi, Exophiala jeanselmii, Pyrenochaeta romeroi* **red**: *Streptomyces pelletierii* **white**: *Actinomyces israelii, Nocardia spp, Streptomyces somaliensis, Pseudallescheria boydii, Cephalosporium spp, Neotestudina rosatii, botryomycosis, Acremonium*
granuloma inguinale	*Calymmatobacterium granulomatis*
hairy leukoplakia	Candida, Epstein-Barr virus, herpesvirus, papillomavirus (associated with HIV)
hand, foot & mouth disease	coxsackievirus A 5, 9, 10, **16**; enterovirus 71
HAV	Giannoti-Crosti s., cutaneous small vessel vasculitis
HBV	cryoglobulinemia, Giannoti-Crosti s., cutaneous small vessel vasculitis
HCV	cutaneous small vessel vasculitis **associations**: PCT
herpangina	coxsackievirus A 1-6, 8, 10, 22 (picornavirus group), coxsackie B, Echovirus 9, 16, 17
herpes zoster	varicella zoster virus
herpes, genital	**HSV 2**, HSV 1
herpes, oral	**HSV 1**, HSV 2
HHV-6	roseola infantum
HHV-8	Castleman's d. (plasma cell variant), Kaposi's sarcoma, primary effusion lymphoma
histoplasmosis	*Histoplasma capsulatum*
hookworm (uncinariasis)	*Ancylostoma duodenale, Necator americanus, A. ceylanicum*
hordeolum	*Staphylococcus*
HSV	cutaneous small vessel vasculitis, paronychia
impetigo contagiosum	group A streptococci, *Staphylococcus aureus*
impetigo of Bockhart	*Staphylococcus aureus*
impetigo, bullous	Staphylococcus aureus (group II phage type 71)
Kaposi's sarcoma	HSV 8

Infectious Diseases and Agents

Klebsiella	folliculitis
larva currens	*Strongyloides stercoralis*
larva migrans	*Hypoderma*-cattle warble fly, *Gastrophilus*-horse botfly
leishmaniasis	**American** (mucocutaneous, espundia): *Leishmania braziliensis, L. panamanesis* vector; *Phlebotemus sandfly, Lutzomyia longipalpis, Psychodopygus wellcomei, Sergeutomyia* **cutaneous**: (oriental sore, Delhi boil, old world cutaneous) *L. tropica, L. major, L. aethiopica, L. infantum* (new world cutaneous); *L. mexicana* complex, *L. braziliensis complex, L. amazonensis* wet form (rural); *L. major* dry form (urban); *L. tropica* chronic (leishmania recidivans) *L. tropica* **diffuse cutaneous** (old world); *L. aethiopica* (new world); *L. braziliensis* complex leishmaniasis recidivans; *L. tropica* post-kala-azar dermal leishmaniasis; L. donovani **visceral**: *L. donovani, L. infantum, L. chagasi* vectors; *Phlebotemus* sandfly, *Lutzomyia longipalpis*
leprosy	*Mycobacterium leprae*
leptospirosis	*Leptospira interrogans*
lice	*Pediculosis humanus corporis, P. humanus capitis, Pthirus pubis*
loiasis	*Loa loa*; vector is *Chrysops dicalis, C. dimidia, C. silacea* deer fly
louse-borne	epidemic typhus, relapsing fever, trench fever
Lyme d.	*Borrelia burgdorferi*, vector is *Amblyoma americanum* (lone star tick), *Ixodes dammini, I. scapulalris, I. pacificus*
lymphogranuloma venereum	*Chlamydia trachomatis*
Majocchi's granuloma	***Trichophyton rubrum***
Malassezia furfur	achromia parasitica, confluent & reticulated papillomatosis of Gougerot & Carteaud, folliculitis, obstructive dacryocystitis, seborrheic dermatitis, tinea versicolor
measles	paramyxovirus
Mediterranean fever	vector is *Rhipicephalus sanguineus* (brown dog tick)
migratory lesions	cutaneous larva migrans, dracunculiasis, fascioliasis, gnathostomiasis, hookworm, loiasis, paragonimiasis, sparganosis, strongyloidiasis
milker's nodule	paravaccinia virus
mite	house dust mite: Dermatophagoides pteronyssinus chiggers: *Trombiculid alfreddugesi, Allodermanyssus splendens*
mite-borne	plague, rickettsialpox, scrub typhus, typhus, viral encephalitis
molluscum contagiosum	poxvirus; MCV I, MCV II
mononucleosis	Epstein-Barr virus
morphea	*Borrellia*

Infectious Diseases and Agents

mosquito-borne	dengue, Eastern equine encephalitis, filariasis, La Crosse encephalitis, malaria, St. Louis encephalitis, Venezuelan equine encephalitis, Western equine encephalitis, yellow fever
mycetoma (Madura foot)	**Actinomycotic**: *Actinomadura maduae, A. pelleteiri, Nocardia asteroides, N. brasiliensis, N. caviae, Streptomyces somaliensis* **Eumycotic:** *Acremonium recifei, A. keliense, A. falciforme, Aspergillus nidulans, Curvularia lunata, C. geniculata, **Exophilia jeanselmei**, Fusarium moniliforme, Leptosphaeria senegalensis, **Madurella mycetomi, M. grisea,** Neotestudina rosati, Petriellidium boydii, **Pseudallescheria boydii,** Pyrenochaeta romeroi*
Mycobacterium	buruli ulcer, cutaneous small vessel vasculitis, fish tank granuloma, leprosy
myiasis	*Callitroga americana* (#1 in US), *Chrysomia bezziana, Cochliomyia hominivorax, Condylobia anthragrophaga, Dermatobia hominis, Wohlfahrtia* spp.
necrotizing fasciitis	Bacteroides, group A, β-hemolytic streptococci, enterococci, mixed aerobic & anaerobic bacteria, *Pseudomonas*, staphylococci
Neisseria	gonorrhea
nodule/cyst (helminthic)	coenurosis, cutaneous larva migrans, cysticercosis, dirofilarisis, dracunculiasis, echinococcosis, fascioliasis, filariasis, gnathostomiasis, loiasis, onchocerciasis, paragonimiasis, schistosomiasis, sparganosis, visceral larva migrans
nucleic acid	**DNA**: Herpes virus family (dsDNA), human papillomaviruses, molluscum contagiosum (poxvirus), paravaccinia virus (milker's nodule), poxvirus (orf) **RNA**: enterovirus (HFM disease), Coxsackie virus (HFM disease), paramyxovirus (rubeola, measles, mumps)
onchocerciasis	*Onchocerca volvulus*, vector is *Simulium* (black fly)
onychomycosis	**dermatophyte fungi** (90%): *Trichophyton rubrum, T. mentagrophytes, Epidermophyton floccosum* **nondermatophyte fungi** (3%): *Acremonium, Aspergillus sp., Fusarium sp., Onycochola canadensis, Scopulariopsis brevicaulis, Scytalidium dimidiatum, Scytalidium hyalinum* **yeast** (7%): *Candida albicans*, others
oral hairy leukoplakia	Epstein-Barr virus
orf	parapoxvirus
otitis externa	*Staphylococcus aureus, Pseudomonas*
paracoccidioidomycosis	*Paracoccidioides brasiliensis*
paragonimiasis	*Paragonimus westermani*
paravaccinia virus	milker's nodule
paronychia	fungal, HSV, *Pseudomonas, Staphylococcus aureus, streptococci* (group A)
pediculosis	*Pediculus humanus capitis, P. humanus corporis, Pthirus pubis*
phaeohyphomycosis	*Exophiala jeanselmei*

Infectious Diseases and Agents

piedra, black	*Piedraia hortae* (ascomycete)
piedra, white	*Trichosporon beigeii*
pinta	*Treponema carateum*
pinworm	*Enterobius vermicularis*
pitted keratolysis	Corynebacterium, *Dermatophilus congolensis, Micrococcus sedentarius*
Pityrosporum ovale	*see Malassezia furfur*
plague	*Yersinia pestis*; vector is *Xenopsylla cheopis* flea
pruritic lesions (helminthic)	cercarial dermatitis, cutaneous larva migrans, dracunculiasis, enterobiasis, fascioliasis, gnathostomiasis, hookworm, loiasis, onchocerciasis, schistosomiasis, strongyloidiasis, visceral larva migrans
Pseudomonas	bacteremia (gram negative), ecthyma gangrenosum, folliculitis, glanders, otitis externa, paronychia
psittacosis	*Chlamydia psittaci*
purpura fulminans	**Group A *Streptococcus pyogenes***, varicella
Q fever	*Rickettsia burnettii*
rat-bite fever	*Spirillum moniliformis, Spirillum minus*
Reiter's syndrome	*Chlamydia trachomatis, Salmonella, Shigella, Yersinia enterocolitica*
relapsing fever	*Borrelia recurrentis, Borrelia duttonii,* vector is *Pediculosis humanis corporis* louse
relapsing fever, tick borne	*Borrelia spp.* Vector is *Ornithodoris* tick
rhinoscleroma	*Klebsiella rhinoscleromatis*
Rickettsia	Q fever, rickettsialpox, Rocky Mountain spotted fever, scrub typhus, trench fever
rickettsialpox	*Rickettsia akari,* vector is *Allodermanyssus sanguineus* (dog mite)
Rocky Mountain spotted fever	*Rickettsia rickettsii* vectors are *Dermacentor variabilis* (eastern US), *Dermacentor andersoni* (Rocky Mountain wood tick-western US), *Amblyoma americanum* (lone star tick)
rosacea	*Demodex* mite (?)
roseola infantum	Herpes virus 6
rubella	togavirus
Salmonella	enteric fever, erythema typhosum, erythema nodosum
salmonellosis	*Salmonella typhi & S. paratyphi*
scabies	*Pediculosis humanis corporis*
scarlet fever	*Streptococcus pyogenes*; pyrogenic exotoxin A, B, or C
schistosomiasis	*Schistosoma mansoni, S. japonicum, S. haematobium, S. mekongi*
scrub typhus	*Rickettsia tsutsugamushi* vector is the *Trombicula deliensis* tick, *Trombiculid akamushi, T. deliense* mite
soduku	*Spirium minus*

Infectious Diseases and Agents

sparganosis	*Spirometra erinaceri, S. mansoni, S. mansonoides, S. proliferum*
sporotrichosis	*Sporothrix schenckii*
staphylococcal	abscess, blistering digital dactylitis, botryomycosis, bullous impetigo, carbuncle, cellulitis, Chediak-Higashi s., chronic granulomatous d., ecthyma, erysipelas, felon, folliculitis, furuncle, hordeolum, impetigo, Job's s., lymphangitis, otitis externa, paronychia, perianal dermatitis, pyoderma, pyomyositis, septic vasculitis, SSSS, stye, toxic shock s., whitlow
staphylococcal scalded skin s.	*Staphylococcus aureus* phage group II
streptococcal	blistering distal dactylitis, cellulitis, ecthyma, erysipelas, erythema elevatum diutinum, erythema nodosum, gangrene, Giannoti-Crosti s., guttate psoriasis, Henoch-Schönlein purpura, impetigo, intertrigo, lymphangitis (acute), paronychia, perianal cellulitis, polyarteritis nodosa, purpura, purpura fulminans, scleredema, streptococcal scalded skin s., subacute nodular migratory tinea amiantacea, toxic shock-like s., vulvovaginitis **associated**: erythema multiforme, erythema nodosum, guttate psoriasis, vasculitis
streptococcal scalded skin s.	*Streptococcus pyogenes*; pyrogenic exotoxin A, B, C
strongyloidiasis	*Strongyloides stercoralis* (larva currens)
stye	*Staphylococcus*
swimmer's itch	*Schistosome cercariae*
syphilis	*Treponema pallidum*
tick paralysis	vector is *Dermacentor variabilis* (American dog tick)
tick-borne	babesiosis, Colorado tick fever, ehrlichiosis, Lyme borreliosis, Powassan encephalitis, Q-fever, relapsing fever, Rocky Mountain spotted fever
tinea barbae	***Trichophyton verrucosum, T. mentagrophytes***
tinea capitis	***Microsporum canis*** (#1 worldwide), ***Trichophyton tonsurans*** (#1 US), ***T. violaceum, M. ferrugineum, T. schoenleinii***
tinea corporis	***T. rubrum***, *M. canis, T. mentagrophytes*
tinea cruris	***T. rubrum, Epidermophyton floccosum***, *T. mentagrophytes*
tinea manum	***E. floccosum, T. rubrum***, *T. mentagrophytes*
tinea nigra	*Exophiala werneckii*
tinea pedis	*T. rubrum, E. floccosum, T. mentagrophytes*
tinea versicolor	*Malassezia furfur (Pityrosporum ovale)*
toxic shock syndrome	*Staphylococcus aureus*; > 90%; toxic shock syndrome toxin-1 (TSST-1)
toxoplasmosis	*Toxoplasma gondii*
trench fever	*Rickettsia quintana, (Rochilemea quintanus)*; vector is *Pediculosis humanis corporis* louse

Infectious Diseases and Agents

trichinosis	*Trichinella spiralis*
trichomycosis axillaris	*Corynebacterium tenuis*
Trichophyton	black dot hair, Majocchi's granuloma, onychomycosis, tinea barbae, tinea capitis, tinea corporis, tinea cruris, tinea manum, tinea pedis
trypanosomiasis	**African**: *Trypanosoma gambiense, T. rhodesiense* vector; *Glossina palpalis*-tsetse fly **American** (Chagas d.): *T. cruzi* vector; assassin bug, kissing bug, reduvid bug Rhodesian vector; *Glossina morsitans*
tuberculosis	*Mycobacterium bovis, M. tuberculosis*
tularemia	*Francisella tularenesis* vectors; *Chrysops dicalis* deer fly, *Dermacentor andersoni* (Rocky Mountain wood tick) *Amblyoma americanum* (lone star tick)
tungiasis	*Tunga penetrans*; sand flea
typhus	**endemic** (murine): *Rickettsia typhi*; vector *Xenopsylla cheopis, Nosopsyllus faasciatus* fleas **epidemic**: *Rickettsia prowazekii* vector is *Pediculosis humanis corporis* louse **scrub**: *Ricketssia tsutsugamushi*
urticaria, acquired cold	EBV
verruca (papovavirus; dsDNA)	actinic keratosis; HPV 36 anogenital intraepithelial neoplasia (precancerous); HPV **16, 18**, 31, 33, 34, 35, 39, 40, 42-45, 51-56, 58, 59, 61, 62, 64, 67-69, 71 anogenital warts, cervical condyloma; HPV 6, 11 butcher's warts; HPV 7 cervical carcinoma; HPV 66 common warts; HPV 2, 4, 27, 29 common warts (immunosuppression); HPV 26 common warts (organ allograft recipient); HPV 77 epidermoid cyst; HPV 60 epidermodysplasia verruciformis, benign & malignant (macular warts); HPV **5, 8**, 9, 12, 14, 15, 17, 19-25, 36, 46, 47, 50 flat warts; HPV 3, 10, 28 flat wart (immunosuppressed); 49 genital warts; HPV 11 keratoacanthoma; HPV 16, 37 laryngeal papillomas; HPV 11 laryngeal carcinoma; HPV 30 melanoma; HPV 38 myrmecia wart; HPV 63 oral focal epithelial hyperplasia; HPV 13, 32 oral papillomas; IIPV 57 oral papillomas (HIV patient); HPV 72, 73 palmoplantar warts; HPV 1 pigmented wart; HPV 65 squamous cell carcinoma (cutaneous); HPV 41, 48 vulvar papilloma; HPV 70
Weil's d.	*Leptospira interrogans serovar icterohemorrhagiae*

Infectious Diseases and Agents

Whipple's d.	*Trophermyma whippleii*
yaws	*Treponema pertenue* vector is *Hippelates* fly
zygomycosis	*Absidia, Apophysomyces, Basidiobolus, Cunninghamella, Mortierellom Mucor, Rhizopus, Saksenaea*

Life-Threatening Dermatoses

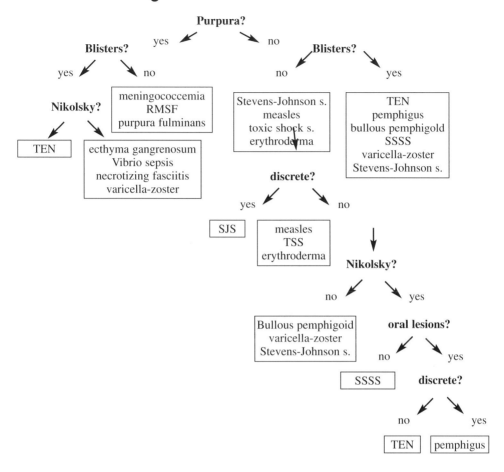

Source: Michael L. Smith, MD

Material, Stain, and Result

acid mucopolysaccharides (AMPS)	alcian blue at pH 0.5 and 2.5 colloidal iron crystal violet toluidine blue	AMPS: light blue AMPS: blue to light green AMPS: matachromatic magenta AMPS: matachromatic magenta
actinomyces	Brown-Brenn Gram-Weigert MacCallam-Goodpasture	organism: blue

amyloid	Congo red
	Congo red and polarized light
	Crystal violet
	Thioflavin-T
	Sirius red
	new cotton dyes:
	   Pagoda red
	   RIT scarlet No. 5
	   RIT cardinal red No. 9
		pale pink to red
		red with green birefringence
		purple red (metachromasia)
		fluoresces yellow with UV radiation
		pink to red
		orange with yellow-green
		   birefringence

bacteria	Brown-Brenn Gram-Weigert MacCallam-Goodpasture	Gram-positive bacteria: blue Gram-negative bacteria: red
basement membrane	periodic acid-Schiff (PAS) Jones methenamine silver	red black
blood cells	Giemsa Chloracetate esterase (Leder)	erythrocytes: red leukocytes: cytoplasm-light blue, nucleus-dark blue, granules-red
blood vessel walls	Verhoeff elastic PAS Gomori's aldehyde fuchsin	elastic membrane: black basement membrane: red elastic fibers, mucin: deep purple
calcium	Alizarin red-S Von Kossa	orange-red calcium salts: black
collagen	Malloy aniline blue Masson trichrome Van Gieson Movat's pentachrome	collagen: blue, elastic fibers: pale yellow collagen, mucin: green Keratin, nuclei, muscle and nerve fibers: dark red collagen: red muscle, nerves: yellow collagen, reticular fibers: yellow, nuclei, elastic fibers: black, muscle: red, ground substance, mucin: blue, fibrinoid: intense red
cryptococcus	Alcian blue mucicarmine PAS	capsule: blue capsule: red cell wall: red
Donovan bodies	Giemsa Warthin-Starry	organism: blue organism: black

Material, Stain, and Result

elastic fibers	Verhoeff-van Gieson	blue-black to black
	Weigert's resorcin-fuchsin	violet to purple
	acid orcein	dark brown
fibrin	phosphotungstic acid-hematoxylin (PTAH)	deep blue
fungi	Gomori methenamine silver (GMS)	fungus wall: black
	PAS	fungus: red
glycogen	Best's carmine	pink to red
	PAS with and without diastase digestion	glycogen is PAS positive (pink) before but not after diastase digestion
Histoplasma capsulatum	Giemsa	reddish blue
leishmania bodies	Giemsa	reddish blue
iron	Perl's potassium ferrocyanide	blue
	Prussian blue	
	Turnbull blue	
	Gomori's iron reaction	
lipids	oil-red O	orange to bright red
	Sudan black B	black
	Scharlack R	bright red
mast cells	Giemsa	metachromatic granules: magenta and blue
	Toluidine blue	
	Leder	
melanin	Fontana-Masson	black granules
mucin	miucicarmine	red
mucoprotein with acid mucopolysaccharides	Alcian blue	blue
	toluidine blue	magenta
	mucicarmine	red
	colloidal iron	blue to light green
with neutral mucopolysaccharides	PAS with diastase digestion	pink; no change after diastase digestion
muscle	Masson trichrome	red
	PTAH	blue to purple
mycobacteria	acid-fast stains: Ziehl-Neelsen, Putt-Fite Kinyoun's carbol fuchsin	bright red
	Wade-Fite	used for *M. leprae*
nerves	Bodian	axons: black
	osmium tetroxide	myelin: black
Nocardia	Gram stains: Brown-Brenn Gram-Weigert MacCallam-Goodpasture	irregularly blue
	GMS	black
	acid-fast stains: Ziehl-Neelsen, Putt-Fite	bright red

Material, Stain, and Result

plasma cells	Giemsa	cytoplasm: blue
	methyl green-pyronin (MGP)	cytoplasm: red
reticulum fibers	Foot	reticulum fibers, melanin, nerves:
(type III collagen)	Foot	black
	Wilder	black
	Gridley	
Rickettsia	Giemsa	blue to violet
spirochetes	modified Steiner	black
	Warthin-Starry	
	Dieterle	

Stain	Uses
acid orcein (Pinkus')	elastic fibers: dark brown, melanin: black, hemosiderin: dark green amyloid: light blue
Alcian blue	pH 0.5-stains strongly acidic substances such as sulfated glycosaminoglycans; chondrotin sulfate, dermatan sulfate,heparin pH 2.5- blue color with glycosaminoglycans and sialomucins, less intense with nucleic acids
aldehyde-fuchsin (Gomori's)	stains elastic tissue, mucosubstances pH<1 stains sulfated acid mucosubstances, not hyaluronic acid pH 1.7 stains sialomucins, elastic fibers, mast cell granules, mucins, cartilage, some fungi: blue-purple
Alizarin red S	specific reaction for Ca++ staining: orange-red can cross react with Ba, Cd, Sr, Pb Ca++ oxalate gives (-) reaction; converted to (+) with incineration
alpha-1-antichymotrypsin	histiocytes
aniline blue	muscle: red collagen: blue
ATPase	Langerhans cells, indeterminate cells, dendritic cells
auramine O immunofluorescent	acid fast bacilli
Bodian	*see silver nitrate*
Calcofluor white	detects fungi in tissue sections and histologically
CAM 5.2	anticytokeratin
carbol fuchsin	acid fast organisms: red
cathepsin B	histiocytes
colloidal iron	binding of colloidal iron by acidic groups; carboxyl and sulfate groups of nucleic acids. AMPS: blue nuclei: red
De Galantha	urate crystals
Dieterle stain	spirochetes
dylon	amyloid

159

Material, Stain, and Result

Stain	Uses
Fite	acid-fast bacilli: red leprosy: useless
Fontana-Masson silver (argentaffin)	melanin, some nerves and reticulum fibers: black nuclei: red cross reacts with argentaffin granules, formalin pigment, iron, lipofuscin
Giemsa	AMPS, mast cell granules: metachromatic purple eosinophils, leishmaniasis, Donovan bodies: red bacteria: blue
gold chloride	Langerhans cells
Gomori's methenamine-silver nitrate	fungus walls: black. *See also Silver nitrate.*
Gram (Brown-Brenn)	Gram-positive bacteria: blue-purple Gram-negative bacteria: red
Gridley	*Coccidioides immitis*
gross cystic disease protein	apocrine cells (Paget's d.)
hematoxylin and eosin	nuclei, Ca++: blue cytoplasm, collagen, nerve, fibrin: red muscle: dark red
Leder (chloracetate esterase)	naphtol-ASD-chloracetate-esterase mast cells and PMNs: red
Leib	amyloid
lipids	bromine-silver, osmic acid, PAS, sudan black: cholesterol esters and triglycerides: blue-black, P-L: gray Oil red O (unsaturated lipids: red, P-L: pink, stains unsaturated and saturated (frozen section only) If negative with bromine-silver but positive with Sudan dye, then you know lipid is exogenous such as paraffin oil granuloma
M241	Langerhans cells, endothelial cells
MAC-1	Langerhans cells
Mallory's phosphotungstic acid and hematoxylin	fibrin, inclusions of infantile digital fibromatosis
Masson's trichrome	hematoxylin, acid fuchsin, and methylene blue
collagen, nuclei: blue	cytoplasm, muscles, fibrin: red
Movat's pentachrome	nuclei: black elastic fibers: dark purple to black collagen: yellow ground substance: blue to bluish green fibrinoid: intense red muscle: red
mucicarmine	epithelial mucins and capsule of cryptococcus/rhinosporidosis: red (pink) acid mucopolysaccharides, Paget's cells
PAS (periodic acid-Schiff)	reactions with glycogens, starches, cellulose, mucosaccharides, gly-colipids, unsaturated lipids, phospholipids. Reactive sites become non-reactive after previous treatment with diastase specific for glycogen. No reaction with hyaluronic acid. Stains basement membranes, fungi: red
Perls	ferric iron
Phorwhite BBU	amyloid

Material, Stain, and Result

Stain	Uses
phosphotugistic acid-hematoxylin	nuclei: red will not demonstrate Fe++ (ferrous), ferritin, or Hb
Pinkus	*see acid orcein*
RIT cardinal red #9	amyloid
RIT scarlet #5	amyloid
scarlet red, Sudan red, Sudan IV, Sudan black	lipid stains
silver bromide/osmium tertoxide	unsaturated lipids (not exogenous oils)
silver nitrate (argyrophilic) Bodian/Gomori's	melanin, reticulum fibers, nerves: black
sirus red	amyloid
thionine	acid mucopolysaccharides
Toluidine blue	AMPS, nucleic acids, mast cell granules: metachromatic purple pH 3.0 most acid mucosubstances show metachromasia pH 1.5 only sulfated substances show metachromasia
Verhoeff-van Gieson	elastic fibers: black collagen: red nuclei: blue muscles, nerves: yellow
von Kossa	Not specific for Ca++. Based on recombination of silver with anion salt, carbonate, phosphate, oxalate, and reduction to metallic silver (black) with light. Ca++ salts usually only salt left after routine processing but urates and uric acids sources of error, can be removed by dissolving in lithium carbonate
Wade stain	atypical mycobacteria
Warthin-Starry	spirochetes and Donovan bodies: black
Ziehl-Neelson	acid fast bacilli: red

Immunofluorescence

biopsy, distant normal skin	leukocytoclastic vasculitis
biopsy, lesional recommended	EM, lichen planus
biopsy, perilesional recommended	bullous lupus erythematosus, bullous pemphigoid, cicatricial pemphigoid, dermatitis herpetiformis, EBA, herpes gestationis, linear IgA dermatosis, pemphigus, PCT
bullous pemphigoid	IgG, complement in homogeneous linear pattern at dermoepidermal junction
cicatricial pemphigoid	1. IgG, complement in homogeneous linear pattern at dermoepidermal junction 2. multiple Igs, complement, and/or fibrin in homogeneous linear pattern at dermoepidermal junction

Material, Stain, and Result

Immunofluorescence

dermatitis herpetiformis	granular, focal IgA at dermoepidermal junction
EB simplex	anti-BP ag: dermal base anti-laminin: dermal base anti-type IV collagen, anti-LDA-1: dermal base
EB, dystrophic	anti-BP ag: epidermal roof anti-laminin: epidermal roof anti-type IV collagen, anti-LDA-1: epidermal roof
EB, junctional	anti-BP ag: epidermal roof anti-laminin: dermal base anti-type IV collagen, anti-LDA-1: dermal base
EBA	1. IgG, complement in homogeneous linear pattern at dermoepidermal junction 2. multiple Igs, complement, and/or fibrin in homogeneous linear pattern at dermoepidermal junction
erythema multiforme	intravascular IgM, complement, &/or fibrin in granular pattern
herpes gestationis	IgG, complement in homogeneous linear pattern at dermoepidermal junction
IgA	DH, linear IgA dermatosis, chronic bullous dermatosis of childhood
IgA dermatosis	IgA at epidermal cell surface
IgG	pemphigus, BP, HG, CP, EBA, LE, LP, PCT
immunofluorescence, indirect	pemphigus foliaceus 70%, bullous pemphigoid >70%, HG factor 25%, linear IgA disease <25%
lichen planus	multiple Ig , complement, &/or fibrin in cytoid bodies in upper dermis
lupus erythematosus, bullous	multiple Igs, complement, and/or fibrin in homogeneous linear pattern at dermoepidermal junction
pemphigus	IgG, complement at epidermal cell surface
porphyria cutanea tarda	multiple Igs , complement, &/or fibrin in interstitial peivascular &/or dermoepidermal junction
split skin findings	**dermis only**: EBA, bullous SLE, cicatricial pemphigoid (some) **epidermis & dermis**: BP (rare) **epidermis only**: BP, cicatricial pemphigoid (some), chronic bullous dermatosis of childhood
vasculitis	intravascular IgM, complement, &/or fibrin in granular pattern

Immunohistochemistry

κ & λ chains	bone-marrow derived
AACT	bone-marrow derived
adnexal carcinoma	sweat gland keratinocyte; keratin, CEA, EMA
AE1/AE3	cytokeratin; malignant peripheral nerve sheath tumor
ALL	CD10
B-cell marker	CD10, CD19, CD20, CD22, CD45RA, light chains

Material, Stain, and Result

Immunohistochemistry

bcl-2	melanocyte
Ber-H2	large cell lymphoma
bone marrow derived	CD68, CD45, CD30, CD20, CD22, CD68, κ & λ chains, CD1-5, 7, 8, HAM56, MAC 387, lysozyme, AACT
CALLA	*see CD10*
CAM 5.2	Merkel cell
carcinoma	cytokeratin +
CD1	bone-marrow derived
CD1a (T6)	thymocyte and Langerhan's cells
CD2	pan T-cell antigen
CD3	pan T-cell antigen
CD4	bone-marrow derived; T cell & macrophages, T helper cells
CD5	T-cell antigen, bone-marrow derived; B-cell subsets
CD7	bone-marrow derived; precursor T cells, T cell subsets, natural killer cells
CD8	bone-marrow derived; T cell subsets, natural killer cells, T suppressor cells
CD10 (CALLA)	precursor B cells, granulocytes; follicular cell lymphoma, ALL
CD19	pan B-cell antigen marker
CD20	pan B-cell antigen, bone-marrow derived
CD22	pan B-cell antigen, bone-marrow derived
CD25	activation & proliferation antigen
CD30 (Ki-1)	activation & proliferation antigen, bone-marrow derived; large cell lymphoma
CD34	DFSP
CD43 (Leu-22)	T cells, macrophages, granulocytes
CD45	bone-marrow derived
CD45RA	pan B-cell marker
CD68	bone-marrow derived
dermal cells	factor XIIIa, vimentin
DFSP	CD34 +, smooth muscle specific actin +/-, smooth muscle actin +/-
EMA	sweat gland keratinocyte, sebocyte
endothelium	CD34, factor VIII-related antigen, *Ulex europaeus*, CD31
epithelial membrane antigen	perineuroma
factor XIIIa	dermal cells; DFSP
fibrous histiocytoma	CD34 +/-, smooth muscle specific actin +/-, smooth muscle actin +/-

Material, Stain, and Result

Immunohistochemistry

follicular center cell lymphoma	CD10
glomus tumor	smooth muscle actin, smooth muscle specific actin +/-
HAM 56	bone-marrow derived
HHF-35	smooth muscle specific actin
HLA-DR	activation & proliferation antigen
keratinocyte, epidermal	cytokeratin, AE-1
keratinocyte, sweat gland	keratin, CEA, EMA
Ki-1	*see CD30*; large cell lymphoma
Ki-1/CD 30 +	anaplastic large cell lymphoma, Reed-Sternberg cells of Hodgkin's d., lymphomatoid papulosis, angioimmunoblastic lymphadenopathy, peripheral T-cell lymphoma, large cell lymphoma, PLEVA, regressing atypical histiocytosis, lymphocytes exposed to phytohemagglutinin, EBV, human T-cell leukemia virus, *S. aureus*
Ki-67	activation & proliferation antigen
Langerhan's cells	S100, Mab 010, CD1a (OKT-6) monoclonal Ab stain, Birbeck granules (electron micrograph), S-100 Ab
Langerhans cell histiocytosis	Langerhans cell; S100, Mab 010
L26	evaluate & confirm B cell presence
large cell lymphoma	Ber-H2
leiomyosarcoma	muscle; actin, desmin
Leu-22	*see CD43*
light chains	monotypic plasma cells
lymphoma	LCA +
lymphoma panels	**fixed tissue**: suspected T-cell lymphoma; UCHL-1, CD30, L26, light chains **frozen tissue**: suspected T-cell lymphoma; CD1a, CD2, CD4, CD7, CD8, CD30, CD43 suspected B-cell lymphoma; CD2, CD20, CD22, kappa, lambda
lysozyme	bone-marrow derived
MAC 387	bone-marrow derived
malignant peripheral nerve sheath tumor	cytokeratin +/-, smooth muscle specific actin +/-, smooth muscle actin +/-, desmin +/-
mast cells	toluidine blue, Giemsa, conjugated avidin
melanocyte	S100 protein, HMB45, cathepsin D, bcl-2
melanoma	melanocyte; S100, HMB45, cathepsin D, bcl-2
Merkel cell	neuron-specific enolase, CAM 5.2, neurosecretory markers

Material, Stain, and Result

Immunohistochemistry

Merkel cell carcinoma	Merkel cell; neuron-specific enolase, CAM 5.2, neurosecretor markers
metastatic cells	thyroglobulin, prostatic acid phosphatase, serotonin
muscle	actin, desmin
myoepithelial cell, myofibroblasts	muscle specific actin, vimentin, glial fibrillary acidic protein
nerve	S100 protein, Leu 7, myelin basic protein
neurofibroma	S100 +/-
neuron-specific enolase	Merkel cell; Merkel cell carcinoma, small cell carcinoma
perineuroma	epithelial membrane antigen
prostatic acid phosphatase	metastatic cells-prostatic carcinoma
rhabdomyosarcoma	muscle; actin, desmin
S-100	adipocytes, apocrine glands, carcinoid, chondrocytes, chondrosarcoma, chondroblastoma, clear cell sarcoma, choroma, eccrine glands (both myoepithelial cells & luminal cells), epithelial sarcoma, folliculostellate cells of adenophypophysis, glial cells, gliomas, Langerhan's cells, liposarcoma, leiomyosarcoma, melanocytes, metastatic breast carcinoma, myxomatous neurothekioma, nerve, nevus cells, osteosarcoma, Schwann cells, synovial sarcoma (some spindle cells)
SCC, poorly differentiated	cytokeratin, AE-1
sebaceous neoplasms	sebocyte; lipase, EMA
sebocyte	lipase, EMZ
serotonin	metastatic cells-carcinoid
schwannoma	S100
small cell carcinoma	neuron-specific enolase, CAM 5.2, neurosecretory markers
solitary fibrous tumor	CD34 +, smooth muscle specific actin +/-, smooth muscle actin +/-
T6	*see CD1a*
TdT	immature B & T cells
thyroglobulin	metastatic cells-thyroid carcinoma
UCHL-1	pan T-cell marker; evaluate & confirm T-cell presence, best marker in paraffin sections
vimentin	dermal cells; DFSP

Medication and Associated Skin Diseases

Medication	Skin Disease
α-adrenergics	xerostomia
β-adrenergic blockers	alopecia, eczema, lichenoid, LE, pityriasiform, pruritus, pseudolymphoma, psoriasis, Raynaud's d., xerostomia
ACE inhibitors	lichenoid, pseudolymphoma, psoriasis, urticaria
acetaminophen	fixed drug eruption, pustular eruption
acetazolamide	hypertrichosis
acetylsalicylic acid	erythroderma, fixed drug eruption, nail bed purpura, pityriasiform, psoriasis, urticaria
ACTH	acneiform eruption, hirsutism, hyperpigmentation, pigmentation (brown), urticaria
actinomycin D	acneiform eruption, hair hyperpigmentation
acyclovir	pruritus
adriamycin	onycholysis, nail pigmentation
alcohol	Raynaud's s., PCT, spider nevus, rosacea
aldactone	SCLE
aldosterone antagonists	xerostomia
alizapride	flushing
alkylating agents	anagen effluvium
allopurinol	alopecia, EM, exanthematous eruption, exfoliative dermatitis, ichthyosiform, LE, pruritus, rash, TEN, vasculitis (leukocytoclastic)
all-trans-retinoic acid	Sweet's s.
amantadine	livedo reticularis
amidopyrine	erythema nodosum
aminocamptothecin	alopecia
aminoglutethimide	capillaritis, LE, psoriasis (pustular)
aminopenicillins	erythema multiforme
aminophylline	eczema, rosacea
aminosalicylic acid	cutaneous small vessel vasculitis, fixed drug eruption, lichenoid, vasculitis (leukocytoclastic)
amiodarone	hyperpigmentation (dermal), linear IgA d., photoallergic drug reaction, photosensitivity, phototoxic drug eruption, pigmentation (slate blue), pruritus
amoxapine	acneiform eruption, TEN, vesiculobullous
amoxicillin	bullous pemphigoid, intertrigo, pustular eruption
amphetamines	Raynaud's d.
amphotericin	exanthematous eruption, nail color change (yellow)

Medication and Associated Skin Diseases

Medication	Skin Disease
ampicillin	exanthematous eruption, fixed drug eruption, Henoch-Schönlein purpura, linear IgA d., pemphigoid, pemphigus foliaceus, pruritus, psoriasis, pustular eruption, rash (morbilliform), TEN, vasculitis
amsacrine	alopecia, stomatitis, urticaria
amyl nitrite	flushing, rosacea
anabolic steroids	acne, hypertrichosis, pruritus
androgens	acneiform eruption, porphyria cutanea tarda
anthracene	phototoxic drug eruption
antibiotics	eczema
anticholinergics	xerostomia
anticoagulants	alopecia
anticonvulsants	fixed drug eruption, pellagra-like, pseudolymphoma, purpura
antidepressants	pellagra-like, photoallergic drug reaction, photosensitivity, pseudolymphoma
antifungals	fixed drug eruption, photoallergic drug reaction
antihistamines	eczema, pseudolymphoma, xerostomia
anti-hypertensives	xerostomia
anti-influenza vaccines	cutaneous small vessel vasculitis
antimalarials	fixed drug eruption, hyperpigmentation (dermal), lichenoid, nail discoloration (blue), ochronosis, photoallergic drug reaction, pruritus, psoriasis
antimetabolites	anagen effluvium
anti-Parkinson	xerostomia
antipsychotics	lichenoid
antithyroid drugs	alopecia
anti-tuberculous	lichenoid, TEN
argyria	nail color change (blue), pigmentation (slate blue)
arsenic	arsenic keratoses, BCC, Bowen's d., bullous eruption, cancer (lung), eczema, exfoliative dermatitis, fixed drug eruption, hyperpigmentation (dermal), lichenoid, lung cancer, nail color change (blue), pigmentation (brown), pityriasiform, psoriasis, Raynaud's d., seborrheic dermatitis, SCC, transverse nail lines, vesiculobullous
asparaginase	flushing, TEN, urticaria
aspirin	dermatomyositis-like, fixed drug eruption, histamine release, petechiae, pruritus, purpura, rash (morbilliform), Reye's s., TEN
astezolamide	hirsutism
atropine	delusion of parasitosis, exanthematous eruption
azathioprine	acneiform eruption

Medication and Associated Skin Diseases

Medication	Skin Disease
AZT	melanonychia
aztreonam	exfoliative dermatitis
barbiturates	bullous eruptions, EM, exanthematous eruption, exfoliative dermatitis, fixed drug eruption, morbilliform eruption, pityriasiform, purpura, TEN, ulcer, urticaria, vesiculobullous
benoxaprofen	phototoxic drug eruption
benzoate	purpura, urticaria
benzodiazepines	exanthematous eruption, fixed drug eruption, photoallergic drug reaction, pseudolymphoma, eruption (morbilliform)
beta-carotene	nail color change (yellow), yellow skin coloration
bismuth	alopecia, hyperpigmentation (dermal), lichenoid, pigmentation (blue-black on gingival margin), pityriasiform
bleomycin	alopecia, anagen effluvium, flushing, hair color change, hair hyperpigmentation, hair pigment loss, hyperpigmentation, hyperpigmentation (linear), melanonychia, neutrophilic eccrine hidradenitis, pigmentation (blue), pruritus, radiation enhancement, Raynaud's d., sclerosis, scleroderma-like, stomatitis, TEN, urticaria
boric acid	alopecia
boron cyclophosphamide	anagen effluvium
brequinar sodium	hyperpigmentation, phototoxic drug eruption
bromides	bullous eruption, erythema nodosum, PG, pustular eruption, vesiculobullous
bromine	panniculitis
bromocriptine	alopecia, erythermalgia, erythromelalgia, flushing, hypertrichosis
busulfan	alopecia (permanent in high dose), EM, erythema nodosum, hyperpigmentation, hyperpigmentation (mucosal), PCT, urticaria, vasculitis (leukocytoclastic)
butorphanol	pruritus
butyl nitrite	flushing
butyrophenones	ichthyosiform
calcium channel blockers	exanthematous eruption, exfoliative dermatitis, pseudolymphoma, urticaria
capsaicin	flushing
captopril	erythroderma, exanthematous eruption, exfoliative dermatitis, LE, lichenoid, linear IgA d., pemphigoid, pemphigus foliaceus, pityriasiform, psoriasis, pruritus, vesiculobullous
carbamazepine	eczema, EM, exanthematous eruption, exfoliative dermatitis, LE, lichenoid, pustular eruption, TEN
carbamides	purpura
carbidopa	scleroderma-like

Medication and Associated Skin Diseases

Medication	Skin Disease
carbimazole	alopecia
carboplatin	flushing, urticaria
carmustine	alopecia, flushing, hyperpigmentation, telangiectasia
cathaxanthin	pigmentation (yellow)
cefaclor	pustular eruption, serum sickness-like
cefamandole	linear IgA d.
cefazolin	intertrigo
cefoxitin	exfoliative dermatitis
cephalexin	acute paronychia
cephalosporins	EM, exfoliative dermatitis, pruritus, serum sickness-like vasculitis, TEN, urticaria
chemotherapeutic agents	acral erythema, alopecia, urticaria, vesiculobullous
chloral hydrate	eczema
chlorambucil	alopecia, EM, neutrophilic eccrine hidradenitis, porphyria (acute intermittent), TEN, urticaria
chloramphenicol	alopecia, exanthematous eruption, onycholysis, pellagra-like, TEN, urticaria
chlordiazepoxide	fixed drug eruption, LE
chloroquine	EAC, exanthem, exfoliative dermatitis, hair pigment loss, lens opacities, lichenoid, photosensitivity, phototoxic drug eruption, pigmentation (blue-gray), PCT, pruritus, psoriasis, purpura
chlorothiazide	purpuric eruption, vasculitis
chlorothiazide	purpura
chlorpromazine	exfoliative dermatitis, LE, lens opacities, nail color change (blue), pigmentation (gray), phototoxic drug eruption, purpuric eruption, eruption (morbilliform)
chlorpropamide	exfoliative dermatitis, pruritus, TEN
chlortetracycline	histamine release, onycholysis
chlorthalidone	LE, psoriasis
cholinergic drugs	flushing
chromium salts	nail color change (yellow)
cimetidine	alopecia, EAC, EM, exfoliative dermatitis, ichthyosiform, LE, seborrheic dermatitis, SLE, urticaria, vasculitis (leukocytoclastic)
ciprofloxacin	EM, fixed drug eruption, TEN
cisplatin	acral erythema, allergic contact dermatitis, exanthematous eruption, exfoliative dermatitis, flushing, hair color change, hyperpigmentation, hyperpigmentation (mucosal), porphyria, urticaria
cladribine	TEN

Medication and Associated Skin Diseases

Medication	Skin Disease
clindamycin	intertrigo, vasculitis (leukocytoclastic)
clofazimine	erythroderma, exfoliative dermatitis, ichthyosiform
clofibrate	LE
clomiphene	alopecia
clonidine	pityriasiform, pruritus, psoriasis, Raynaud's d.
cocaine	pruritus
codeine	erythema multiforme, exfoliative dermatitis, histamine release, psoriasis
colchicine	alopecia, pruritus
colistin	pruritus
color film processors	lichenoid eruption
corticosteroids	acanthosis nigricans, acneiform eruption, hirsutism, hypertrichosis, striae, vasculitis (leukocytoclastic)
corticotropin	urticaria
coumadin	chilblains-like erythema, pruritus, purpura
curare	urticaria
cyanamide	Raynaud's d.
cyanocobalamin (Vitamin B12)	acneiform eruption
cyclohexylamines	scleroderma-like
cyclophosphamide	acral erythema, alopecia, EM, flushing, hair color change, hair hyperpigmentation, hyperpigmentation, hyperpigmentation (mucosal), hyperpigmentation (palms & soles), melanonychia, neutrophilic eccrine hidradenitis, PCT, porphyria (acute intermittent), stomatitis, urticaria, vasculitis (leukocytoclastic)
cyclosporine	acneiform eruption, flushing, gingival hyperplasia, hirsutism, hypertrichosis, linear IgA d., psoriasis, rosacea
cyproterone acetate	flushing
cytarabine	acral erythema, alopecia, neutrophilic eccrine hidradenitis, stomatitis, TEN, urticaria, vasculitis (leukocytoclastic)
cytosine arabinoside	acral erythema
dacarbazine	alopecia, fixed drug eruption, flushing, phototoxic drug eruption, radiation photosensitivity
dactinomycin	acneiform eruption, alopecia, folliculitis, hyperpigmentation, phototoxic drug eruption, radiation enhancement, radiation recall, stomatitis
danazol	erythema multiforme, hypertrichosis
dapsone	Beau's lines, eruption (morbilliform), exfoliative dermatitis, fixed drug eruption, hemolysis, lichenoid, methemoglobinemia, porphyria cutanea tarda, TEN

171

Medication and Associated Skin Diseases

Medication	Skin Disease
daunorubicin	acral erythema, allergic contact dermatitis, alopecia, folliculitis, hair hyperpigmentation, hyperpigmentation, stomatitis, urticaria
demeclocycline	lichenoid
desipramine	exfoliative dermatitis
detoconazole	melanonychia
dexamethasone	pruritus
dextran	urticaria
dextromethorphan	fixed drug eruption
diazacholesterol	ichthyosiform
diaziquone	urticaria
diazoxide	alopecia, hirsutism, hypertrichosis, pruritus, rosacea
diclofenac	dermatomyositis-like, linear IgA d.
dicloxacillin	TEN
didemnin B	flushing, urticaria
diethylstilbestrol	acanthosis nigricans, erythema multiforme, erythema nodosum, flushing, hirsutism, LE, PCT, urticaria
diflunisal	exanthem, fixed drug eruption
digoxin	hypertrichosis, psoriasis
dilantin	acneiform eruption, alopecia, exanthem, hirsutism, pseudolymphoma, exanthematous eruption, LE, pseudolymphoma, serum sickness-like, SLE, TEN
diltiazem	exanthematous eruption, exfoliative dermatitis, flushing, gingival hyperplasia, vasculitis (leukocytoclastic)
dimercaprol	exfoliative dermatitis
dinitrophenol	nail color change (yellow)
diphenhydramine	fixed drug eruption
diphenoxylate	pruritus
diphenylhydantoin	erythema multiforme, hypertrichosis
dipyridamole	rosacea, vesiculobullous
disulfiram	eczema, TEN
diuretics	eczema
dixyrazine	ichthyosiform
DNCB	nail color change (yellow)
dobutamine	pruritus
docetaxel	acral erythema, flushing, hyperpigmentation, scleroderma-like, urticaria
doxifluridine	acral erythema

Medication and Associated Skin Diseases

Medication	Skin Disease
doxorubicin	acral erythema, allergic contact dermatitis, alopecia, cellulitis, flushing, hair hyperpigmentation, hyperpigmentation, hyperpigmentation (mucosal), hyperpigmentation (palms & soles), neutrophilic eccrine hidradenitis, onycholysis, phototoxic drug eruption, radiation enhancement, radiation recall, TEN, urticaria (localized)
doxycycline	onycholysis, phototoxic drug eruption, TEN
dyazide	hypertrichosis
dyrazine	ichthyosiform
edatrexate	stomatitis
enalapril	pruritus
epirubicin	alopecia, stomatitis, urticaria (localized)
ergocalciferol	ichthyosiform
ergotamine	Raynaud's d., ulcer
erythromycin	eruption (morbilliform), exanthematous eruption, fixed drug eruption, Henoch-Schönlein purpura, pruritus, pustular eruption, TEN
erythropoietin	hypertrichosis
estrogen	acanthosis nigricans, EAC, erythema nodosum, histamine release, hyperpigmentation (melasma-like), hypertrichosis, porphyria cutanea tarda, pruritus, spider nevus
ethambutol	acneiform eruption
ethionamide	acneiform eruption, alopecia
ethosuximide	LE
EtOH	histamine release, porphyria cutanea tarda, Raynaud's d., rosacea
etoposide	acral erythema, alopecia, erythema multiforme, flushing, Raynaud's d., urticaria
etretinate	erythroderma, pili torti, pruritus, psoriasis
fansidar	TEN
fenbufen	erythroderma
fenoterol	hypertrichosis
fentanyl	pruritus
fiorinol	fixed drug eruption
floxuridine	acral erythema, stomatitis
fluorescein	nail color change (yellow)
fluorobutyrphenone	alopecia
fluoroquinolones	fixed drug eruption, photosensitivity
fluorouracil	acral erythema, allergic contact dermatitis, alopecia, BP, cellulitis, eczema, flushing, folliculitis, hyperpigmentation, hyperpigmentation (mucosal), pellagra-like, photosensitivity, phototoxic drug eruption, radiation enhancement, radiation photosensitivity, stomatitis, TEN, urticaria

Medication and Associated Skin Diseases

Medication	Skin Disease
fluoxetine	urticaria
fluoxymesterone	acneiform eruption, furuncle, hirsutism
flutamide	flushing
fotemustine	hyperpigmentation
furosemide	lichenoid, pemphigoid (bullous), phototoxic drug eruption, PCT, pruritus, pseudoporphyria, vesiculobullous
G-CSF	pyoderma gangrenosum, Sweet's s.
gentamicin	alopecia, erythroderma, exanthematous eruption, rash (morbilliform)
glibenclamid	linear IgA d.
glucocorticoids	acanthosis nigricans
glucophage	linear IgA d. (?)
glutamate	rosacea
glutethimide	erythema multiforme
GM-CSF	erythroderma, exanthematous eruption, PG, Sweet's s.
gold	eczema, erythema nodosum, exanthematous eruption, exfoliative dermatitis, fixed drug eruption, hyperpigmentation (dermal), LE, lichenoid, pityriasiform, psoriasis, purpuric eruption, seborrheic dermatitis, SCLE, TEN, vasculitis (leukocytoclastic)
gold salts	exfoliative dermatitis, exanthematous eruption, keratoderma, lichenoid eruption, pityriasis rosea-like eruption, rash (morbilliform)
griseofulvin	exfoliative dermatitis, erythema multiforme, LE, photoallergic drug reaction, photosensitivity, phototoxic drug eruption, pityriasiform, porphyria cutanea tarda, purpuric eruption, rash (morbilliform), SCLE, TEN, urticaria, vasculitis (leukocytoclastic), vesiculobullous
halides	bullous eruption, pustular eruption
halofantrine	pruritus
halogens (see each also)	acneiform eruption, erythema nodosum, TEN
haloperidol	acneiform eruption, hair pigment loss
HCTZ	ichthyosiform, phototoxic drug eruption, pruritus
heavy metals	alopecia, Raynaud's d.
heparin	petechiae, pruritus, purpura, vasculitis (leukocytoclastic)
heroin	fixed drug eruption, pemphigus foliaceus, pruritus
hexachlorobenzene	hirsutism, porphyria cutanea tarda
hexamethylene bisacetamide	vasculitis (leukocytoclastic)
HMG-CoA reductase inhibitors	eczema

Medication and Associated Skin Diseases

Medication	Skin Disease
hydantoin	acanthosis nigricans, alopecia, cutaneous small vessel vasculitis, EM, exanthematous eruption, exfoliative dermatitis, hypertrichosis, LE, TEN, urticaria, vasculitis (leukocytoclastic)
hydralazine	rosacea, SLE, urticaria, vasculitis (leukocytoclastic)
hydroquinone	ochronosis
hydroxychloroquine	exfoliative dermatitis, porphyria cutanea tarda
hydroxyurea	acral erythema, alopecia, dermatomyositis-like (long term), erythema multiforme, fixed drug eruption, hyperpigmentation, hyperpigmentation (mucosal), LE, lichenoid, phototoxic drug eruption, stomatitis, telangiectasia, ulcers (leg), vasculitis (leukocytoclastic)
hypnotics	xerostomia
hypocholesterolemics	alopecia
hypoglycemics	eczema, exanthematous eruption, lichenoid, photoallergic drug reaction, TEN
ibuprofen	fixed drug eruption, psoriasis
idarubicin	acral erythema, alopecia, stomatitis, urticaria (localized)
ifosfamide	alopecia, hyperpigmentation
imipenem	pustular eruption
imipramine	exfoliative dermatitis, pruritus, TEN, urticaria
indomethacin	alopecia, psoriasis, urticaria, vasculitis (leukocytoclastic)
insulin	acanthosis nigricans, cutaneous small vessel vasculitis, keloid, lipoatrophy, urticaria, vasculitis (leukocytoclastic)
interferon	alopecia, flushing, linear IgA d., psoriasis
interleukins	linear IgA d., psoriasis
iodides	bullous eruption, dermatitis herpetiformis (worsens), exfoliative dermatitis, PG, purpuric eruption, pustular eruption, rosacea, vasculitis (leukocytoclastic), vesiculobullous
iodine	linear IgA d., panniculitis, psoriasis
irinotecan	alopecia
iron	hyperpigmentation (dermal)
isoniazid (INH)	acanthosis nigricans, acneiform eruption, cutis laxa, exanthematous eruption, exfoliative dermatitis, lichenoid, LE, pellagra-like, pityriasiform, rash (morbilliform), striae
isoprel	rosacea
isordil	rosacea
isotretinoin	erythema nodosum, exfoliative dermatitis, pili torti, pityriasiform, pruritus, PG, pyogenic granuloma, xanthomas (eruptive)
ketoconazole	erythroderma, melanonychia, nail color change (blue), pruritus, vasculitis (leukocytoclastic)

Medication and Associated Skin Diseases

Medication	Skin Disease
ketoprofen	pityriasiform
lead	hyperpigmentation (dermal)
leuprolide	flushing, LE
levamisole	lichenoid, vasculitis (leukocytoclastic)
levodopa	alopecia, LE, pemphigus foliaceus
lithium	acneiform eruption, erythema multiforme, exanthematous eruption, exfoliative dermatitis, LE, lichenoid, linear IgA d., pseudolymphoma, psoriasis
lomefloxacin	photosensitivity, pruritus
lomustine	acral erythema, flushing, neutrophilic eccrine hidradenitis
lovastatin	LE
mechlorethamine	allergic contact dermatitis, alopecia, erythema multiforme (IV), hyperpigmentation, stomatitis, urticaria
meclofenamate	eruption
medroxyprogesterone	acneiform eruption
mefloquine	exfoliative dermatitis
mellaril	vesiculobullous
melphalan	acral erythema, alopecia, hair hyperpigmentation, urticaria
meperidine	histamine release
mephenesin	hair pigment loss
mephenytoin	hyperpigmentation (melasma-like)
meprobamate	eczema, fixed drug eruption
mercaptopurine	acral erythema, pellagra-like, stomatitis, vasculitis (leukocytoclastic)
mercury	acrodynia, bullous eruption, eczema, exfoliative dermatitis, hyperpigmentation (dermal), nail color change (blue), vesiculobullous
mesna	urticaria
methaqualone	fixed drug eruption
methazolamide	exanthematous eruption
methotrexate	accelerated rheumatoid nodule development, acral erythema, alopecia, erythema multiforme, erythroderma, exfoliative dermatitis, folliculitis, furuncle, hair color change, hyperpigmentation, photosensitivity, phototoxic drug eruption, porphyria cutanea tarda, purpura, radiation enhancement, reactivation of ultraviolet light induced erythema, stomatitis, TEN, ulcers (leg), urticaria, UV recall, vasculitis (leukocytoclastic)
methoxsalen	psoriasis
methoxypromazine	pityriasiform
8-methoxypsoralen	onycholysis

Medication and Associated Skin Diseases

Medication	Skin Disease
6-methylcoumarin	photoallergic drug reaction
methyltestosterone	acanthosis nigricans
methyldopa	alopecia, black hairy tongue, lichenoid, seborrheic dermatitis, SLE
methylphenidate	delusion of parasitosis
methysergide	LE, pigmentation (red), Raynaud's d.
metoclopramide	flushing
metoprolol	alopecia
metronidazole	fixed drug eruption, intertrigo, pityriasiform, pruritus
metyrapone	hypertrichosis
miconazole	pruritus
minipress	TEN
minocycline	exfoliative dermatitis, fixed drug eruption, hyperpigmentation (dermal), melanonychia, onycholysis, pigmentation (blue, brown, gray), Sweet's s.
minoxidil	eczema, erythema multiforme, erythroderma, hirsutism, hypertrichosis
mithramycin	cellulitis, flushing, stomatitis, TEN
mitomycin	acral erythema, allergic contact dermatitis, alopecia, erythema multiforme, phototoxic drug eruption, radiation photosensitivity, stomatitis, urticaria
mitotane	acral erythema, erythema multiforme, urticaria
mitoxantrone	acral erythema, alopecia, hyperpigmentation, neutrophilic eccrine hidradenitis, urticaria, vasculitis (leukocytoclastic)
morphine	flushing, histamine release, pruritus, psoriasis
musk ambrette	persistent light reaction, photoallergic drug reaction
nafoxidine	hair pigment loss
naftizone	pruritus
nalidixic acid	photosensitivity, phototoxic drug eruption, PCT, pseudoporphyria, vesiculobullous
naproxen	fixed drug eruption, phototoxic drug eruption, porphyria cutanea tarda
neomycin	contact dermatitis, eczema, exfoliative dermatitis
neuroleptics	seborrheic dermatitis
niacin	flushing, pruritus
niacinamide	acanthosis nigricans
nicardipine	erythermalgia
nickel	ear lobe dermatitis, pompholyx
nicotinic acid	acanthosis nigricans, flushing, ichthyosiform, rosacea

Medication and Associated Skin Diseases

Medication	Skin Disease
nifedipine	erythermalgia, erythromelalgia, exfoliative dermatitis, flushing, gingival hyperplasia, pemphigus foliaceus, pustular eruption, telangiectasia, vasculitis (leukocytoclastic)
nitrate	rosacea
nitrofurantoin	exanthematous eruption, exfoliative dermatitis, LE, TEN
norfloxacin	fixed drug eruption
NSAIDs	alopecia, erythema multiforme, exanthematous eruption, fixed drug eruption histamine release, photoallergic drug reaction, photosensitivity, phototoxic drug eruption, pityriasiform, pruritus, pseudolymphoma, psoriasis, purpura, thrombocytopenic purpura, TEN, urticaria, vasculitis (leukocytoclastic), vesiculobullous
nystatin	eczema, erythroderma, fixed drug eruption
OCPs (oral contraceptive pills)	acanthosis nigricans, acneiform eruption, acrodermatitis enteropathica, alopecia, androgenetic alopecia, chloasma, cutaneous small vessel vasculitis, erythema nodosum, fixed drug eruption, Fox-Fordyce d., herpes gestationis, hyperpigmentation (dermal), melasma, monilethrix (improves), photoallergic drug reaction, pigmentation (brown), progressive mesangiocapillary glomerulonephritis of partial lipodystrophy, pruritus, spider nevus, subacute nodular migratory panniculitis, Raynaud's d., SLE, Sweet's s., telangiectasia, telogen effluvium (upon stopping), vasculitis (leukocytoclastic), zinc deficiency
opiates	fixed drug eruption, flushing, urticaria
organic solvents	POEMS s., sclerodermatous changes
oxadiazolopyrimidine	hypertrichosis
oxicam derivatives	TEN
oxyphenbutazone	erythema multiforme, fixed drug eruption
oxytetracycline	erythroderma
PABA esters	photoallergic drug reaction, phototoxic drug eruption
paclitaxel	acral erythema, alopecia, EM, fixed drug eruption (bullous), flushing, stomatitis, urticaria
papaverine	rosacea
paracetamol	exfoliative dermatitis, fixed drug eruption
paraphenylenediamine	lichenoid
penicillamine	anetoderma, cutis laxa, dermatomyositis-like, DLE, elastosis perforans serpiginosa, erythema multiforme, hirsutism, hypertrichosis, LE, lichenoid, morphea, nail color change (yellow), onychoschizia, pemphigus foliaceus, pemphigus vulgaris, pemphigoid, psoriasis, SCLE, scleroderma-like, TEN, vesiculobullous
penicillin	black hairy tongue, bullous eruption, bullous pemphigoid, cutaneous small vessel vasculitis, eczema, erythema annulare centrifugum, EM, erythema nodosum, exanthematous eruption, exfoliative der-

Medication and Associated Skin Diseases

Medication	Skin Disease
	matitis, fixed drug eruption, Henoch-Schönlein purpura, linear IgA d., panniculitis, pemphigus foliaceus, pemphigus vulgaris, pemphigoid, pityriasiform, pustular eruption, rash, serum sickness-like vasculitis, SLE, TEN, urticaria, vasculitis (leukocytoclastic), vesiculobullous
pergolide	erythromelalgia
phenacetin	erythema nodosum, fixed drug eruption, panniculitis, pemphigoid
phenazopyridine	pigmentation (yellow)
phenelzine	delusion of parasitosis
phenindione	chilblains-like erythema, exfoliative dermatitis
phenobarbital	acneiform eruption, bullous eruption, erythema multiforme, erythroderma, exfoliative dermatitis, pemphigus foliaceus, TEN
phenol	ochronosis
phenolphthalein	erythema multiforme, bullous eruption, fixed drug eruption, TEN, urticaria, vesiculobullous
phenothiazines	cutaneous small vessel vasculitis, eczema, erythema multiforme, exanthematous eruption, exfoliative dermatitis, hyperpigmentation (dermal), hypertrichosis, LE, lichenoid, photoallergic drug reaction, photosensitivity, phototoxic drug eruption, pruritus, pseudolymphoma, purpura, rash (morbilliform), seborrheic dermatitis, thrombocytopenic purpura, urticaria, vasculitis (leukocytoclastic)
phenylbutazone	cutaneous small vessel vasculitis, erythema multiforme, exanthematous eruption, exfoliative dermatitis, fixed drug eruption, LE, pemphigus foliaceus, purpuric eruption, rash, TEN, urticaria, vasculitis (leukocytoclastic)
phenytoin	acneiform eruption, erythema multiforme, exanthematous eruption, exfoliative dermatitis, gingival hyperplasia, hirsutism, hyperpigmentation, hyperpigmentation (melasma-like), hypertrichosis, hypopigmentation, LE, lichenoid, linear IgA d., pigmentation (brown), pseudolymphoma, TEN, vasculitis, vesiculobullous
pindolol	psoriasis
piroxicam psoralens	alopecia, fixed drug eruption, leukopenia, pemphigus foliaceus, phototoxic drug eruption, rash, SCLE
pituitary extract	acanthosis nigricans
plaquenil	erythema annulare centrifugum, pigmentation (blue-black), psoriasis (exacerbation)
plicamycin	flushing, hyperpigmentation, TEN
polymyxin antibiotics	histamine release, pruritus, urticaria
polyvinylchloride	sclerosis
porphyrins	phototoxic drug eruption
potassium thiocyanates	alopecia

Medication and Associated Skin Diseases

Medication	Skin Disease
practolol	dermatomyositis-like, psoriasis
prazosin	erythema multiforme
probenecid	pruritus
procainamide	eczema, SCLE, SLE, urticaria, vasculitis (leukocytoclastic)
procarbazine	fixed drug eruption, flushing, hyperpigmentation, hyperpigmentation (palms & soles), phototoxic drug eruption, stomatitis, TEN, urticaria
progesterone	erythema annulare centrifugum, hypertrichosis, pruritus
propranolol	alopecia, lichenoid, pemphigus foliaceus, psoriasis
propylthiouracil	vasculitis (leukocytoclastic)
psoralen	acneiform eruption, hypertrichosis, melanonychia, pemphigoid, phototoxic drug eruption
PUVA	bullous pemphigoid, vesiculobullous
pyrazolon derivatives	exfoliative dermatitis
pyribenzamine	pityriasiform
pyridoxine	porphyria cutanea tarda
pyrimethamine	lichenoid
pyritinol	erythema multiforme, panniculitis, pemphigus foliaceus
quinacrine	alopecia, eczema, exfoliative dermatitis, ochronosis, pigmentation (yellow)
quinidine	eczema, erythroderma, exanthematous eruption, exfoliative dermatitis, fixed drug eruption, Henoch-Schönlein purpura, LE, lichenoid, livedo reticularis, petechiae, phototoxic drug eruption, porphyria cutanea tarda, pruritus, psoriasis, purpuric eruption, pustular eruption, thrombocytopenic purpura, urticaria, vasculitis (leukocytoclastic)
quinine	acneiform eruption, cutaneous small vessel vasculitis, fixed drug eruption, Henoch-Schönlein purpura, histamine release, lichenoid, livedo reticularis, petechiae, porphyria cutanea tarda, purpura, TEN, vasculitis (leukocytoclastic)
radiocontrast media	histamine release
reserpine	LE, rosacea
resorcinol	eczema, ochronosis
13-cis-retinoic acid	erythema nodosum
retinoids	alopecia, ichthyosiform, mucositis
rifampin	erythema multiforme, exfoliative dermatitis, flushing, pemphigus foliaceus, pemphigus vulgaris, porphyria cutanea tarda, TEN
salazopyrin	erythema multiforme
salicylanilides	persistent light reaction
salicylates	bullous eruption, erythema annulare centrifugum, erythema multiforme, erythema nodosum, fixed drug eruption, urticaria, vesiculobullous

Medication and Associated Skin Diseases

Medication	Skin Disease
scopolamine	histamine release
sedatives	purpura, purpura pigmentosa chronica, xerostomia
serum	vasculitis (leukocytoclastic)
silver	hyperpigmentation (dermal)
somatostatin	linear IgA d.
sotalol	vasculitis (leukocytoclastic)
spironolactone	hypertrichosis
steroids	pseudolymphoma
streptokinase	vasculitis (leukocytoclastic)
streptomycin	cutaneous small vessel vasculitis, eczema, EM, exanthematous eruption, exfoliative dermatitis, hypertrichosis, LE, lichenoid, TEN, urticaria, vasculitis (leukocytoclastic)
sulfa	nail color change (blue), pemphigoid, serum sickness-like vasculitis
sulfadiazine	exfoliative dermatitis
sulfanilamide	phototoxic drug eruption
sulfapyridine	pellagra-like
sulfasalazine	bullous pemphigoid, erythroderma
sulfathiazole	panniculitis
sulfonamides	cutaneous small vessel vasculitis, eczema, erythema multiforme, erythema nodosum, erythroderma, exanthematous eruption, exfoliative dermatitis, fixed drug eruption, nail changes, photoallergic drug reaction, photosensitivity, phototoxic drug eruption, pruritus, purpuric eruption, serum sickness-like, SLE, TEN, urticaria, vasculitis (leukocytoclastic), vesiculobullous
sulfones	erythema nodosum
sulfonylureas	erythema multiforme, erythema nodosum, exfoliative dermatitis, lichenoid eruption, photoallergic drug reaction, photosensitivity, phototoxic drug eruption, porphyria cutanea tarda, SCLE
sulindac	chilblains-like erythema, fixed drug eruption
suramin	acral erythema, erythema multiforme, flushing, papules (keratotic), pruritus, TEN, UV recall
tacrolimus	hypertrichosis
tamoxifen	cutaneous small vessel vasculitis, dermatomyositis-like, flushing, hair color change, hirsutism, vasculitis (leukocytoclastic)
tar	acneiform eruption, folliculitis, nail color change (yellow)
tartrazine	purpura
tegafur	acral erythema, dermatomyositis-like, hyperpigmentation, hyperpigmentation (mucosal), LE, lichenoid, phototoxic drug eruption, stomatitis

Medication and Associated Skin Diseases

Medication	Skin Disease
teniposide	alopecia, flushing, urticaria
terbutaline	exfoliative dermatitis
testosterone	alopecia, hypertrichosis, pruritus
tetracycline	black hairy tongue, candidiasis, EM, erythema nodosum, exanthematous eruption, fixed drug eruption, lichenoid, nail color change (yellow), onycholysis, photosensitivity, phototoxic drug eruption, PCT, pseudoporphyria, SLE, splinter hemorrhage, TEN, urticaria, vasculitis (leukocytoclastic)
thallium	alopecia, anagen effluvium
theophylline	rosacea
thiamin	histamine release
thiazides	cutaneous small vessel vasculitis, eczema, erythema nodosum, exanthematous eruption, exfoliative dermatitis, lichenoid, onycholysis, photoallergic drug reaction, photosensitivity, phototoxic drug eruption, rash (morbilliform), purpura, SCLE, serum sickness-like vasculitis, thrombocytopenic purpura, vasculitis (leukocytoclastic), vesiculobullous
thiobendazole	TEN
thioguanine	stomatitis
thiol derivatives	pemphigoid
thiopronine	elastosis perforans serpiginosa, pemphigus vulgaris
thioridazine	vesiculobullous
thiotepa	alopecia, hyperpigmentation, urticaria
thiouracil	alopecia, anagen effluvium, rash, SLE, vasculitis
thyroid hormones	hypertrichosis
thyrotropin-releasing hormone	flushing
timolol	erythroderma
tobacco	Raynaud's d.
tolbutamide	phototoxic drug eruption, pruritus
tolmetin	fixed drug eruption
tomudex	stomatitis
topotecan	alopecia, stomatitis
trazodone	exanthematous eruption, exfoliative dermatitis, urticaria
triazinate	acanthosis nigricans
2,4,5-trichlorophenol	porphyria cutanea tarda
tricyclic antidepressants	xerostomia
trimethadione	acneiform eruption, alopecia, erythema multiforme, SLE

Medication and Associated Skin Diseases

Medication	Skin Disease
trimethoprim	erythema multiforme, urticaria
trimethoprim/sulfadoxine	TEN
trimethoprim- sulfamethoxasole	erythema multiforme, erythroderma, exanthematous eruption, exfoliative dermatitis, fixed drug eruption, leukocytoclastic vasculitis, linear IgA d., TEN, urticaria
trimetrexate	flushing, urticaria
triparanol	alopecia, ichthyosiform
tripelennamine	pityriasiform
tryptophan	dermatomyositis-like, eosinophilic fasciitis (contaminated), sclerosis
vaccines	erythema nodosum, vasculitis (influenza)
valproic acid	alopecia, scleroderma-like, TEN
vancomycin	exfoliative dermatitis, histamine release, linear IgA d., "red man" s., TEN, vasculitis (leukocytoclastic)
vasodilators	rosacea
verapamil	erythermalgia, flushing, gingival hyperplasia
vigabatrin	linear IgA d.
vinblastine	acneiform eruption, alopecia, photoallergic drug reaction, photosensitivity, phototoxic drug eruption, stomatitis
vincristine	acral erythema, alopecia, Raynaud's d., stomatitis, urticaria
vindesine	alopecia
vinorelbine	alopecia, hyperpigmentation
vinyl chloride	Raynaud's d., scleroderma-like
vitamin A	alopecia
vitamin B complex	pruritus
vitamin B12 (cyanocobalamin)	acneiform eruption
vitamin K (IM)	sclerosis
vitamins	vasculitis (leukocytoclastic)
zidovudine	exfoliative dermatitis, hyperpigmentation (nail), hyperpigmentation (linear)
zinostatin	urticaria

Mouth and Mucous Membranes

alcoholism	beefy tongue, black hairy tongue, glossitis, leukoplakia, parotid swelling
beefy tongue	glossitis due to vitamin B deficiency; alcoholism, pernicious anemia
Biederman's sign	dark red color of anterior pillars of throat; syphilitics (some)
black hairy tongue	hyperplasia of filiform papillae with bacterial overgrowth; alcoholism, systemic illnesses
burning tongue	iron deficiency, pernicious anemia
carp's mouth	narrowed mouth width; Plummer-Vinson s.
cerebriform tongue	deep rugate fissures of tongue; pemphigus vegetans (Hallopeau)
Chadwick's sign	dark blue or purple color of vaginal mucosa; pregnancy
cheilitis	actinic prurigo, artichokes, beta blockers, dentrifices, glucagonoma s., idiopathic calcinosis cutis, oranges, Kawasaki's d., lipstick, mangos
chelitis, angular	acrodermatitis enteropathica, atopic dermatitis, *Candida*, Down s., hypersalivation, mechanical, Plummer-Vinson s., protein deficiency, riboflavin deficiency, *S. aureus* infection, Streptococcal infection
cobblestone, lips	idiopathic calcinosis cutis
cobblestone, oral mucosa	Cowden d., Darier's d.
Corrigan's sign	purple line at junction of teeth & gum; chronic copper poisoning
erosions	erythema multiforme, lichen planus, pemphigoid, pemphigus
fissured tongue	geographic tongue (20%), Melkersson-Rosenthal triad
Forscheimer spots	pinpoint rose colored macules & petechiae on soft palate; rubella
gingival hyperplasia	epilepsy, HSM, leukemia, medications, mental retardation, nail hypoplasia, sensorineural hearing loss, Zimmerman-Laband s.
gingival pigmentation	amalgam tattoo, azidothymidine, betel nut chewing, bismuth, heavy metals, minocycline, phenolphthalein, quinacrine, silver nitrate, tattooing, tobacco chewing,
gingivitis	Chediak-Higashi s., diabetes mellitus, Herpes simplex, Letterer-Siwe d., leukocyte adhesion s., lichen planus, lupus erythematosus, neutropenia, rosacea, scurvy
gingivitis, desquamative	cicatricial pemphigoid, lichen planus, pemphigus vulgaris
gingivitis, marginal	cyclic neutropenia
glossitis	alcoholism, biotin deficiency, *Candida*, carcinoid s., secondary lues, folic acid deficiency, geographic tongue, giant cell arteritis, griseofulvin ingestion, hypertrichosis lanuginosa, median rhomboid glossitis, necrolytic migratory erythema, Plummer-Vinson s., primary amyloidosis, tricyclic administration, penicillamine, vitamin B1 deficiency, vitamin B2 deficiency, vitamin B12 deficiency, zinc deficiency
glossodynia	painful tongue; folate deficiency, geographic tongue, vitamin B12 deficiency
glossopyrosis	burning tongue
gum hypertrophy	Cross-McKusick-Breen s., Darier's d., dilantin administration, juvenile hyaline fibromatosis, mercury administration

Mouth and Mucous Membranes

hairy leukoplakia	**HIV**, immunosuppression
Koplik spots	white spots on buccal mucosa; **measles**, coxsackievirus A16, echovirus 9
Krisovski's sign	cicatricial lines radiating from the mouth; congenital syphilis
lead lines	blue-black macule on gingiva margin from insoluble sulfide salts; bismuth therapy, lead intoxication
lentigo; labial	Albright's s., Laugier-Hunziger s., neurofibromatosis, Peutz-Jeghers s., labial melanotic macule
leukokeratosis	gray-white thickening of oral mucous membrane; pachyonychia congenita (60%)
leukoplakia	alcoholism, dyskeratosis congenita
macroglossia	acromegaly, hypothyroidism, mucopolysaccharidoses, sarcoidosis
oral melanosis	Addison's d., Albright's s., amalgam tattoo, bismuth, lead, Peutz-Jeghers s., Riehl's melanosis
oral pain	pemphigus vulgaris
pigment, intraoral	amalgam tattoos, oral melanoacanthoma, Peutz-Jeghers s., Addison's d., hemochromatosis, neurofibromatosis
raspberry tongue	strawberry tongue
scrotal tongue	Cowden's d., Down s., idiopathic (autosomal dominant), Melkersson-Rosenthal s.
smooth tongue	vitamin B deficiency
sore tongue	pernicious anemia
stomatitis	acute atrophic oral candidiasis, cancrum oris, glucagonoma, griseofulvin, Kawasaki's s., lazy leukocyte s., 6-mercaptopurine, methotrexate, penicillamine, Reiter's s., Stevens-Johnson s., tricyclic antidepressants
stomatodynia	painful mouth
stomatopyrosis	burning mouth
strawberry gingivitis	Wegener's granulomatosis (pathognomonic)
strawberry tongue	hyperplastic lingual papillae; Kawasaki's s., scarlet fever, TSS
thrush	oral candidiasis; diabetes mellitus, HIV, corticosteroids, antibiotics
tongue, atrophic	achlorhydria, ariboflavinosis, cardiac disease, iron deficiency anemia, malabsorption, megaloblastic anemia, pellagra, Plummer-Vinson s., pernicious anemia
tongue, beefy red	cobalamin deficiency, glucagonoma s.
tooth pit	punctate tooth enamel defect; tuberous sclerosis (>4 teeth)
white strawberry tongue	white coating with reddened hypertrophied papillae protruding through; scarlet fever
Wickham's striae	reticulate white lines on papules & buccal mucosa; lichen planus
xerostomia	aging, medications, RA, Sjögren's s.

Nails

age-related changes	koilonychia, lamellar dystrophy, longitudinal pigment (blacks), onychodystrophy (10-66%), onychogryphosis, onychomadesis, onychorrhexis, pitting, pressure changes, red spotted lunula, slowed growth, Terry's nails, thickened plate, thinned plate, trachyonychia
alcoholism	clubbing, koilonychia, red lunulae, Terry's nails
alopecia areata	Beau's lines, brittle nails, koilonychia, leukonychia punctata, longitudinal ridging, onycholysis, onychomadesis, pits, red nails, spotted lunulae, thickened nails
angel wing deformity	deformity of nail; lichen planus
anonychia	absent of all or portion of nail; congenital, lichen planus
AZT	melanonychia
azure lunulae	agyria, Wilson's d.
bands; longitudinal pigmented	acrodermatitis enteropathica, Addison's d., AIDS, amyloid (primary), arsenic, carcinoma of breast, carpal tunnel s., Cushing's s., fluorosis, gastrointestinal disease, hemosiderosis, hyperbilirubinemia, hyperthyroidism, hypopituitarism irradiation, Laugier-Hunziger s., malnutrition, melanoma (metastatic), ochronosis, Peutz-Jeghers s., porphyria, pregnancy, syphilis (secondary)
bands; longitudinal white	Hailey-Hailey d.
beading	rheumatoid arthritis
Beau's lines	transverse depression of nail plate; alopecia areata, β-blockers, cytotoxic drugs, dysmenorrhea, MI, nutritional deficiency, post fever, psoriasis
beta-blockers	Beau's lines, digital ischemia, leukonychia (apparent), onychomadesis
blue nails	antimalarials, AZT, 5-flouracil, hematoma, Wilson's d.
brachydactyly	pseudohypoparathyroidism
brachyonychia	AD; greater width than length of nail plate AKA racquet nail
brittle nails	dehydration, elderly, irritant contact, lichen planus, Marinesco-Sjögren s., nail polish, onychomycosis, psoriasis, retinoids
brown/black nails	AZT (esp. blacks), antimalarials, Peutz-Jeghers s.
canal	single wide groove from matrix pressure; myxoid cyst
chevron nail	V-shaped longitudinal ridging in children
chromonychia	abnormal nail color; external contactant, methemoglobinemia, systemic chemical absorption
clubbing	cuticle (Lovibond's) angle greater than 180 degrees due to fibrovascular hyperplasia; acrocyanosis, alcohol, amyloidosis (secondary), angiectasis, arsenic, *Ascaris* infection, beryllium, biliary cirrhosis, bronchitis, bronchiectasis, cardiopulmonary disease, CHF, chilblains, chronic myelogenous leukemia, Clouston's s., collagen vascular disease, congenital dysplasia, congenital heart d., citrullinemia, cretinism, diarrhea (chronic-sprue), cyanotic heart disease, emphysema, endocarditis (subacute bacterial), familial, fibrosarcoma, GI neoplasm, Gottron's s., Graves' d., hepatic cirrhosis,

Nails

hereditary sclerosing poikiloderma, Hodgkin's d., hypertrophic hypervitaminosis A, hypothyroidism (thyroid acropathy), osteoarthropathy, idiopathic, Kaposi's sarcoma, leprosy, liver disease, lung abscess, lung cyst, lymphoma, Maffucci's s., mercury, mesoendothelioma, myxedema, myxoid tumor, neutropenia (chronic familial), pachydermoperiostosis, Peutz-Jeghers s., phosphorus, pneumonia, POEMS s., post-thyroidectomy, primary polycythemia, pseudotumor, pulmonary fibrosis, **pulmonary neoplasm** (<5%), Raynaud's d., rheumatic fever, scleroderma, SLE, sprue, syphilis, syringomyelia, tuberculosis, ulcerative colitis

clubbing-unilateral or unidigital	arterial aneurysm, brachial arteriovenous fistula, erythromelalgia, felon, gout (tophaceous), lymphangitis, median nerve injury, Pancoast's tumor, sarcoidosis, shoulder subluxation, trauma
Darier's d. (Darier-White d.)	distal V-shaped notch, red longitudinal subungual streaks, wedge-shaped subungual hyperkeratosis, white longitudinal subungual streaks
discoloration, topical agents that cause	**black**: phenol sulfate hydroquinone, red wine, silver nitrate **blue**: cyanide, oxalic acid, silver **gray-blue**: ammoniated mercury, mercuric chloride (with UV) **green**: chlorophyll, copper salts **orange-brown**: anthralin, Arning's tincture, burnt sugar, chromium salts, chrysarobin, dinitrotoluene, dithranol, formaldehyde, flutaraldehyde, henna, hydroquinone, iodohydroxyquinolene, iron, mepacrine, nicotine, paraquat, pecan, picric acid, potassium permanganate, pyrogallol, resorcin, rivanol, roasted coffee, thermal injury, vioform, walnuts **purple**: gentian violet **red**: carbol-fuchin **yellow**: amphotericin, dinitro-orthocresol, dinubuton, fluorescein, hydrofluoric acid
dyschromia	white/red longitudinal streaks; Darier-White d., SCC in situ proximal nail bed white, absent lunula; Terry's nail double white translucent bands; Muehrcke's lines distal brown; Lindsay's nail
dysplasia, toenails	popliteal web s.
dystrophy	amyloidosis, Clouston's s., exfoliative erythroderma, glucagonoma s., KID s., Olmsted's s., Rabson-Mendenhall s., Rothmund-Thompson s., Sabinas s., trauma, Zinsser-Cole-Engman s.
dystrophy, median	habit tic, mucous cyst
dystrophy, occupational	motor oils, permanent wave solutions, solvents, trauma
eggshell nails	dull gloss, brittle, easily split nail
friable	nail enamel use, onychomycosis (superficial)
groove, longitudinal	Schopf-Schulz-Passarge s. (*see median canaliform dystrophy of Heller*)
groove, oblique	Schopf-Schulz-Passarge s.

Nails

groove, transverse	AKA Beau's line
growth, decrease rate of nail	acute infection, aging, antimitotoic drugs, cold climate, congestive heart failure, decreased circulation, females, hypothyroidism, paralysis, immobilization, lactation, malnutrition, measles, mumps, nighttime, peripheral neuropathy, pneumonia, smoking, systemic disease, yellow nail s.
growth, increase rate of nail	dominant hand, hyperpituitarism, hyperthyroidism, AV shunt, local repetitive trauma, longer digits, males, onycholysis, periungual inflammation, pregnancy, premenstrual, psoriasis, regeneration, warm climate
half and half nails	white proximal & brown distal nail (melanin); chronic renal failure, uremia AKA Lindsay's nails
hard nails	pachyonychia congenita
harlequin nail	distal yellow stained nail & proximal clear nail after abrupt smoking cessation
Heller's median canaliform dystrophy	split midline nail with proximal angled ridges esp. on thumbs
hemionychia	nail-patella s.
Hippocratic nail	onychogryphosis
hook nail	bowing of nail due to lack of support of the short bony phalanx
Hutchinson's sign	pigment leaching into nail fold; melanoma
hyperkeratosis, subungual	crusted scabies, Darier-White d., lichen planus, onychomycosis, PRP, psoriasis, Reiter's s.
hyperpigmentation	acrokeratosis verruciformis of Hopf, Laugier-Hunziger s., panhypopituitarism
hyperpigmentation, chemotherapeutic agents	aminoglutethimide, bleomycin, busulfan, cisplatin, cyclophosphamide, cytarabine, dacarbazine, dactinomycin, daunorubicin, docetaxel, doxorubicin, etoposide, fluorouracil, hydroxyurea, idarubicin, ifosfamide, melphalan, methotrexate, mitomycin, mitoxantrone, tegafur, vincristine
ingrown	retinoids
koilonychia	alkalis & acids, acanthosis nigricans, acromegaly, alopecia areata, anemia (chronic), Bantis s., cachexia, chondroectodermal dysplasia (Ellis-van Creveld s.), coronary artery disease, Darier's d., ectodermal dysplasia, familial, focal dermal hypoplasia, frostbite, Gottron's s., hemochromatosis, hypothyroidism, hypovitaminosis B2 & C, idiopathic, incontinentia pigmenti, **iron deficiency**, LEOPARD s., lichen planus, malnutrition, monilethrix, nail-patella s., Nezelof's s., normal children, occupational, onychomycosis, palmar hyperkeratosis, palmoplantar keratoderma, pellagra, petroleum products, Plummer-Vinson s., polycythemia vera, porphyria cutanea tarda, post-gastrectomy, primary amyloid, psoriasis, Raynaud's d., renal transplant, scleroderma, sideropenic anemia, steatocystoma multiplex, syphilis, thyrotoxicosis, thermal burns, thioglyoclate contact (hairdressers) AKA spoon nail

Nails

leukonychia	white spots on nail plate due to matrix dysfunction; β-blockers, chilblains, dysmenorrhea, Hodgkin's d., idiopathic, leprosy, metastatic carcinoma, nephritis, psoriasis, tuberculosis **longitudinal**: Darier's disease **punctate**: minor trauma **total**: inherited **transverse**: systemic disorder
lichen planus	angel wing deformity, atrophy, onycholysis, onychomadesis, onychorrhexis, pterygium, shedding, subungual hyperkeratosis, subungual hyperpigmentation, thinning
Lindsey's nails	white proximal, red/brown distal nail; chronic renal failure AKA half & half nails
liver disease	brittleness, clubbing, flat nails, striations, watch-glass deformity, white bands, white nails
Lovibond's angle	cuticle angle; greater than 180(indicates clubbing (*see clubbing*)
lunula, absent	endocrine, collagen vascular reticuloendothelial d., normal variant
lunula, dyschromia	azure: hepatolenticular degeneration (Wilson's d.) blue: agyria red: heart failure, collagen vascular d. white: ischemia yellow: tetracycline
lunula, red spotted	alopecia areata
lunula, triangular	nail-patella s.
lunula, ulceration	GVH d.
median canaliform dystrophy of Heller	split midline nail with fir tree-like appearance at backward angle; myxoid cyst
Mees' lines	paired narrow white transverse nail lines; antimony poisoning, arsenic exposure, cachectic state, carbon monoxide poisoning, carcinoid, cardiac insufficiency, childbirth, chemotherapy, crush injury, cryotherapy, endemic typhus, erythema multiforme, fluorosis, fracture, glomerulonephritis, gout, herpes zoster, Hodgkin's d., hyperalbuminemia, lead poisoning, leprosy, malaria, measles, menstruation, myocardial infarction, parathyroid insufficiency, pellagra, pneumonia, protein deficiency, psoriasis, renal failure, renal transplant, shock, sickle cell anemia, syphilis, systemic disease, thallium poisoning, tuberculosis, ulcerative proctitis, vitamin B12 deficiency, warm-reacting antibody immunohemolytic anemia, zinc deficiency
melanonychia	AZT, bleomycin, cyclophosphamide, ketoconazole, melanoma, minocycline, psoralen, PUVA
melanonychia, fungal	*Aspergillus, Scitolytium, Scopulariopsis*
melanonychia, longitudinal multiple	Addison's d., AIDS, Cushing's s., folic acid deficiency, hyperthyroidism, vitamin B12 deficiency
melanonychia, transverse	cytotoxic drugs
micronychia	nail-patella s.

Nails

Morton's toe	2nd toe longer than great toe, may become injured by shoes
Muehrcke's nails, lines	paired white parallel transverse bands; hypoalbuminemia ($2°$ to chemotherapy)
nail plate thickening	chronic trauma, Darier-White d., lichen planus, onychomycosis, pachyonychia congenita, psoriases, PRP, scabies (crusted)
nicotine sign	yellow discoloration of distal fingers & fingernails; smokers
notch, distal	Darier's d.
oil drop sign	yellow-brown lesions under nail plate; psoriasis AKA salmon patch
onychochauxis	thickening, darkening, and irregular surface; diabetes mellitus, HIV, hypogonadism
onychodystrophy	alopecia areata, psoriasis
onychogryphosis	brown, thickened spiraled nail; footwear trauma, ichthyoses, impaired circulation, onychomycosis, poor hygiene, psoriasis AKA ram's horn nails
onychoheterotopia	ectopic nails
onycholysis	distal irregular separation of nail plate from nail bed; acrylic nail cement, **allergic contact dermatitis**, amyloid, anemia, bacteria, Bantu porphyria, bronchiectasis, carcinoma of lung, circulatory disorders, Cronkhite-Canada s., CTCL, dermatitis, diabetes mellitus, drug reaction, eczema, erythropoietic porphyria, erythropoietic protoporphyria, formaldehyde, **fungus**, Graves' d., histiocytosis X, ischemia (peripheral), leprosy, lichen planus, lupus erythematosus, neuritis, panhypopituitarism, pellagra, pemphigus vulgaris, plasticizers, pleural effusion, porphyria, pregnancy, pseudoporphyria of hemodialysis, **psoriasis**, pustular eruption of pregnancy, Raynaud's phenomenon, Reiter's s., scleroderma, Sezary s., SCC, syphilis, **thyroid d., trauma**, Vitamin C deficiency, warts, yellow nail s.
onychomadesis	shedding of nail plate; alopecia areata, β-blockers, thrombosis
onychomycosis	**proximal & proximal white superficial**: HIV, immunosuppression, hyperhidrosis, diabetes mellitus, aging **proximal subungual onychomycosis (HIV)**: *Trichophyton rubrum, T. megninii* **white superficial onychomycosis**: *T. mentagrophytes* **nondermatophytes**: *Candida, Scopulariopsis brevicaulis, Hendersonula toruloidea (Scytalidium dimidiatum), Aspergillus sydowii*
onychorrhexis	longitudinal grooves & ridges of nail plate; alopecia areata, lichen planus, normal with aging (mild)
onychoschizia	metabolic acidosis
Osler's toe	onychogryphosis
paronychia, acute	infection, manicuring, retinoids, trauma
paronychia, chronic	biting, contactants, dermatitis, infection, psoriasis, sucking
parrot-beaking	widening onychocorneal band of finger nails; Unna-Thost d.
periungual infarcts	Wegener's granulomatosis

Nails

photo-onycholysis	mercaptopurine, PUVA
pincer (trumpet) nails	footwear pressure, idiopathic, osteoarthritis, psoriasis, subungual exostoses
pitting	**alopecia areata**, atopy, basal cell nevus s., chronic paronychia, Darier's d., **eczema**, fungal infection, lichen nitidus, lichen planus, normal variant, **psoriasis**, Reiter's d., reticulate acropigmentation of Kimura, rheumatoid arthritis, trauma
pseudo-Hutchinson's sign	discoloration of matrix; subungual hematoma
pseudopyogenic granuloma	retinoids
psoriasis	grooves, leukonychia, oil drop sign, onychodystrophy, onycholysis, pitting, salmon patch, splinter hemorrhage, spooning, subungual hyperkeratosis
pterygium	scarring nail bed separation from matrix; familial, idiopathic, **lichen planus**, progressive systemic sclerosis, Raynaud's d., Stevens-Johnson s., trauma, vascular insufficiency
Quincke's pulse	aortic insufficiency
racquet nail	AD; greater width than length of nail plate AKA brachyonychia
ram's horn	onychogryphosis
rheumatoid d.	atrophy, capillary dilation, proximal erythema
ridging	CIE, Darier's d., lichen planus, normal elderly, peripheral vascular d., RA
ridging; longitudinal	acrokeratosis verruciformis of Hopf, panhypopituitarism
salmon patch	yellow-brown subungual discoloration, psoriasis, AKA oil drop sign
splinter hemorrhages	damaged longitudinal vessel of nail bed which exudes blood; **dermatologic**: alopecia mucinosa, Darier's d., eczema, exfoliative dermatitis, keratosis lichenoides chronica, mycosis fungoides, onychomatricoma, pemphigoid, pemphigus, pen-push purpura, psoriasis, pterygium, purpura, polyarteritis nodosa, pityriasis rubra pilaris, porphyria, Raynaud's d. **infectious: bacterial endocarditis**, fungi, HIV, onychomycosis, psittacosis, trichinosis **medications**: drug reaction, methoxsalen, tetracycline **miscellaneous**: altitude (high), irradiation, normal variants, radial artery puncture, radiodermatitis, trauma, Vitamin C deficiency **systemic**: amyloid, anemia, antigen-antibody complex disease, **antiphospholipid coagulopathy**, antiphospholipid s., Behçet's s., Buerger's d., cirrhosis, cryoglobulinemia, cystic fibrosis, **diabetes mellitus** (10%), dialysis, emboli (arterial), histiocytosis X, Letterer-Siwe d., leukemia, Osler-Weber-Rendu d., malignancy, mitral stenosis, multiple sclerosis, glomerulonephritis, heart disease, hemochromatosis, hepatitis, hypertension, hypoparathyroidism, illness (chronic), peptic ulcer d., pulmonary d., rheumatic fever, rheumatoid arthritis, sarcoid, scurvy, septicemia, SLE, thrombocytopenia, transplant patients, trauma, thyrotoxicosis, vasculitis, Wegener's granulomatosis

Nails

spoon nails	AKA koilonychia
telangiectasia, periungual	cystic fibrosis
telangiectasia, posterior nail fold	SLE, systemic sclerosis, dermatomyositis, RA, Raynaud's s.
tennis toe	Morton's toe distally injured by sporting events or small shoes
Terry's nails	white proximal, distal pink nail (onychodermal band); CHF, diabetes mellitus, liver cirrhosis, normal elderly
thickening	alopecia areata, congenital ectodermal defects, congenital malalignment of the great toe nails, Darier's d., Fischer-Jacobsen-Clouston s., fungal infection, pachyonychia congenita, pityriasis rubra pilaris, psoriasis, trauma
thinning	alopecia areata
trachyonychia	rough, dull, brittle nails with frayed edges; alopecia areata, chemical exposure, eczema, idiopathic, lichen planus, psoriasis, twenty nail dystrophy
trumpet nail	AKA pincer nail
tumors in children	angiokeratoma, digital fibroma, enchondromas of Maffucci's s., exostoses, Koenen's (angiofibromas of tuberous sclerosis), hemangiomas of blue rubber bleb nevus or Klippel-Trenaunay-Weber s., incontinentia pigmenti, juvenile xanthogranuloma, osteochondroma, pyogenic granuloma
turtle back nail	Fabry's d.
twenty nail dystrophy	see trachyonychia
verrucae, nail region	HPV-1, 2, 4
washboard nails	longitudinal depression affecting one or both thumb nails; habitually pushing back cuticle
watch glass deformity	mild clubbing with slight convex surface of nail; *see clubbing*
white	cirrhosis, cryoglobulinemia, Raynaud's s., selenium deficiency, systemic sclerosis
yellow	oxalic acid, *Pneumocystis* infection in AIDS, smoking, Touraine-Solente-Golè s.
yellow nail s.	yellow nails, absent cuticles, increased curvature, diminished lunulae, onycholysis, slowed growth; bronchiectasis, carcinoma of larynx, chronic bronchitis, chronic lymphedema, pulmonary d., rheumatoid arthritis, sinusitis, thyroid disease

Scales, Tests,and Techniques

ABO linkage	nail-patella s.
acetowhitening	application of 5% acetic acid solution to detect condyloma (false + common)
albuminuria	serum sickness s.
aldolase, elevated	dermatomyositis
alopecia areata scale	**I**: 83%, common, good prognosis, <6% progress to alopecia totalis **II**: 10%, round/reticular patches, asthma, rhinitis, dermatitis, frequent childhood onset, > 75% alopecia totalis **III**: 4%, reticular hair loss, continuous disease activity, hypertension in 1 or both parents, 39% alopecia totalis **IV**: 3%, combined type, age usually >40, prolonged course, 10% alopecia totalis
alpha-fetoprotein	ataxia telangiectasia
aminoaciduria	agrinosuccinicaciduria, Hartnup's d., hydroxydynurenuria, Netherton's s., peeling skin s.
ANA (false positives)	alcoholism, aging, leprosy, thyroid d., substrate differences
ANCA (anti neutrophilic cytoplasmic antibodies)	Churg-Strauss s., polyarteritis nodosa, Sweet's s., Wegener's granulomatosis
androgenetic alopecia scale, female	**I**: mild crown hair density loss, frontal hair line retained **II**: moderate crown hair density loss, frontal hair line retained **III**: extensive hair density decrease; sparse frontal hairline
androgenetic alopecia scale, male	**I**: normal frontal-parietal hairline **II**: symmetric triangular recession in frontal-parietal regions **III**: borderline cases **IV**: deep frontal-temporal recession with hair loss along mid-frontal scalp **V**: extensive frontal-parietal and frontal recession in association with sparse hair on vertex **VI**: vertex separated from anterior hair loss area by region of sparse hair **VII**: loss of area dividing crown with anterior hair loss **VIII**: vertex baldness with occipital and temporal hair band
anemia	exfoliative erythroderma,
anemia, hemolytic	brown recluse spider bite, runting s.
anemia, hypochromic	Plummer-Vinson s.
angry back s.	patch testing; false + reactions (up to 40%), hypersensitivity caused by strong + reaction to one allergen AKA excited skin s.
anticardiolipin Ab, elevated	anticardiolipin Ab s., Behçet's d., Degos' d., livedo vasculitis
antithyroid antibodies	DLE (women)
Broders system	malignancy grading system for SCC (undifferentiated cells); **grade 1** < 25% undifferentiated cells, **grade 2** < 50%, **grade 3** < 75%, **grade 4** > 75%

Scales, Tests,and Techniques

c-ANCA	connective tissue disease, infection, malignancy, Wegener's granulomatosis
chemotactic deficiencies/ chemotactic abnormalities	acrodermatitis enteropathica, C3 deficiency, familial chemotactic deficiency, hyperimmunoglobulin E s., immunosuppression, pyoderma gangrenosum **leukocytes**; Wiskott-Aldrich s. **neutrophils**; Chediak-Higashi s., hyperimmunoglobulin E s., lazy leukocyte s., Shwachman s.
cholesterol, decreased	*see hypocholesterolosis*
cold agglutinins	PSS, SLE

complement deficiencies	**C1q**: no hereditary deficiency; seen in Bruton's and SCIDS, may have SLE, urticaria and EM-like lesions, urticaria is non-pruritic
	C1r: AR; collagen vascular disease, vasculitis, bronchitis, paronychia, SLE-like syndrome
	C1s: SLE and +ANA, infectious endocarditis with meningitis
	C2: AR; most common inherited deficiency, 1:1000, usually healthy, autoimmune disorders, increased infections?
	C3: 1) hereditary; infections gram positive and negative
	    2) C3b inactivator deficiency; infections
	    3) C3 nephritogenic factor; antibody to C3bBb protects from degradation, glomerulonephritis, partial lipodystrophy, SLE
	C4: AR; infected skin lesions, decreased CH50, typical SLE
	C5: infections, SLE

creatinine phosphokinase	increased; dermatomyositis, toxic shock s.
cryoglobulins	acrodermatitis chronica atrophicans, atrophie blanche, leg ulcers, lymphoma, myeloma, pernio, plane xanthomas, SLE, Sjögren's s., Wegener's granulomatosis
Cat scratch d. skin test (CSD)	cat scratch d. skin test; aspirate lymph node, heat inactivate pus 3 days at 60° C, dilute with sterile saline, freeze. Inject intradermally into forearm of patient with suspected d. Raised nodule >5 mm in 2-3 days is diagnostic.
dermatomyositis	elevated serum creatinine phosphokinase, elevated serum aldolase, electromyography (low amplitude, short duration, polyphasic potentials)
diascopy	two slides used to visualize a lesion under pressure to differentiate red color from capillary dilatation versus blood extravasation; GA, lymphoma, sarcoidosis, TB, vasculitis
Dick test	intracutaneous inoculation of 0.1 mL of standard diluted preparation of pyrogenic exotoxin leading to 1 cm or greater area of local erythema at 24 hours; historic test for scarlet fever
electrocardiographic abnormalities	LEOPARD s.
eosinophilia	**dermatologic**: angiolymphoid hyperplasia with eosinophilia, atopic dermatitis, Behçet's s., BP, chronic acral dermatitis, DH, distinctive eruptive discoid and lichenoid eruption (oid-oid), eosinophilic cellulitis, eosinophilic granuloma, eosinophilic pustular folliculitis, ery-

thema nodosum, erythema toxicum neonatorum, exfoliative dermatitis, granuloma faciale, GVH d., herpes gestationis, hypereosinophilic s., incontinentia pigmenti, pansclerotic morphea of children, pemphigus, plasmacytoma, polyarteritis nodosa, prurigo agyria, pseudolymphoma, sarcoidosis, urticaria, urticaria pigmentosa, Well's s.

infectious: chronic mucocutaneous candidiasis, coccidioidomycosis, crusted scabies, cutaneous larva migrans, dracunculosis, erythema infectiosum, eosinophilic pustular folliculitis, eosinophilic fasciitis, hookworms, infectious urticaria, larva migrans, larva currens, leprosy, loiasis, myiasis, onchocerciasis, parasites, pinta, scabies, scarlet fever, schistosomiasis, secondary syphilis, toxocariasis, trichinosis

neoplastic: angioimmunoblastic lymphadenopathy, lymphomatoid papulosis, malignant histiocytosis, mycosis fungoides, Waldenstrom's macroglobulinemia

other: drug hypersensitivity, gold administration, insect bite, Letterer-Siwe d., Loeffler's s., mastocytosis, NERD s., nodular fat necrosis, PSS, relapsing polychondritis, sarcoid, Sjögren's s., systemic nodular panniculitis (Weber-Christian),

vascular: allergic granulomatosis, angioedema, periarteritis nodosa, systemic mastocytosis, urticaria, vasculitis, Wegener's granulomatosis

estrogen receptors	giant nevi, dysplastic nevi, nevi of pregnancy
Ferriman & Gallwey scale	scale to measure hirsutism of a woman; 11 locations graded 1-4. Score of 8+ denotes hirsutism
Frei test	historic test for lymphogranuloma venereum
FTA-ABS	fluorescent treponemal antibody absorption; serological diagnostic test for syphilis
Goeckerman regime	coal tar followed by suberythermic UV light doses; psoriasis treatment
GVH d. scale; histopathology	**0**: normal epidermis or epidermal changes of other cutaneous disorders **1**: focal or diffuse vacuolar alteration of the basal cell layer **2**: dyskeratotic squamous cells in epidermis or hair follicle epithelium **3**: subepidermal cleft or microvesicle formation **4**: complete separation of the epidermis from the dermis
grattinage	light scraping & scratching which may reveal scaling
hair pull	gentle traction to 25 to 50 terminal scalp hairs; 2-3 shed hairs per pull is pathologic, anagen hairs are pathologic
hair window	shaving of hair, then patient returns 3 to 30 days later to evaluate regrowth
HGA elevation, urine	alkaptonuria
5-hydroxy-indoleacetic acid (5HIAA) excretion, urinary	acetanilid, chlorpromazine, glyccryl guaiacolate, Lugol's solution, mephenesin carbamate, methenamine, methocarbamol, methyldopa, monoamine oxidase inhibitors, phenacetin, phenothiazines, promazine, promethazine, reserpine
hydroxyproline	acetylcholinesterase, C1q, collagen, elastin, hyperthyroidism, Marfan's s. (increased amount in urine), sarcoidosis

Scales, Tests,and Techniques

hypercalcemia	hyperparathyroidism, sarcoidosis, subcutaneous fat necrosis of the newborn
hypercholesterolemia	familial, cyclosporine, lupus erythematosus
hyperglobulinemia	acrodermatitis chronica atrophicans, AIDS, anticonvulsants, asparaginase, pyoderma gangrenosum, dermatomyositis, DLE, EED, ethanol abuse, eosinophilic fasciitis, hydralazine, lepromatous leprosy, LE, MCTD, malnutrition, narcotics, necrobiotic xanthogranuloma, nodular vasculitis, oral contraceptives, pansclerotic morphea of children, parasitic infestations, phenytoin administration, phenylbutazone, sarcoidosis, Sjögren's s., SLE, Waldenstrom's macroglobulinemia, Wegener's granulomatosis
hyperlipidemia	familial, retinoid induced
hypocholesterolosis	glucagonoma, Tangier's d.
hypocomplementemia	serum sickness s.
hypoglobulinemia	chronic mucocutaneous candidiasis with thymoma, steroid, dextran, methotrexate, zinc deficiency, gluten-sensitive enteropathy
immune complexes	MCTD, PSS, Reiter's d., sarcoidosis
immunoglobulins	**IgE**: decreased; Louis-Bar s. increased; atopic dermatitis, erosive pustular folliculitis **IgA**: decreased; ataxia-telangiectasia, Louis-Bar s. **IgG**: decreased; ataxia-telangiectasia
Ingram method	coal tar bath, UVB & anthralin; psoriasis treatment
iron deficiency	*Candida* susceptibility, glossodynia, hair loss, perleche
Kveim test	historic test for sarcoidosis; intradermal injection of homogenized tissue from a patient with sarcoidosis
latex allergen solution preparation	1. Place 20 one cm^2 pieces of latex glove in 5 ml sterile saline 2. shake occasionally over 2 hour period 3. transfer to sterile container without rubber top 4. discard after 1 week
latex allergy testing	If step is −, continue; if step is +, discontinue 1. closed patch test with 1 cm piece of latex glove 20 minutes (or less if +) on forearm 2. cut out one finger of glove, place on finger for 20 minutes (or less if +) 3. wear whole glove for 20 minutes (or less if +) 4. prick test with latex allergen solution, use histamine & saline controls
leukocytosis	acne fulminans, cold urticaria, erysipelas, pustular bacterid of Andrews, Sweet's s.
leukopenia	plaquenil, generalized DLE, necrobiotic xanthogranuloma, sarcoidosis, serum sickness s., silver sulfadiazine
light chain diseases	massive cutaneous hyalinosis, nodular amyloidosis, primary amyloidosis
lupus anticoagulant	anticardiolipin antibody s.

Scales, Tests,and Techniques

lupus band test	unaffected (normal) skin biopsy for immunoreactants at dermal-epidermal junction; IgG, IgM, IgA (50% in SLE)
Lyme d. (false +)	infectious mononucleosis, RA, SBE, SLE, spirochetoses
lymphopenia	Louis-Bar s., Nezelof's s., sarcoidosis, severe combined immunodeficiency s.
M protein	POEMS s.
Maltese cross crystals	urine sediment shape; Fabry's d.
Mazotti test	hypersensitivity, severe pruritus, occasional anaphylaxis after treatment with diethylcarbamazine; onchocerciasis (diagnostic)
melanoma signs and history	**A:** asymmetric shape; **B:** border irregularity and scalloping; **C:** color mottling; brown, black, gray, red, white; **D:** diameter; **E:** elevation, enlargement (history of increase in size); **F:** family history
microhemagglutination (MHA-TP) test	serological diagnostic test for syphilis
monoclonal gammopathy	necrobiotic xanthogranuloma
Montenegro test	delayed-type hypersensitivity skin test; leishmaniasis

mycosis fungoides, staging

	T	N	M
IA:	T1	N0	M0
IB:	T2	N0	M0
IIA:	T1-2	N1	M0
IIB:	T3	N0-1	M0
III:	T4	N0-1	M0
IVA:	T1-4	N2	M0
IVB:	T1-4	N0-2	M1

mycosis fungoides, TNM classification	**cutaneous involvement** (T); **T0** lesion clinically and/or histologically suspicious but not diagnostic **T1** plaques involving 10% or < **T2** plaques involving > 10% **T3** tumors and/or ulcers **T4** erythroderma covering 70% or > **lymph nodes** (N); **N0** clinically and pathologically normal **N1** clinically enlarged but benign microscopically **N2** microscopically malignant **viscera** (M); **M0** no visceral involvement **M1** visceral involvement
National Psoriasis Foundation (NPF) psoriasis score	1) Assessment of induration of two target lesions at each visit Target lesion A rated 0 (clear) to 5 Target lesion B rated 0 (clear) to 5 2) Body Surface Area (BSA) covered with psoriasis Scoring = change in BSA *relative to baseline* expressed as a percent 0% = 0 and 100% = 5 (no improvement or worse) 3) Physician's global assessment = 0 (clear) to 5 4) Patient's global assessment = 0 (clear) to 5 5) Itching = 0 (clear) to 5 Added score = X / 30 possible points
natural killer cells	decreased; Cowden's s., Fanconi's anemia increased; cartilage hair hypoplasia
neutrophil chemotaxis, decreased	Chediak-Higashi s., hyperimmunoglobulin E s., lazy leukocyte s., Shwachman s., Wiskott-Aldrich s.,

Scales, Tests,and Techniques

neutrophilia	Sweet's s., Von Zambusch pustular psoriasis
neutropenia	necrobiotic xanthogranuloma, Schwachman's s., Wiskott-Aldrich s.

Overall Lesion Severity (OLS) scale for psoriasis	Score		Description
	0	Clear	Plaque = 0 (no elevation over normal skin) Scaling = 0 (no scale) Erythema = +/– (hyperpigmentation, pigmented macules, diffuse faint pink or red coloration)
	1	Minimal	Plaque = +/– (difficult to ascertain but possible elevation) Scaling = +/– (surface dryness with some white coloration) Erythema = up to moderate (up to definite red coloration)
	2	Mild	Plaque = slight (but definite, edges indistinct or sloped) Scaling = fine (partly or mostly covering lesions) Erythema = up to moderate (up to definite red coloration)
	3	Moderate	Plaque = moderate (elevation with rough or sloped edges) Scaling = coarser (covering most or all lesions) Erythema = moderate (definite red coloration)
	4	Severe	Plaque = marked (elevation with hard or sharp edges) Scaling = coarse (non-tenacious scale covers most or all lesions) Erythema = severe (bright red coloration)
	5	Very severe	Plaque = very marked (elevation with hard, sharp edges) Scaling = very coarse (thick, tenacious scale, rough surface over most or all lesions) Erythema = very severe (dusky to deep red coloration)

pancytopenia	Seckel's s., Zinsser-Cole-Engman s.
Papanicolaou smear	technique for detection of HPV induced cervical dysplasia or carcinoma AKA Pap smear
paper test	paper strip between tooth & marginal gingiva; lead or bismuth line persists above paper
paraproteinemia	amyloidosis, cold hemolysins, cryoglobulins, cryofibrinogens, EED, EM, necrobiotic xanthogranuloma, planar xanthoma, plasmacytoma, POEMS s., pyoderma gangrenosum, Schnitzler's s., scleredema, scleromyxedema, subcorneal pustular dermatosis, Sweet's s.
patch testing	?; doubtful reaction, faint macular erythema +; weak positive reaction- erythema, infiltration, possible papule ++; strong positive

Scales, Tests,and Techniques

	reaction; erythema, infiltration, papules, vesicles +++; extreme positive bullous reaction –; negative reaction IR; irritant reaction NT; not tested
phototrichogram	hair shaving with subsequent comparative photographs 3-5 days later
prolidase deficiency	annular erythema, atrophie blanche, eczematous eruptions, keratosis pilaris, leg ulcers, lymphedema, macular and papular lesions, photosensitivity, premature graying of hair, purpuric lesions, scar formation, simian crease, skin fragility, telangiectasias, xerosis
polyarteritis nodosa (ARA criteria)	1. Weight loss >/= 4 kg. 2. Livedo reticularis 3. Testicular pain or tenderness 4. Myalgia, weakness, or leg tenderness 5. Mononeuropathy or polyneuropathy 6. Diastolic BP > 90 mm Hg 7. Elevated BUN/creatinine 8. Hepatitis B virus 9. Arteriographic abnormality 10. Neutrophils on biopsy of small or medium sized artery

Psoriasis Area and Severity Index (PASI) scale (scale for erythema, thickness and scaling is 0–4; degree involvement = %)

		Head	Trunk	Upper Limbs	Lower Limbs
1	Erythema				
2	Thickness				
3	Scaling				
4	Total				
5	Degree involvement				
6	Multiply row 4 and row 5				
7		$\times 0.10$	$\times 0.30$	$\times 0.20$	$\times 0.20$
8	Multiply row 6 and row 7				
9	Total (add columns in 8)				

Physician Global Assessment (PGA) scale for psoriasis

	Improvement	
Cleared	100%	Remission of all clinical signs & symptoms compared to baseline, except for residual erythema, pigmentation
Excellent	75-99%	Improvement of all clinical signs & symptoms compared to baseline, except for residual erythema, pigmentation
Good	50-74%	Improvement of all clinical signs & symptoms compared to baseline
Fair	25-49%	Improvement of all clinical signs & symptoms compared to baseline
Slight	1-24%	Improvement of all clinical signs & symptoms compared to baseline
Unchanged		Clinical signs & symptoms unchanged from baseline
Worse		Clinical signs & symptoms deteriorated from baseline

Scales, Tests,and Techniques

Prausnitz-Kustner reaction test	test for physical urticaria
protein C deficiency	DIC, myeloma, purpura fulminans neonatorum
provocative use test (PUT)	screening for allergy to cosmetics; cosmetic applied BID up to 2 weeks to 5 cm area of antecubital forearm AKA repeat open application test (ROAT)
PRP classification	**I:** classic adult **II:** atypical adult **III:** classic juvenile **IV:** circumscribed juvenile **V:** atypical juvenile
psoralen dosing	
psoriasis, common lab abnormalities	anemia (mild), IgA (increased), α_2-macroglobulin (increased), C-reactive protein (increased), immunoglobulin aberrations, immune complexes (increased), nitrogen balance (negative), sedimentation rate (prolonged), uric acid (elevation)
rapid plasma reagin (RPR) test	a non-specific (non-treponemal) antibody test (for syphilis)
repeat open application test (ROAT)	screening for cosmetic allergy; cosmetic applied BID to 5 cm area of antecubital forearm up to 2 weeks AKA provocative use test (PUT)
rheumatoid factor +	dermatomyositis, PSS, Sjögren's s.
riboflavin deficiency	perleche
Ro antibody +	complement deficiency, lupus in Asians, late onset lupus, neonatal LE, Sjögren's s., SCLE, SLE, ANA negative SLE
Rumpel-Leede test	sign of capillary fragility; pressure (tourniquet) produces petechiae, seen in RMSF, scarlet fever AKA tourniquet test
salt-split skin	DIF performed on sodium chloride cleavage of skin along lamina lucida; in BP, IF is on the epidermal side, in EB, IF is on the dermal side
Schirmer test	measurement of wetness of filter paper strip pressed to conjunctiva, used in Sjögren's s.
Schwartzman reaction	intensified response in experimental animals to bacteria containing LPS or purified LPS
serologic test for syphilis (STS)	often (-) in primary syphilis, (+) in secondary syphilis, false negative may occur with HIV d.
skin types	**I:** sensitive, always burns easily, never tans, light pigment, red hair, freckled, Celtic, erythrodermic **II:** sensitive, burns easily, tans minimally, light pigment, blue eyed, Slavic, Germanic **III:** normal, burns moderately, tans gradually, darker pigmentation **IV:** normal, burns minimally, tans always, dark pigmentation, Mediterranean **V:** insensitive, rarely burns, tans profusely, dark pigmentation; Middle Eastern, Latin light African **VI:** insensitive, never burns, deeply pigmented, most dark pigmentation, dark Africans

psoralen dosing

Weight (Kg)	<30	30-50	51-65	66-80	81-90	91-115	>115
Weight (Lbs)	<65	65-100	101-145	146-175	176-200	201-250	>250
Dose (mg)	10	20	30	40	50	60	70

Scales, Tests,and Techniques

squash preparation	flattened, unstained biopsy tissue to observe viable micracidia in schistosomiasis
syphilis, test for	**non-specific**: VDRL (Venereal Disease Research Laboratory), RPR (rapid plasma reagin) **specific**: FTA-ABS (fluorescent treponemal antibody absorption), MHA-TP (microhemagglutination), TPI *Treponema pallidum* immobilization
T cells	**decreased helper** (serum): ataxia telangiectasia, DLE, HIV, malnutrition, MCTD, PUVA, sarcoidosis, vitiligo **increased helper** (lesional): alopecia areata, early lichen planus, Jessner's lymphocytic infiltrate, sarcoidosis, tuberculoid leprosy, ENL lesions, granuloma annulare, lymphomatoid granulomatosis **increased helper** (serum): Kawasaki's d.
T4/T8 ratio, decreased	AIDS, lepromatous leprosy, GVHD (chronic), pre-active Beçhet's d., rheumatoid arthritis (lymph nodes), sarcoidosis (serum elevation), sun tanning, hepatitis B, rhinoscleroma
thrombocytopenia	Albright's s., drugs (acetaminophen, allopurinol, chlorothiazide, digoxin, furosemide, gold salts, lidocaine, loxoscelism, methyldopa, penicillin, phenylbutazone, quinine, quinidine, rifampin, sulfonamides), kala-azar, Gaucher's s., Good's s., Hermansky-Pudlak s., qualitative defect, SLE with anticoagulant, TORCH s., toxic shock s., Wiskott-Aldrich s., Zinsser-Cole-Engman s.
Tine test	old tuberculin test
touch preparation	slide prepared from direct touch on involved skin
tourniquet test	see Rumpel-Leede test
toxic shock s., criteria	1. Fever >/= 38.9° 2. Diffuse macular erythema 3. Desquamation 1-2 weeks after onset 4. Hypotension 5. Three organ systems affected; GI (N/V), muscular (myalgia, elevated CPK), mucous membrane (conjunctival, oropharyngeal, vaginal hyperemia), renal (BUN/creatinine > twice normal, pyuria), hepatic (bilirubin, SGOT, SGPT > twice normal), hematologic (thrombocytopenia), neurologic (disorientation, altered consciousness, focal findings) 6. Absence of evidence of other cause of illness
Treponema pallidum immobilization (TPI) test	serological diagnostic test; syphilis
Tzanck prep	blisters unroofed, contents smeared on slide, dried, then stained with Sedi-stain giant cells seen histologically; herpes virus family acantholytic cells; pemphigoid
ulcer, decubitus grade	**1:** epidermal; blanchable erythema, minimal swelling and warmth, discrete border **2:** dermal; inflammation partial thickness skin loss; blistering, erythema, induration, abrasion, moist pink wound base, pain but no necrosis **3:** subcutaneous ulcer; exposed muscle, fat, tendons, down to fascia deep crater may be undermined, sinus tract, exudate, infection may be present **4:** beyond deep fascia, usually to bone full thickness loss with extensive necrosis and muscle, tendon, joint capsule damage, undermining, sinus tracts, exudate, infection

urticaria, physical (tests)	**aquagenic**: apply water compress at 35° C to upper body 30 minutes *positive*; pinpoint pruritic hives within 2-30 minutes. **cholinergic**: half immerse pt. in 42° bath to raise oral temperature 0.7° or more *positive*; pruritus, warmth, tingling, burning preceding onset of pinpoint wheals with large halos in 2-30 minutes alternative 1) exercise; does not distinguish from EIA, 2) methacholine skin challenge + in 33% of patients with cholinergic urticaria **delayed pressure**: 15 lb. weight across shoulder or thigh for 15 minutes *positive*; deep painful erythematous swelling at pressure site within 2 hours **dermatographism**: firm stroking of forearm or back with instrument *normal*; immediate blanching followed by red flare for 10 minutes *simple dermatographism*; linear wheal and flare, lasting 10-15 minutes *symptomatic dermatographism*; local pruritus with linear wheal and flare lasting _ to 3 hours **exercise**: treadmill for 5-10 minutes, consider food challenge *positive*; four phase response-fatigue, warmth, pruritus, erythema followed by urticaria and +/- respiratory/GI/CV abnormalities episodes are sporadic and may not be reproducible **solar**: expose 1 x 1 cm back/buttocks to light wavelengths at 10 cm for 10 minutes *positive*; pruritus, erythema, edema within minutes, followed by papule or wheal **vibration**: forearm stimulation with vortex for 4 minutes *positive*; local pruritus, erythema, edema within minutes

UVA dosing

Skin type	I	II	III	IV	V	VI
Initial dose (J/cm^2)	0.5	1.0	1.5	2.0	2.5	3.0
Increment (J/cm^2)	0.5	0.5	0.5-1.0	0.5-1.0	1.0-1.5	1.0-1.5

UVB dosing

Skin type	I	II	III	IV	V	VI
Initial dose (mJ/cm^2)	20	25	30	40	50	60
Increment (mJ/cm^2)	5	10	15	20	25	30

Vancouver burn scale	**height** (depression): normal (flat)=0, <2 mm=1, <5 mm=2, >5 mm=3 **pigmentation**: normal=0, hypopigmentation=1, hypopigmentation=2 **pliability**: normal=0, supple (flexible with minimal resistance)=1, yielding (giving way to pressure, moderate resistance but not solid scar mass)=2, firm (solid inflexible unit, resistant to manual pressure)=3, banding (rope like tissue, blanches with scar extension, does not limit ROM if at joint)=4, contracture (permanent shortening of scar producing deformity/distortion, limits ROM)=5 **vascularity**: normal=0, pink (slight increase in blood supply)=1, red (significant increase local blood supply=2, purple (excessive local blood supply)=3
VDRL (false +)	anticardiolipin antibody s., infectious mononucleosis, lepromatous leprosy, leptospirosis, Lyme d., malaria, relapsing fever, SLE
Venereal Disease Research Laboratory	(VDRL) a nonspecific (non-treponemal) antibody test; syphilis
Weil-Felix reaction	nonspecific test; epidemic typhus (*Rickettsia typhi*)

Scales, Tests, and Techniques

Wood's lamp exam

exam using 360 nm wavelength (long wave) UV light

infectious: *Pseudomonas*, *Corynebacterium minutissimum*-coral red (erythrasma), *Pityrosporum ovale* (tinea versicolor)-yellow-orange

nevus anemicus; becomes invisible

pigment: accentuates epidermal pigment, dermal pigment is not accentuated

tinea capitis: *M. canis*, *M. audouinii*, *M. ferrugineum*, *M. distortum*, *M. gypseum*-green

urine; PCT

skin; ash-leaf spots

miscellaneous: ephelides, melasma accentuation, "invisible" lichen planus

Signs and Symptoms and Associated Conditions

Signs/Symptoms	Conditions
abdominal pain	acanthosis nigricans, angioedema, Canada-Cronkhite s., carcinoid s., collagen vascular d., Crohn's d., Degos' d., dermatomyositis, Fabry's d., Gardner's s., Henoch-Schönlein purpura, herpes zoster, IBD, malignant atrophic papulosis, neurofibromatosis, Peutz-Jeghers s., porphyria (acute intermittent porphyria, ALA dehydratase deficiency porphyria, hereditary coproporphyria, variegate porphyria), ulcerative colitis, Whipple's d.
abscess, perirectal	chronic granulomatous d.
absent skin findings	*see invisible dermatoses*
achalasia	Rozychi's s.
acrocyanosis	familial dysautonomia, oxalic acid
acrodynia	mercury poisoning
acromegaly	acanthosis nigricans, coarse hair, cutis verticis gyrata, hyperpigmentation
acroosteolysis	distal phalangeal necrosis; acrodermatitis continua, Buerger's d., carpal tunnel s., cervical rib, diabetes, familial mandibulo-acral dysplasia, juvenile dermatomyositis, hypertrophic osteoarthropathy, leprosy, myelopathy, perniosis, polyvinyl chloride exposure, psoriatic arthritis, PSS, Raynaud's d., SLE, systematized mesodermal dysplasia, syringomyelia, systemic sclerosis, tabes dorsalis
adrenal atrophy	Siemerling-Creutzfeldt d.
adrenal failure	histoplasmosis, mucocutaneous candidiasis, paracoccidiodomycosis, tuberculosis, vitiligo
aged appearance	Cockayne's s., progeria
albopapuloid lesion	generalized dominant dystrophic epidermolysis bullosa (Pasini)
allergic shiners	allergic rhinitis, atopic dermatitis
alopecia	*see hair section*
anemia	ancylostomiasis, blue rubber bleb s., dermatomyositis, dermatitis herpetiformis, dyskeratosis congenita, erythroderma, erythrocytic porphyria, exfoliative dermatitis, Fabry d., Felty's s., glossitis, glucagonoma, Hallopeau-Siemens s., hookworm disease, hypothyroidism, kala-azar, Kawasaki d., koilonychia, Letterer-Siwe d., loxoscelism, lupus erythematosus, Osler-Weber-Rendu s., psoriasis, sarcoidosis, scleroderma, toxic epidermal necrolysis
anesthesia	NLD
angel's kiss	fading macular stain
angioedema	ACE inhibitors, adenocarcinoma, anti-C1INH autoantibodies, autoimmune, CLL, cryoglobulinemia (essential), cutaneous necrotizing venulitis, histiocytic lymphoma, non-Hodgkin's lymphoma, **idiopathic**, IgA myeloma, lymphosarcoma, lymphocytic lymphoma, monoclonal gammopathy, myelofibrosis, serum sickness, Waldenstrom's macroglobulinemia

Signs and Symptoms and Associated Conditions

Signs/Symptoms	Conditions
angioid streaks ("apples") of eyes	retinal change-tears in Bruch's membrane of eye; acromegaly, Cowden's d., Ehlers-Danlos s., hyperphosphatemia, intracranial disorders, lead poisoning, Paget's d., pituitary disorders, PXE, sickle cell anemia, trauma
anhidrosis	anhidrotic ectodermal dysplasia, anticholinergic drugs, atopic dermatitis, congenital ectodermal defect, diabetes mellitus, diabetic neuropathy, Fabry's d., Franceschetti-Jadassohn s., Guillain-Barre s., Helweg-Larssen s., idiopathic, miliaria profunda, multiple myeloma, myxedema, orthostatic hypotension, progressive segmental anhidrosis, quinacrine anhidrosis, Ross s., Sjögren's s., SLE, systemic sclerosis
annular	drug eruptions, erythema marginatum, LE, mycosis fungoides, secondary syphilis
annular with papules	dermatophytosis, erythema migrans, erythema multiforme, figurate erythemas, GA, LE, lichen planus, lupus vulgaris, mycosis fungoides, sarcoid, syphilis (secondary & tertiary), urticaria
annular with scales	dermatophytosis, pityriasis rosea, psoriasis, seborrheic dermatitis
anodontia	Christ-Siemens-Touraine s.
anorexia	Whipple's d.
anosmia	Kallmann's s.
anovulation	Stein-Leventhal s.
aortic stenosis	Williams s.
aphthae	Behçet's d., Crohn's d., dermatitis herpetiformis, gluten sensitive enteropathy, HIV, iron deficiency, regional enteritis, ulcerative colitis, vitamin B12 deficiency
aplasia, dermal	MIDAS s.
apple jelly color	red-brown plaque on diascopy; lupus vulgaris
arachnodactyly	Marfan s.
arrhythmias	phenol, Refsum's d.
arteriovenous fistulas	Klippel-Trenaunay-Weber s.
arteriovenous malformations	hereditary hemorrhagic telangiectasias (pulmonary), proteus s.
arthritis/arthralgias	**dermatologic**: acne conglobata, acne fulminans, allergic granulomatosis, benign cutaneous polyarteritis nodosa, cold urticaria, EED, erysipelas, erythema multiforme, erythema nodosum, Henoch-Schönlein purpura, hidradenitis suppurativa, ochronosis, Sweet's s. **infectious**: atypical mycobacteriosis, cellulitis, dengue, gonococcal arthritis, erythema infectiosum, hepatitis, Lyme d., metastatic gonorrhea, meningococcemia, mononucleosis, necrotizing fasciitis, Reiter's s., rheumatic fever, rubella (adults), schistosomiasis, sporotrichosis **systemic**: alkaptonuria, Behçet's d., cyclic neutropenia, dermatomyositis, gout, familial Mediterranean fever, familial cold urticaria,

Signs and Symptoms and Associated Conditions

Signs/Symptoms	Conditions
	familial hypertriglyceridemia (type V), glanders, gout, Haverhill fever, hemochromatosis, Henoch-Schönlein purpura, hypocomplementemic urticarial vasculitis s., juvenile rheumatoid arthritis, Katayama fever, Kawasaki's d., Lofgren's s., lupus erythematosus, lymphogranuloma venereum, lymphomatoid granulomatosis, mixed connective tissue d., morphea, Muckle-Wells s., multicentric reticulohistiocytosis, pancreatic fat necrosis, pansclerotic morphea of children, phytosterolemia, polyarteritis nodosa, post-cardiotomy s., pseudolymphoma, psoriatic arthritis, PSS, RA, Reiter's s., sarcoidosis, Schnitzler's s., self-healing juvenile cutaneous mucinosis, serum sickness, SLE, Stevens-Johnson s., Still's d., systemic nodular panniculitis (Christian-Weber d.), thrombotic thrombocytopenia purpura, Weber-Christian s., Wegener's granulomatosis, Werner's s., Whipple's d.
arthrogryposis	Johnston's s.
Asboe-Hansen sign	blister extension when pressure is applied to top of blister; pemphigus vulgaris
ash leaf spots	hypopigmented leaf-shaped macules; **1:** normal persons **2:** neurologic disorder **3** or more: tuberous sclerosis (70-90%)
asthma	atopy, Buckley's s., Churg-Strauss s.
ataxia	ataxia telangiectasia, biotin dependent carboxylase deficiency, Hartnup d., Louis-Bar s., multiple carboxylase deficiency, Refsum's d., Shapira's s., Wyburn-Mason's s.
atherosclerosis	progeria
athletes' nodules	fibrous tissue mass or cystic lesion from trauma AKA surfer's nodules
atrichia	*see hair section*
atrophie blanche	arteriosclerosis, connective tissue d., diabetes mellitus, dysproteinemia, hypertension, idiopathic, stasis dermatitis
atrophoderma, perifollicular	Bazex s., Conradi-Hunermann s., keratosis pilaris
atrophy	acrodermatitis chronica atrophicans, anetoderma, atrophoderma, atrophic LP, BCC (morphea-like), corticosteroid use, Cushing's d., dermatomyositis, DLE, LE, lichen sclerosis, morphea, necrobiosis lipoidica, radiodermatitis (chronic), sarcoid, scleroderma, striae
atrophy, dermal	Parry-Romberg s.
axillary freckling	LEOPARD s., Moynahan's s., **neurofibromatosis**, progeria, Watson's s. AKA Crowe's sign
bag of worms	appearance; angioma arteriole endothelioma, Dercum's d., plexiform neurofibroma
baker's itch	pruritus due to mite bites
balanitis	Reiter's s.
barber's pole umbilical cord	alternating red, blue, and white umbilical cord; congenital syphilis

Signs and Symptoms and Associated Conditions

Signs/Symptoms	Conditions
bath itch	water induced pruritus occurring after bathing or showering; hypereosinophilic s., myelodysplasia, **polycythemia vera**
beak nose	chronic granulomatous d., Hallermann-Streiff s., leishmaniasis, lupus vulgaris, pangeria (Werner's s.), sclerodermoid GVH d.
birth, lesions presenting at	acrogeria, acrokeratosis verruciformis, aggressive infantile fibromatosis, aplasia cutis, ash leaf macule, blue rubber bleb nevus s., congenital self-healing reticulohistiocytoma, congenital total lipodystrophy, cutis marmorata telangiectatica congenita, diffuse and macular atrophic dermatosis, endovascular papillary angioendothelioma of childhood (Dabska tumor), epidermolysis bullosa (Koebner), erythema toxicum neonatorum, fibrous hamartoma of infancy, fibromatosis colli, follicular atrophoderma, generalized congenital fibromatosis, hemangiomas, herpes gestationis, incontinentia pigmenti, infantile myofibromatosis, inflammatory linear verrucous epidermal nevus, infundibulofolliculitis, juvenile hyaline fibromatosis, juvenile xanthogranuloma, lymphangiomas of the alveolar ridges in neonates, mastocytoma, multiple lentigines s., nevus comedonicus, nevus lipomatosus cutaneous superficialis (Hoffman-Zurhelle), Peutz-Jeghers s., piebaldism, pili torti, pseudoainhum, self-healing reticulohistiocytosis, stiff skin s., smooth muscle hamartoma, transient neonatal pustular melanosis, verrucous nevus, Waardenburg's s., white forelock, white sponge nevus
birthmarks	albinism, aplasia cutis congenita, blue rubber bleb s., café au lait spots, cutis marmorata telangiectatica congenita, epidermal nevi, hemangiomas, hemangiomatosis, hypopigmentation, junctional nevocellular nevi, lymphangioma, Mongolian spot, nevocellular nevi, nevus comedicus, phenylketonuria, sebaceous nevi
black dot infection	tinea capitis
black dots, punctate	thrombosed dermal capillaries from transepithelial elimination seen after paring lesion; clots, connective tissue chromoblastomycosis, fungal elements, wart
black heel	shearing injury to heel AKA talon noir
black race, decreased incidence	pediculosis capitis, secondary anaphylactic reactions to insect stings
black race, increased incidence	acne keloidalis, AZT induced nail pigmentation, adult T cell leukemia/lymphoma, alveolar ridge lymphangioma in neonates, disseminated infundibulofolliculitis, focal acral hyperkeratosis, follicular eczema, infantile acropustulosis, lipedematous alopecia, Kawasaki's s., keratotic papules of palmar creases, Mal de Meleda s., mucinous carcinoma, mycosis fungoides, oral melanoacanthoma, papillary eccrine adenoma, papular pityriasis rosea, penile thromboses, proximal trichorrhexis nodosa, pseudofolliculitis barbae, sarcoidosis, Sezary's s., sinus histiocytosis with massive lymphadenopathy, tinea capitis, transient neonatal pustular melanosis, verrucous sarcoidosis

Signs and Symptoms and Associated Conditions

Signs/Symptoms	Conditions
black toe	shearing sports injury to distal (usually 2nd) toe
blepharitis	atopic dermatitis, contact dermatitis, EEC s., psoriasis, rosacea, seborrheic dermatitis
blepharochalasis	Ascher's s.
blindness	cicatricial pemphigoid, onchocerciasis
bloodhound appearance	premature aged hanging skin folds; cutis laxa
blue dermal lesions	BCC, cylindroma, eccrine spiradenoma, desmoplastic trichoepithelioma, hidradenoma papilliferum, infantile neuroblastoma, sudoriparous angioma
blue sclera	agyria, Ehlers-Danlos (Type I and VII, A, B, and C), incontinentia pigmenti, osteogenesis imperfecta (type I and II in children), pseudoxanthoma elasticum (40%), Russell-Silver s.
blue toes	anticardiolipin antibody s., antiphospholipid s., atheromatous emboli, connective tissue d., malignancy, polyarteritis, polycythemia, Raynaud's d, thrombocytosis, vasculitis
blueberry muffin lesion	petechiae & ecchymoses of newborns; AIDS, congenital CMV inclusion disease, congenital leukemia, congenital rubella, congenital toxoplasmosis, congenital varicella
bombshell eruption	large central papule surrounded by smaller satellite papules; secondary syphilis
bone cysts	basal cell nevus s., keratosis follicularis (Darier's d.), neurofibromatosis, tuberous sclerosis
bone lesions	Letterer-Siwe d., Hand-Schüller-Christian d., syphilis
bone pain	histiocytosis X, mastocytosis, metastatic melanoma
bossing, frontal	basal cell nevus s., congenital lues, prolidase deficiency, Rothmund-Thomson s.
bottlenose	sign of alcoholic liver d.
brachydactyly	Nicolaides-Baraitser s.
breakfast, lunch, and dinner	three lesions in a row; bedbug bites
bronzing of skin	Elejalde s. (after sun exposure), tuberous sclerosis
buboes	enlarged inguinal lymph nodes; chancroid
bullae, dermoepidermal	**dermolytic**: dermatitis herpetiformis, epidermolysis bullosa acquisita, epidermolysis bullosa dystrophicans, porphyria cutanea tarda **junctional**: bullous pemphigoid, junctional epidermolysis bullosa
bullae, flaccid	bullous EM, DH, EB, PCT, pemphigus foliaceus, pemphigus vulgaris
bullae, hands and feet	arthropod bites, BP, bullous fixed drug, bullous LP, contact, DLE, EB, EM, hand foot and mouth d., herpetic whitlow, hydroa, PCT, photoallergic, phytophotodermatitis, PMLE, Sweet's s., tinea, Weber-Cockayne s.

Signs and Symptoms and Associated Conditions

Signs/Symptoms	Conditions
bullae, intraepidermal	**basal**: epidermolysis bullosa simplex, erythema multiforme, lichen planus, lupus erythematosus **granular layer**: bullous impetigo, friction blister, pemphigus foliaceus, SSSS, subcorneal pustular dermatosis **spinous layer**: eczematous dermatitis, herpesvirus, pemphigus (familial benign) **suprabasal**: Darier's d., pemphigus vulgaris
bullae, neonatal	acrodermatitis enteropathica, bullous congenital ichthyosiform erythroderma, bullous impetigo, bullous pemphigoid, epidermolysis bullosa, incontinentia pigmenti, urticaria pigmentosa
bullae, tense	EBA, herpes gestationis, pemphigoid
bulldog jaw	mandibular protuberance; late congenital syphilis
burning skin sensation	causalgia, dermatitis herpetiformis, epidermolysis bullosa, erythema chronicum migrans, erythropoietic protoporphyria, familial cold urticaria, glossodynia, heat urticaria, Hodgkin's d., hydroa estivale, meralgia paresthetica, pellagra, perioral candidiasis, phototoxicity, phytodermatitis, reflex sympathetic dystrophy (causalgia), vulvodynia
burns; lesions arising in	BCC, malignant fibrous histiocytoma, SCC
burrow	scabies (pathognomonic)
butterfly configuration	postinflammatory hyperpigmentation sparing the mid back; hepatobiliary disease
butterfly rash	erythema of nose & cheeks in butterfly shape; Bloom's s., bromoderma, complement deficiency, dermatomyositis, erythema infectiosum, GVH, homocystinuria, pellagra, pemphigus erythematosus, seborrheic dermatitis, **SLE**, Sweet's s.
button hole sign	invagination of lesion with pressure; neurofibroma
café-au-lait macules	sharply defined brown macules; Albright's s., ataxia-telangiectasia, Bannayan-Zonana s., basal cell nevus s., Bloom's s., Cowden's s., dyskeratosis congenita, epidermal nevus s., Fanconi's s., Gaucher's s., Hunter's s., juvenile xanthogranuloma, Leschke's d., Louis-Bar s., McCune-Albright s., multiple lentigines s., **neurofibromatosis**, nevus spilus, normal persons, Russell-Silver s., Ruvalcaba-Myhre-Smith s., Tay's s., tuberous sclerosis, Turner's s., von Hippel-Lindau d., Watson's s., Westerhof's s.
calcification/calcinosis	calciphylaxis, CREST, dermatomyositis (15% adults, 50% children), Down s., Ehlers-Danlos s., hypervitaminosis D, infection, IV calcium infusion milk-alkali s., neoplasms, nevoid basal cell s., panniculitis, PCT, PSS, PXE, Rothmund-Thomson s., sarcoidosis, SLE, subepidermal calcified nodule, trauma, Werner's s.
calcinosis	COPS s., CREST s., dermatomyositis, scleroderma
candidiasis	*see under Eponyms and Syndromes*
capillary malformations	proteus s.
caput medusae ***	dilated periumbilical veins secondary to portal hypertension; alcoholism

Signs and Symptoms and Associated Conditions

Signs/Symptoms	Conditions
cardinal signs of inflammation	dolor (pain), calor (heat), rubor (erythema), tumor (swelling), & functio laesa (loss of function)
cardiomyopathy	Fabry d., Hermansky-Pudlak s., hypereosinophilic s., LEOPARD s.
cardiopulmonary d.	amyloidosis, collagen vascular d., cystic fibrosis, LE, LEOPARD s., lipoid proteinosis, lymphomatoid granulomatosis, multicentric reticulohistiocytosis, PXE, relapsing polychondritis, RA, sarcoidosis, scleroderma, SLE, yellow nail s.
cardiovascular d.	Kawasaki d., Lyme borreliosis, Marfan's s., Reiter's s., syphilis
carotenemia	anorexia nervosa, diabetes mellitus, hepatic disease, hypothyroidism, hypopituitarism, inborn errors of metabolism
carp's mouth	narrowed mouth width; de Lange s., Plummer-Vinson s.
cartilage inflammation	MAGIC s.
cat bite sign	osteochondritis of medial proximal tibial metaphysis; congenital syphilis AKA Wimberger sign
cataracts	Albright's s., atopic dermatitis (8%, usually posterior & shield shaped), Behçet's d., cerebrotendinous xanthomatosis, congenital rubella, Christ-Siemens-Touraine s., Clouston's s., Cockayne's s., Conradi's s., Cross-McKusick-Breen s., DeBarsy's s., Fabry's d., Hallermann-Streiff s., hidrotic ectodermal dysplasia, incontinentia pigmenti, Marinesco-Sjögren s., nail-patella s., pachyonychia congenita, pangeria, Rothmund-Thomson s., thymic hypoplasia (DiGeorge s.), thymoma with immunodeficiency, Werner's s., Wiskott-Aldrich s.
cayenne pepper spots	minute red petechiae on lesion borders; Schamberg's d.
ceruloderma	drugs, Mongolian spot, nevus of Ota
chagasids	morbilliform or erythema marginatum-like eruption; acute phase of Chagas d.
chagoma	erythematous subcutaneous nodule; Chagas d.
chancre	painless ulcer; primary syphilis
cheilosis	Candida, riboflavin deficiency
chelitis	AK, Bloom's s., contact chelitis, factitial chelitis, Gamborg-Nielson PPK, granulomatosis chelitis, necrotizing sialometaplasia, plasma cell chelitis, Plummer-Vinson s.
chicken skin	*see peau d'orange*
Christmas tree pattern	papules & plaques following skin tension lines on the back; erythema dyschromicum perstans, KS, lichen planus, lichenoid reaction, pityriasis lichenoides, **pityriasis rosea**, syphilis (secondary)
cigarette paper skin	epidermal & dermal atrophy; acrodermatitis chronica atrophicans, Ehlers-Danlos s., parapsoriasis (large plaque), mycosis fungoides (patch stage)
claw hand	leprosy

Signs and Symptoms and Associated Conditions

Signs/Symptoms	Conditions
cleft lip/palate	EEC s., popliteal web s., Rapp-Hodgkin s.
clinodactyly	nail-patella s.
CNS calcification	BCC s., lipoid proteinosis, Papillon-Lefevre s., toxoplasmosis, tuberous sclerosis
coast of California	smooth bordered café-au-lait spots; neurofibromatosis
coast of Maine	jagged pigmented café-au-lait spots, may be dermatomal; McCune-Albright s.
cobblestone knuckles	hyperkeratosis; Unna-Thost d.
cobblestone papules, mouth	Darier's d.
cobblestone skin	appearance; Crohn's d., Cowden d., Darier's d., lichen amyloidosis, lipoid proteinosis, MEN IIb, tuberous sclerosis
cold agglutinins	acrocyanosis, elderly, gangrene, Raynaud's
colic	Peutz-Jeghers s.
collarette	peripheral lesional scale; EAC, mycoses (superficial), pityriasis rosea, PLC, syphilis (secondary)
collarette, necrolytic	pemphigus foliaceus
collodion membrane	Gaucher's d., ichthyosis (**congenital erythrodermic** [67%], lamellar recessive), Johnston's s., Netherton's s., self-healing collodion baby, trichothiodystrophy
condyloma lata	moist verrucous genital plaques; secondary syphilis
confetti macules	chemical leukoderma, tuberous sclerosis, vitiligo, leukoderma punctatum, tinea versicolor, IGH, photoaging
congestive heart failure	progeria
conjunctivitis & conjunctival involvement	actinic prurigo, Behçet's d., bullous dyskeratosis congenita, cat scratch d., cicatricial pemphigoid, erythema multiforme, erythema nodosum, Fabry d., iodides, Kawasaki's s., lamellar ichthyosis, LP, Lyme d., molluscum contagiosum, moth dermatitis, psoriatic arthritis, Reiter's s., rosacea, sarcoidosis, Sweet's s., trichinosis, Wegener's granulomatosis, X-linked aggamaglobulinemia, Zinsser-Cole-Engman s.
cool skin	arterial insufficiency, hypothyroidism, venous stasis
copper colored papules	secondary syphilis
copra itch	pruritus due to mite bites
corn flake sign	flaking keratinous papules; legs in Flegel's d.
cornea, clouding	chlorpromazine, Tangiers' d.
cornea, dystrophy	anhidrotic ectodermal dysplasia, angiokeratoma corporis diffusum, Darier's d., epidermolysis bullosa of the polydysplastic type, Hurler's s., keratosis follicularis spinulosa, non-bullous ichthyosiform erythroderma, PRP, Rothmund-Thomson s., xeroderma pigmentosum

Signs and Symptoms and Associated Conditions

Signs/Symptoms	Conditions
cornea, erosion	cicatricial pemphigoid, DEB (Hallopeau-Siemens), DEB-inversa
cornea, opacities	antimalarials, chlorpromazine, cicatricial pemphigoid, Fabry's d., Lawrence-Seip d., lepromatous leprosy, Morquio's s., mucopolysaccharidoses, Richner-Hanhart s., PUVA, prolidase deficiency, Winchester s., xeroderma pigmentosa, X-linked ichthyosis
coup de sabre	linear, atrophic depression of central forehead; scleroderma
cracked skin	fine desquamation with cracking along natural skin lines; kwashiorkor
crazy paving dermatitis	erosive, peeling skin; kwashiorkor
crust, honey-colored	thick, dried fluid; eczematous dermatitis, impetigo
crust, varnish-like	dried exudate; bullous impetigo
cryptorchidism	Cockayne's s., popliteal pterygium s., Tay's d., X-linked ichthyosis
cutaneous horn	AK, basal cell epithelioma, granular cell tumor, Kaposi's sarcoma, KA, renal carcinoma (metastatic), sebaceous carcinoma, SCC, SK, trichilemmal keratosis, verrucae vulgaris
cutis laxa	loose, redundant skin; amyloidosis, cutis laxa s., DeBarsy's s., geroderma osteodysplastica, Patterson's s., plasma cell dyscrasias, PXE, SCARF s., wrinkly skin s.
cutis marmorata	physiologic reaction to cold exposure; Cushing's s., de Lange s., Down s., normal persons (children), trisomy 18
cutis verticis gyrata	acromegaly, amyloidosis
cysts, multiple	basal cell nevus s., congenital leukonychia, Dowling-Degos d., Gardner's d., hexachlorobenzene-induced PCT, steatocystoma multiplex
deafness	knuckle pads, pili torti, relapsing polychondritis **congenital**: albinism, Alezzandrini's s., BADS s., Bart-Pumphrey s., Björnstad's s., Cockayne's s., congenital lues, congenital rubella, congenital syphilis, Crandall's s., ectodermal dysplasia, Fisch's s., HID s., hypomelanosis of ITO, JEB-progressiva, KID s., LEOPARD s., Marfan's s., Morquio's s., Moynahan s., Muckle-Wells s., multiple lentigines s., osteogenesis imperfecta, palmoplantar keratoderma (AD), Pallister-Killian s., Ramsay-Hunt s., Refsum's d., Rozychi's s., Tietze's s., TORCH s., Waardenburg's s., Wegener's s., Woolf's s., xeroderma pigmentosum, Ziprowski-Margolis s.
death, premature	Proteus s., Sanfilippo's s., SCIDs, Siemerling-Creutzfeldt d., xeroderma pigmentosa
delirium	erysipelas
dell	central depression in papule; anetoderma, lichen sclerosis, molluscum contagiosum, sebaceous hyperplasia
dermal thinning	Cushing's s.
dermatoglyphic absence	Rapp-Hodgkin s.
dermographism	urticaria due to physical allergy—response to firm stroking with dull instrument; hypereosinophilic s. (>75%), mastocytosis, NERD s., normal persons, urticaria

Signs and Symptoms and Associated Conditions

Signs/Symptoms	Conditions
dermographism, white	blanch at sites of stroking; atopic dermatitis, GVHD
desquamation	dermatophyte infection, GVHD, ichthyosis, Kawasaki d., kwashiorkor, PR, syphilis, SSSS, TEN, vitamin A deficiency, vitamin A toxicity
desquamation, latent	scale that appears only after scratching; parapsoriasis, psoriasis, PR (early), tinea versicolor
dew drop on a rose petal	vesicle on pink base; varicella (chickenpox)
diaphoresis, nocturnal	acromegaly, carcinoid s., diabetes mellitus, lymphoma, vasculitis
diarrhea	acrodermatitis enteropathica, carcinoid s., chronic granulomatous d., dermatitis herpetiformis, Leiner's d., lymphopenic agammaglobulinemia, mastocytosis, Nezelof's s., runting s., SCIDS, Whipple's d.
digitate dermatosis	fingerprint shape yellowish patches on trunk; SPP
dimple sign	lateral pressure results in depression; dermatofibroma
dirty appearance	skin (especially nuchal) appears dirt covered; Darier's d., ichthyosis
dollar paper markings	minute telangiectasia similar to paper money fibers; chronic liver d.
drumstick fingers	finger shape with wider proximal portion; Fischer-Jacobsen-Clouston s.
dryness	aged skin, atropine-like drugs, cholesterol reducing drugs, chronic nephritis, ichthyosis, myxedema, niacin, retinoids
dwarfism	de Lange s., Moynahan's s., trichomegaly
dysphagia	acanthosis nigricans, Behçet's s., bullous pemphigoid, celiac d., Darier's d., DEB, dermatitis herpetiformis, dermatomyositis, lichen planus, Plummer-Vinson s., PSS, PV, Steven-Johnson s., systemic sclerosis, tylosis
ear nodules	chondrodermatitis nodularis chronica helices, collagenous papules of the aural conchae, elastotic nodules of the antihelix, multicentric reticulohistiocytosis, Unverricht's s.
ear pit	preauricular cyst
earlobe creases	risk factor for cardiovascular death (1.5x)
ecchymoses	actinic purpura, amyloidosis, anticoagulants, benign hypergammaglobulinemic purpura, Cushing's s., DIC, Ehlers-Danlos s., glucocorticoid use, Hermansky-Pudlak s., hemophilia, hepatic insufficiency, psychogenic purpura, PXE, scurvy, vitamin K deficiency
eclabion	Neu-Laxova s.
ectopia lentis	homocystinuria, Marfan's s.
ectropion	Neu-Laxova s., Rapp-Hodgkin s.
edema, eyelid	aldosteronism, dermatomyositis, MEN 3 (nodular swelling) trichinosis, urticaria
edema, facial	Melkersson's s.
edema, hands & feet	NERD s.

Signs and Symptoms and Associated Conditions

Signs/Symptoms	Conditions
edema, periorbital	Chagas' d., trichinosis
elderly	**actinic**: photoaging, cutis rhomboidalis nuchae, solar lentigo, Favre-Racouchot d., solar purpura, venous lakes, stellate scars, radiodermatitis **autoimmune**: amyloidosis, cryoglobulinemia, dermatomyositis, giant cell arteritis, hypersensitivity vasculitis, LE, livedo reticularis, morphea, pemphigus vulgaris, progressive psoriatic arthritis, sarcoidosis, systemic sclerosis, Wegener's granulomatosis **eczema**: nummular, gravitational, asteatotic, lichen simplex chronicus, atopic, auto-sensitization, prurigo nodularis **feet**: bunions, calluses, clavi, corns, onychauxis, onychocryptosis, onycholysis, onychogryphosis, onychophosis, subungual exostosis **infections**: acrodermatitis chronica obliterans, Candida, dermatophyte, cellulitis, herpes simplex, herpes zoster, pyoderma **lymphoma**: CTCL, cutaneous B cell lymphoma, leukemia cutis, multiple myeloma, macroglobulinemia, parapsoriasis en plaque, Sezary s. **mucous membranes**: cheilitis, perleche, leukoplakia, oral cancer **nails**: dystrophy **neoplasia, benign**: acrochordons, cherry angioma, clear cell acanthoma, colloid millium, cutaneous horns, fibroepithelioma, KA, sebaceous adenoma, seborrheic keratosis **neoplasia**: actinic keratoses, angiosarcoma, BCC, Bowen's d., cutaneous metastases, melanoma (desmoplastic, lentigo maligna, nodular, superficial spreading), lentigo maligna, Merkel cell carcinoma, Paget's d., SCC
en coup de sabre	forehead lesion; linear scleroderma
enamel paint spot	darkened plaques; kwashiorkor
enchondromatosis	Maffucci's s.
endocrine abnormalities	Carney's s., POEMS s.
ephelides	NAME s.
epicanthal fold	Down s., Dubokowitz's s., Klinefelter's s., Turner's s.
epidermal translucency	Cushing's s.
epiphora	Rapp-Hodgkin s.
epistaxis	glanders, hereditary hemorrhagic telangiectasia, Henoch-Schönlein purpura, Hermansky-Pudlak s., idiopathic thrombocytopenic purpura, kala-azar, Lucio's phenomenon, polyarteritis nodosa, polycythemia rubra vera, PXE, SLE, systemic mastocytosis, universal telangiectasia, Waldenstrom's macroglobulinemia, Wegener's granulomatosis
erythroderma	**dermatologic**: actinic reticuloid, airborne contact dermatitis, atopic dermatitis, candidiasis, contact dermatitis (generalized), crusted scabies, hypereosinophilic s., ichthyosis, Leiner's d., lichen planus, LE, mastocytosis, nummular eczema, peeling skin s., pemphigus foliaceus, phytophotodermatitis, PRP, **psoriasis** (20%), Reiter's d., scalded skin s., seborrheic dermatitis, stasis dermatitis

Signs and Symptoms and Associated Conditions

Signs/Symptoms	Conditions
	neoplastic: carcinoma (colon, lung, liver, pancreas, prostate, stomach, thyroid), CTCL, Hodgkin's d., lymphoma (30%), mycosis fungoides, Sezary s., T-cell leukemia, T-cell lymphoma **systemic**: complement deficiency, dermatomyositis, erythrodermic mastocytosis, sarcoidosis **other**: GVH disease, drug reactions
erythroderma, exfoliative	**skin disease**: atopic dermatitis, chronic actinic dermatitis, contact dermatitis, CTCL, dermatophytosis, drug allergy, Hailey-Hailey d., ichthyosis (hereditary), LE, Leiner's d., lichen planus, mycosis fungoides, pemphigoid, pemphigus foliaceus, pityriasis rubra pilaris, psoriasis, Reiter's s., Sarcoid, seborrheic dermatitis, SSSS, stasis dermatitis **systemic disease**: AML, CML, fallopian tube carcinoma, GVH d., HIV infection, lung carcinoma, lymphoma, multiple myeloma, rectal carcinoma, reticulum cell sarcoma
erythroderma, neonatal	Chanarin-Dorfman s., infantile atopic dermatitis, Netherton's s.,
esophageal abnormality	CREST s., PACK s., PSS
esophageal cancer	arsenic, Plummer-Vinson s., tylosis
esophageal strictures	Zinsser-Cole-Engman s.
ethnic groups	**American Indians**: actinic prurigo, cutaneous diphtheria, oral focal epithelial hyperplasia (Heck's s.), PMLE **Amish**: Ellis van Creveld s., yellow mutant albinism **Asian**: macular amyloidosis, Kawasaki d. **Canadian Indians**: PMLE (lip involvement) **Chinese**: lichen amyloidosis **Dutch**: Hermansky-Pudlak s. **French Canadian**: Clouston's hidrotic ectodermal dysplasia **Hispanic**: lichen planus pigmentosis, melasma **Japanese**: Behçet's d., congenital onychodysplasia of the index finger, HTLV-1, lipodystrophia centrifugalis abdominalis infantalis, Rieh's melanosis, syringomas **Jews (Ashkenazi)**: Bloom's s., distinctive exudative discoid & lichenoid dermatitis (oid-oid), familial Mediterranean fever, Gaucher's d., Niemann Pick d., pemphigus foliaceus, pemphigus vulgaris, Riley-Day s., thromboangiitis obliterans, vitiligo, Ziprokowski-Margolis s. **Mediterranean**: Chanarin-Dorfman s., KS (classic) **Middle Eastern**: Behçet's d.. Chanarin-Dorfman s., macular amyloidosis **Puerto Rican**: Hermansky-Pudlak s. **South American**: macular amyloidosis **South African**: pseudomonilethrix
excoriation	atopy, contact dermatitis, DH, infestations, neurodermatitis, stasis dermatitis
exfoliation, palmar	Kawasaki d., scarlet fever, TSS
exophthalmos	Hand-Schüller-Christian d., hyperthyroidism, Langerhan's cell histiocytosis, rhinoscleroma

Signs and Symptoms and Associated Conditions

Signs/Symptoms	Conditions
expressionless appearance	panhypopituitarism, scleredema, scleroderma
eyelid lesions	multiple clear cell hidradenomas, primary mucinous carcinoma of the skin, sebaceous carcinoma, signet ring cell carcinoma, syringomas
facial abnormalities	Ambras s., Bloom's s., cardio-facio-cutaneous s., DiGeorge s., Gorlin's s., Hallermann-Streiff s., Neu-Laxova s., Pallister-Killian s., Rubinstein-Taybi s., Russell-Silver s., Ruvalcaba-Myhre-Smith s., Sotos' s., PIBIDS s., Williams s.
facial palsy/paralysis	Heerfordt s., Melkersson-Rosenthal s., mycosis fungoides, Melkersson's s., Ramsay-Hunt s.
failure to thrive	chronic granulomatous d., homocystinuria, Leiner's d., Netherton's s., Omenn's s., Partingtons s., SCIDs
feet	black heel, black toe, callous, clavus, contact dermatitis, digital fibromatosis, eccrine poroma, hyperkeratosis plantaris, infantile digital fibroma, mal perforans, myxoid cyst, piezogenic papules, pitted keratolysis, pompholyx, PPK, pustulosis plantaris, pyoderma, tinea pedis, verrucae
fertility abnormalities	IBIDS s.
fever	acne fulminans, carbuncle, cold urticaria, cytophagic histiocytic panniculitis, dermatomyositis, erythema nodosum, erythema multiforme, familial Mediterranean fever, familial cold urticaria, LE, Lofgren's s., lymphomatoid granulomatosis, malignant histiocytosis, Muckle-Wells s., pustular psoriasis, of Reiter's d. (arthritis), sarcoidosis, Schnitzler's s., serum sickness s., Stevens-Johnson s., Sweet's s., systemic nodular panniculitis, TEN, toxic shock s., ulceronecrotic PLEVA, Weber-Christian d., Whipple's d.
fever and rash, child	dengue, dermatomyositis, erysipelas, gonococcemia, Henoch-Schönlein purpura, hepatitis (acute), hypersensitivity vasculitis, juvenile RA, Kawasaki's d., leptospirosis, Lyme d., meningococcemia, mononucleosis, rheumatic fever, RMSF, scarlet fever, SLE, Still's d., SSSS, viral exanthem
figurate erythema	annular erythema of infancy, annular urticaria, bullous pemphigoid, chronic granulomatous d. (carrier mothers),erythema annulare centrifugum, erythema gyratum repens, erythema marginatum, erythema migrans, erythema multiforme, familial annular erythema, LE (annular), mycosis fungoides, necrolytic migratory erythema, psoriasis (annular), tinea
fingerpad infarcts	scleroderma, SLE
fish-mouth wound healing	Ehlers-Danlos s.
fistulas	amebiasis, chronic granulomatous d., Crohn's d., LGV, lobomycosis, nevus comedonicus, scrofuloderma, sporotrichosis, tuberculosis fistulosa subcutanea
flag sign	bands of light & dark dyspigmented hair; kwashiorkor

Signs and Symptoms and Associated Conditions

Signs/Symptoms	Conditions
flaky paint dermatitis	erosion & peeling skin; kwashiorkor
fleur de lis nose	flattened nasal bridge; congenital syphilis AKA saddle nose
flushing	alcoholism, anxiety, blushing, cancer (bronchus, pancreas, renal, small bowel, stomach, teratoma, thyroid), carcinoid s., cardiopulmonary d., cholinergic erythema, disulfiram-like medications, drugs, emotional, foods, harlequin s. (unilateral), horseshoe kidneys (Rovsing's s.), hyperthermia, leukemia (basophilic chronic granulocytic), male hypogonadism, mastocytosis, menopause, migraine headaches, Parkinson's d., pheochromocytoma, rosacea, spinal cord lesions
formication	sensation like bugs crawling across skin; delusions of parasitosis
freckling, axillary	neurofibromatosis AKA Crowe's sign
frog spawn	clustered vesicles; lymphangioma circumscriptum
fugitive swellings	see Calabar swellings
gangrene, digital	arteriosclerosis obliterans, atheromatous embolism, RA, Raynaud's d.
genital abnormalities	LEOPARD s., Moynahan's s.
genital ulceration	chancroid, eosinophilic granuloma of bone, fusospirillary infection (erosive balanitis), Hand-Schüller-Christian d., herpes simplex, leukemia cutis, primary histoplasmosis, syphilis
genital, female	allergic contact dermatitis, aphthae, bullous erythema multiforme, Candida vulvitis, Candida vulvovaginitis, chancres, chancroid, cicatricial pemphigoid, Crohn's d., cysts, eczema, fixed drug eruption, granuloma inguinale, HSV, hidradenitis suppurativa, irritant contact dermatitis, lichen planus, lichen sclerosis, Paget's d., pemphigus vulgaris, pruritus vulvae, psoriasis SCC, syringoma, vulvar fissure, vulvodynia, verrucae
genital, male	acquired nevomelanocytic nevi, acrochordon, fibroepithelial polyp, acute scrotum, allergic contact dermatitis, amebiasis, amyloidosis, angiokeratoma, aphthosis, atopic dermatitis, bacterial infection, balanitis, balanoposthitis, BCC, Becker's nevus, Behçet's d., benign epidermal tumor, benign penile melanosis, benign penile lentiginosis, cicatricial pemphigoid, contact urticaria, cutaneous larva migrans, CTCL, dartoic leiomyoma, ecthyma gangrenosum, ectopic sebaceous glands, edema, epithelioid hemangioendothelioma, erythema multiforme, erythrasma, extramammary Paget's d., fixed drug eruption, Fournier's gangrene, fungal infection, genital verrucous carcinoma, glomangioma, glomus tumor, granular cell tumor, herpes simplex, hidradenitis suppurativa, human papillomavirus, idiopathic calcinosis of scrotum, idiopathic pain, irritant contact dermatitis, juvenile xanthogranuloma, Kaposi's sarcoma, leiomyosarcoma, rhabdomyosarcoma, lichen nitidus, lichen planus, lichen sclerosis lichen simplex, lymphangioma circumscriptum, lymphatic filariasis, malignant fibrous histiocytoma, malignant melanoma, molluscum contagiosum, neurilemmoma, neurofibroma, pediculosis pubis, pemphigus vulgaris, Peyronie's d., phimosis, paraphimosis, pityriasis

Signs and Symptoms and Associated Conditions

Signs/Symptoms	Conditions
	rosea, priapism, pruritus ani, micaceous balanitis of Civatte, psoriasis vulgaris, Reiter's s., sarcoma, scabies, schistosomiasis, sclerosing lymphangitis, scrotal cyst, seborrheic dermatitis, seborrheic keratoses, SCC, squamous intraepithelial lesion, syringoma, trichomycosis pubis, tuberculosis, varicella-zoster virus, verruciform xanthoma, vitiligo
gigantism	Beckwith-Wiedemann s., EMG s.
gingival hypertrophy	Cross-McKusick-Breen s., dilantin, Zimmerman-Laband s.
glaucoma	cutis marmorata telangiectatica congenita
glistening dots	retinoscopic finding; Sjogren-Larsson's s.
glossitis	*see mouth & mucous membrane section*
goose flesh, permanent	hard nodules around hair follicles; starvation
goose skin	prickled skin; pellagra
grained leather	yellow to tan lichenified plaques; infiltrative mastocytosis
gray patch	discrete, gray, lusterless hair; tinea capitis
gray skin	chlorpromazine administration
grocer's itch	pruritus due to mite bites
groove sign	groove between two muscle bundles; eosinophilic fasciitis
growth, increased	acromegaly, Berardinelli's s., Marfan's s., total lipodystrophy
growth, stunted	AEC s., Albright's s., autosomal recessive cutis laxa, BIDS s., Bloom's s., cardio-facio-cutaneous s., Cockayne's s., DeBarsy's s., De Sanctis-Cacchione s., dominant dystrophic epidermolysis bullosa, (Cockayne-Touraine), dystrophic epidermolysis bullosa (Albopapuloidae type), Ehlers-Danlos s. type VII (arthrocholasis multiplex), Fabry's d., Fischer-Jacobsen-Clouston s., IBIDS, incontinentia pigmenti, juvenile hyaline fibromatosis, keratosis follicularis (Darier's), LEOPARD s., leprechaunism, Maffucci's s., Marinesco-Sjögren s., Morquio, Moynahan's s., Noonan's s., Olmsted's s., pangeria, peeling skin s., progeria, Rothmund-Thomson s., Rubinstein-Taybi s., Rud's s., Satoyoshi's s., Schwachman's s., Shapira's s., systematized mesodermal dysplasia, Turner's s., Werner's s., Winchester s., xeroderma pigmentosa
gumma	ulcerative reaction to treponemes; tertiary syphilis
gynecomastia	aging, Basex s., cimetidine, hemodialysis, hepatic failure, Klinefelter's s., leprous orchitis, myotonic dystrophy, Nizoral, obesity, paraplegia, penicillamine, physiologic, POEMS s., Silvestrini-Corda s., spironolactone, starvation, systemic steroids, testicular failure, testicular tumors (interstitial cell tumor, seminoma, Sertoli cell tumor, teratomas)
gyrate erythema	*see figurate erythema*
halo phenomenon	blue nevi, compound nevi, congenital nevi, epithelioid nevi, intradermal nevi, melanoma, neurofibroma, seborrheic keratoses, spindle nevi

Signs and Symptoms and Associated Conditions

Signs/Symptoms	Conditions
hamartomatous polyps	Cowden's s.
hanging groin	folds of inelastic inguinal skin with LAD; onchocerciasis
harlequin sign	reddened lower half of body & blanching of upper half; infancy (temporary vasomotor disturbance)
head light sign	sparing of nose and surrounding skin; atopic dermatitis
headaches	anti-phospholipids of SLE, cold urticaria, cyclosporine, familial cold urticaria, giant cell arteritis, griseofulvin, indomethacin, nalidixic acid, OCPs, Raeder's s., TMP-SMX, vasodilators
heart block	atrophoderma vermiculata, Chagas d., Lyme d., neonatal LE, PSS, Reiter's d., sarcoidosis, SLE
heat intolerance	congenital ichthyosiform erythroderma, Franceschetti-Jadassohn s., lamellar ichthyosis
heliotrope rash	violaceous color of eyelids; aldosterone-producing tumors, dermato-myositis, toxoplasmosis, trichinosis
hemangioma	epidermal nevus s., Klippel-Trenaunay-Weber s., Maffucci's s.
hematuria	Henoch-Schönlein purpura, roseola
hemidysplasia	CHILD s.
hemihypertrophy	Beckwith-Wiedemann s.
hemiparesis	Sturge-Weber s.
hemiplegia	Partingtons s.
hemorrhage	Hermansky-Pudlak s., Letterer-Siwe d.
hemorrhage, gastrointestinal	Peutz-Jeghers s., pseudoxanthoma elasticum
hepatomegaly	exfoliative erythroderma, Sanfilippo's s., Schnitzler's s.
hepatosplenomegaly	Beckwith-Wiedemann s., Chediak-Higashi s., exfoliative erythro-derma, Griscelli s., hemochromatosis, hypereosinophilic s., Langerhan's cell histiocytosis, Letterer-Siwe d., mastocytosis s., runting s., TORCH s., Wiskott-Aldrich s.
herald patch	first appearing erythematous plaque; pityriasis rosea AKA mother patch, plaque primitive, primary medallion, primary plaque
heterochromic irides	Fisch's s., infantile neuroblastoma, nail-patella s., piebaldism, Romberg's s., Waardenburg's s.
hirsuitism	*see hair section*
hoarseness	dominant dystrophy epidermolysis bullosa (Cockayne-Touraine), endemic syphilis (bejel) early secondary stage, Farber's d., keratosis lichenoides chronica, lipoid proteinosis, pachyonychia congenita, xanthoma disseminatum
hypercarotenemia	dietary, hypothyroidism
hypercortisolism	acanthosis nigricans, acne, atrophic skin, hyperpigmentation, hyper-trichosis, poor wound healing, striae, telangiectasia

Signs and Symptoms and Associated Conditions

Signs/Symptoms	Conditions
hyperesthesia	brown recluse spider bite, diabetes mellitus, erythema nodosum, erythromelalgia, herpes zoster, Melkersson-Rosenthal s., paroxysmal finger hematoma, Raynaud's phenomenon, temporal arteritis, thrombophlebitis
hyperhidrosis, generalized	acrocyanosis, acrokeratoelastoidosis, acromegaly, atopic dermatitis, acrodynia, acroangiodermatitis, AV malformations, Böök's s., causalgia, dermatomyositis, diabetes mellitus, drug withdrawal, EBS-Weber-Cockayne, epidermolysis bullosa (Koebner), familial autonomia (Riley-Day s.), Gamborg-Nielson PPK, Hines & Bannick s., hyperpituitarism, hyperthyroidism, hypoglycemia, incontinentia pigmenti, lymphoma, malaria, mal de Meleda, menopause, palmar-plantar keratoderma, Papillion-Lefevre s., pheochromocytoma, pitted keratolysis, pompholyx, pregnancy, shock, syringomyelia, tar melanosis, tuberculosis, Unna-Thost s., Weber-Cockayne s.
hyperhidrosis, localized	blue rubber bleb nevus, eccrine angiomatous hamartoma, eccrine nevus, frostbite, glomus tumor, nevus sudoriferous, reflex sympathetic dystrophy, tinea corporis, tinea versicolor, trichomycosis axillaris
hyperhidrosis, palms & soles	Böök's s., chloracne, emotional stress, onycholysis, plantar warts, shoe dermatitis, tinea pedis, Unna-Thost s., Zinsser-Cole-Engman s.
hyperkeratosis	Neu-Laxova s., Omenn's s., peeling skin s., Refsum's d.
hyperkeratosis, palms & soles	peeling skin s., Zinsser-Cole-Engman s.
hyperlipidemia	biliary cirrhosis (primary), diabetes mellitus, isotretinoin, multiple myeloma, myxedema, nephrotic s., OCPs, pancreatitis (chronic), paraproteinemia
hypermelanosis	see hyperpigmentation
hyperostosis	SAPHO s., Schnitzler's s.
hyperparathyroidism	central giant cell granuloma, racket nail
hyperpigmentation	acromegaly, Addison's d., AIDS, acromegaly, amyloidosis, arsenic ingestion, asthma, carcinoid s., cirrhosis, Cushing's d., dermatomyositis, drugs, ependymoma, erythema dyschromicum perstans, erythema multiforme, folate/B12 deficiency, Grave's d., GVHD, hemochromatosis, hemodialysis, Hodgkin's d., hyperthyroidism, hypothyroidism, IVDA, infection (malaria, kala-azar, tuberculosis, schistosomiasis), kwashiorkor, lichen planus, lymphoma, melasma, menses, metastatic malignant melanoma, morphea, Nelson's s., neoplasia, nevus of Ito/Ota, pellagra, pemphigus vulgaris, pheochromocytoma, phynoderma, POEMS s., porphyria cutanea tarda, pregnancy, PSS, rheumatoid arthritis, SLE, Schilder's d., schizophrenia, scurvy, sprue, Still's d., Vagabond's d., variegate porphyria, visceral leishmaniasis, vitamin B12 deficiency, Whipple's d., Wilson's d.
hyperpigmentation, Addison d.-like	Addison's d., ACTH administration, acromegaly, AIDS, carcinoid, cirrhosis, Cushing's s., hepatolenticular degeneration, hyperthyroidism, lymphoma, Nelson's s. (ACTH producing), pheochromocy-

Signs and Symptoms and Associated Conditions

Signs/Symptoms	Conditions
	toma, POEMS s., PCT, Schilder's d., scleroderma, Siemerling-Cruezfeldt d., Still's d.
hyperpigmentation, blue	blue nevus, Carleton-Biggs s., Levene's s., melanoma, Mongolian spots, nevus of Ota, nevus of Ito
hyperpigmentation, dermal	**melanocytotic**: blue melanocytotic nevus, Carleton-Biggs s., Levene's s., Mongolian spot, nevus of Ito, nevus of Ota **melanotic**: chronic nutritional deficiency, erythema ab igne, erythema dyschromicum perstans, fixed drug eruption, Franceschetti-Jadassohn s., hemochromatosis, incontinentia pigmenti, macular amyloidosis, melanoma, melasma, Parry-Romberg s., pinta, postinflammatory, Riehl's melanosis **non-melanotic**: alkaptonuria, drugs, heavy metals, ochronosis, tattoos
hyperpigmentation, melanocytotic	centrofacial neurodysraphic lentiginosis, lentigines, lentigo, LEOPARD s., Moynahan's s., Peutz-Jeghers s., PUVA tan, solar lentigo, Sotos' s., UV tan
hyperpigmentation, melanotic	**chemical**: arsenic, berloque dermatitis, bleomycin, busulfan, cyclophosphamide, 5-fluorouracil (systemic), nitrogen mustard (topical), psoralen, tar **developmental**: acropigmentation of Dohi, acropigmentation of Kitamura, Becker's melanosis, café-au-lait macule (Albright's s., Bloom's s., gastrocutaneous s., neurofibromatosis, Silver-Russell s., Watson's s., Westerhof's s.), carbon baby s., dermatopathia pigmentosa reticularis, Dowling-Degos d., dyskeratosis congenita, ephelides, familial periorbital hyperpigmentation, familial progressive hyperpigmentation, Fanconi's s., human chimera, ichthyosis nigricans, LAMB s., NAME s., neurocutaneous melanosis, nevus spilus, POEMS s., Siemerling-Creutzfeldt d. **endocrine**: ACTH and MSH producing tumors, ACTH therapy, Addison's d., Carney's complex s., estrogen therapy, melasma, pregnancy **inflammatory**: atopic dermatitis, DLE, lichen planus, lichen simplex, postinflammatory melanosis, psoriasis, tinea versicolor **metabolic**: Gaucher's d., hemochromatosis, hepatolenticular degeneration, Niemann-Pick d., PCT **miscellaneous**: chronic hepatic insufficiency, Cronkhite-Canada s., scleroderma, Whipple's s. **neoplastic**: acanthosis nigricans (associated with adenocarcinoma, lymphoma), mastocytosis, melanoma **nutritional**: kwashiorkor, pellagra, sprue, vitamin B_{12} deficiency **physical**: trauma, UV tan
hyperpigmentation, postinflammatory	atopic dermatitis, contact dermatitis, exanthems, drug eruptions, primula, rhus dermatitis, stasis dermatitis
hyperpigmentation, reticulated	Dowling-Degos d., dyskeratosis congenita, Franceschetti-Jadassohn s., Kitamura s., Partingtons s., progeria, Zinsser-Cole-Engman s.
hypersplenism	Tay's s.
hypertelorism	basal cell nevus s., cri du chat s., LEOPARD s., neurofibromatosis, Noonan's s., thymic hypoplasia, Pallister-Killian s.

Signs and Symptoms and Associated Conditions

Signs/Symptoms	Conditions
hypertension	cyclosporine, giant cell arteritis, livedo reticularis, neurofibromatosis, nodular vasculitis, polyarteritis nodosa, pseudoxanthoma elasticum, SLE
hyperthyroidism	acanthosis nigricans, alopecia, alopecia areata, clubbing, dermatographism, flushing, herpes gestationis, hyperhidrosis, koilonychia, onycholysis, pigmented eyelids, onycholysis, palmar erythema, hyperpigmentation, myxedema (pretibial), McCune-Albright s., Plummer's nail, pruritus, reticulated erythematous mucinosis, telangiectasia, urticaria, vitiligo
hypertrichosis	*see hair section*
hypocortisolism	hyperpigmentation, loss of axillary hair, mucocutaneous candidiasis, vitiligo
hypodontia	Schopf-Schulz-Passarge s., Seckel's s.
hypogonadism	ataxia telangiectasia, Bloom's s., Crandall's s., DeSanctis-Cacchione s., Fanconi's s., hemochromatosis, Kallmann's s., Klinefelter's s., Moynahan's s., Noonan's s., pangeria (Werner's s.), Prader-Willi s., Rothmund-Thomson s., Rud's s., Silvestrini-Corda s., xeroderma pigmentosa
hypohidrosis	acquired ichthyosis, Basex s., congenital sensory neuropathy, cretinism, Fabry's d., Franceschetti-Jadassohn s., hypothyroidism, leprosy, lichenoid drug eruption, NLD, PSS, post-miliarial hypohidrosis, progeria, sciatic injury, Sjögren's s., striate keratoderma, sunburn, trench foot
hypohidrosis, localized	blue rubber bleb nevus, causalgia, glomus tumor, Goplan's d., pachydermoperiostosis, painful pretibial myxedema, POEMS s.
hypomelanosis	*see hypopigmentation*
hypoparathyroidism	Rothmund-Thomson s.
hypopigmentation	Addison's d., antimalarials, chronic protein deficiency, GVHD, halo nevus, hypopituitarism, Kwashiorkor, malignant melanoma, monobenzyl ether of hydroquinone, para-tertiary butyl phenol, pernicious anemia, post-inflammatory hypopigmentation, post kala-azar dermal leishmanoid, SCLE, selenium deficiency, systemic steroid administration, thyroid d., vitiligo
hypopigmentation, melanocytopenic	**chemical**: catechols, monobenzylether of hydroquinone, *p*-substituted phenols, sulfhydryls **dietary**: vitamin B_{12} deficiency **genetic**: ataxia telangiectasia, piebaldism, phenylketonuria, vitiligo (Alezzandrini's s., idiopathic, Vogt-Koyanagi-Harada s.), Waardenburg's s., Woolf's s., xeroderma pigmentosa, Ziprokowski-Margolis s. **inflammatory**: actinic reticuloid, mycosis fungoides, onchocerciasis, pityriasis lichenoides chronicus, pinta, yaws **miscellaneous**: alopecia areata, scleroderma **neoplastic**: halo nevus, leukoderma acquisitum centrifugum **physical**: burns, trauma

Signs and Symptoms and Associated Conditions

Signs/Symptoms	Conditions
hypopigmentation, melanopenic	**albinism**: Type I OCA; A; tyrosinase negative, B; yellow, MP; minimal pigment, TS; temperature sensitive Type II OCA; tyrosinase positive, unclassified Type III OCA; Chediak-Higashi s., Cross-McKusick-Breen s., Griscelli s., Hermansky-Pudlak s., rufous, BADS s., canities premature, Fanconi's s., histidinemia, homocystinuria, Horner's s., hypomelanosis of Ito and mosaicism, Menkes' kinky hair, nevus depigmentosus, tuberous sclerosis **chemical**: arsenic, chloroquine, glucocorticoids, hydroxychloroquine, hydroquinone, mercaptoethylamines, retinoids **endocrine**: Addison's d., hypopituitarism, hypothyroidism **iatrogenic**: post dermabrasion, post laser **inflammatory**: leprosy, pityriasis alba, postinflammatory (discoid lupus, eczema, psoriasis), post Kala-azar, sarcoidosis, syphilis, tinea versicolor **metabolic**: Alpert's s., chromosomal 5p defect, osteopathic striae, prolidase deficiency **miscellaneous**: canities, Horner's s., idiopathic guttate hypomelanosis, Vagabond's leukoderma **neoplastic**: melanoma **nutritional**: chronic protein loss, Kwashiorkor, malabsorption, nephrosis, ulcerative colitis
hypopigmentation, non-melanotic	anemia, edema, nevus anemicus, Woronoff's ring
hypopigmentation, perifollicular	Darier's d., Grover's d., tinea versicolor, vitiligo
hypopigmentation, postinflammatory	alopecia mucinosa, atopic dermatitis, CTCL, DLE, eczema, psoriasis, guttate parapsoriasis, lichen planus, lichen sclerosis, lichen striatus, pityriasis lichenoides chronica, seborrheic dermatitis
hypopyon	pustule with clear fluid above dependent pus; Sneddon-Wilkinson d.
hypotension	Addison's d., toxic shock s.
hypothermia	Hines & Bannick s.
hypothyroidism	acanthosis nigricans, cutis verticis gyrata, dermatographism, eruptive xanthoma, erythema ab igne, hypercarotenemia, keratosis pilaris, macroglossia, myxedema, onycholysis, POEMS s., reticulated erythematous mucinosis
hypotonia	Elejalde s.
hystrix	porcupine-like (hyperkeratosis); ichthyosis hystrix of Curth & Macklin
ice pick scars	post acne scarring
ichthyosis linearis circumflexa	migratory polycyclic double-edged scale; Netherton's s. (pathognomonic)
immune deficiency	Griscelli s.
induration	amyloidosis, lichenification, myxedema, scleroderma

Signs and Symptoms and Associated Conditions

Signs/Symptoms	Conditions
infections, recurrent	Omenn's s., prolidase deficiency, Schwachman's s., severe combined immunodeficiency s., Wiskott-Aldrich s.
infertility	keratosis follicularis (Darier's d.), trichothiodystrophy
insect bites	dermatofibromatosis, granuloma annulare, lymphocytoma cutis, papular urticaria, prurigo nodularis
intussusception	Peutz-Jeghers s.
invisible dermatoses	adrenoleukomyeloneuropathy, agyria, anhidrotic ectodermal dysplasia, anetoderma, atrophoderma, connective tissue nevus, dermal melanocytosis, dystonic juvenile lipidoses, epidermal hyperpigmentation, ganglioside storage d., hypopigmentation, ichthyosis, inclusion cell d., lipoatrophy, macular amyloidosis, mastocytosis, mucopolysaccharidoses, neuronal ceroid lipofuscinosis, onchocerciasis, porokeratosis, psychiatric disorders, tinea, urticaria
iritis	Behçet's d., leprosy, relapsing polychondritis, Reiter's s., rosacea, sarcoidosis, secondary lues, Sweet's s.
ironed out appearance	epidermal atrophy leading to flattening; DLE, injury
ischemia, cutaneous	kidney, leukemia, lymphoma, myeloma, ovary, pancreas, polycythemia rubra vera, small bowel, stomach
island sparing	uninvolved skin in erythrodermic plaques; PRP
isomorphic response	lesion appearance at sight of trauma; AKA Koebner phenomenon (see eponym section)
jaundice	bile duct stricture/tumor, congenital toxoplasmosis, drugs, hepatic d., hepatitis, hemolysis, leptospirosis (Weil's d.), pancreatitis, Q fever, TORCH s., yellow fever
jazz ballet bottom	buttock cleft abscess
jogger's nipples	eroded, swollen, painful hyperkeratotic nipples from shirt rubbing
joint hypermobility	Job s.
keratitis	erythema multiforme, gold administration, lepromatous leprosy, Richner-Hanhart s., rosacea
keratodermic sandal	hyperkeratosis of soles extending up sides of feet; PRP
keratoses	Graham-Little s., xeroderma pigmentosum
keratotic papules, palms	Cowden's s.
keratotic pits, palms	nevoid BCC s.
keratotic plaques	Papillon-Lefevre s.
kidney shaped plaque	large plaque parapsoriasis, mycosis fungoides
kissing lesions	verrucae
knotty cypress	lesion appearance; erythema gyratum repens
knuckle pads	thickened extensor surface of IP joints; Dupuytren's contracture, diffuse epidermolytic PPK, esophageal cancer, hyperkeratosis, **idiopathic**, oral leukoplakia, Peyronie's d., pseudoxanthoma elasticum, trauma

Signs and Symptoms and Associated Conditions

Signs/Symptoms   Conditions

Signs/Symptoms	Conditions
kyphoscoliosis	epidermal nevus s.
lacrimation abnormalities	Riley-Day s.
lead lines	blue-black macule on gingiva margin from insoluble sulfide salts; bismuth, lead intoxication
lentigines	Carney's s., centrofacial lentiginosis, Danoff's s., generalized lentiginosis, LAMB s., LEOPARD s., Laugier-Hunziger s., Louis-Bar s., Moynahan's s., NAME s., Peutz-Jeghers s., Tay's s. , unilateral lentiginosis
lentigines, genital	Sotos' s.
leonine facies	folds of facial skin giving lion-like appearance; actinic reticuloid, amyloidosis, kala-azar, leprosy, leukemia cutis, lepromatous leprosy, mucinosis, multicentric reticulohistiocytosis, mycosis fungoides, pachydermoperiostosis, progressive nodular histiocytoma, Sezary s., scleromyxedema
leopard skin	hypopigmented areas in darkly pigmented Africans; onchocerciasis
leopard spotting	yellow mottling of posterior pole of eye; PXE
leukocytosis	EM, erythroderma, pustular miliaria, pustular psoriasis
leukoderma	metastatic melanoma, Rozychi's s., vitiligo
leukodystrophy	Siemerling-Creutzfeldt d.
leukopenia	varicella, Felty's s., leishmaniasis, measles, rickettsial pox, RMSF, rubella, SLE
leukoplakia	Zinsser-Cole-Engman s.
lichenification	atopic dermatitis, Chanarin-Dorfman s. (dorsal hands), eczema, lichen simplex chronicus, neurodermatitis, stasis dermatitis
limb defects	Adams-Oliver s., CHILD s., epidermal nevus s., Maffucci's s., Neu-Laxova s., proteus s., Roberts phocomelia s.
livedo reticularis	anticardiolipin s., arteriosclerosis, cryoglobulinemia, cutis marmorata, dermatomyositis, drugs, emboli, idiopathic, LE, lymphoma, PAN, pancreatitis, RA, syphilis, TB
liver palms	palmar erythema: 1) warm hands & exaggerated palmar mottling, 2) well-demarcated hypothenar erythema (more common); alcoholism
liver spots	solar lentigines
lizard skin	atrophy of skin; onchocerciasis
lumpy jaw	nodular submandibular swelling; cervicofacial actinomycosis
lymphadenopathy, generalized	**connective tissue d.**: dermatomyositis, LE, RA, Still's d. **infectious**: brucellosis, cat-scratch d., Chagas d., HIV, kala-azar, mononucleosis, plague, rubella, rubeola, scarlet fever, toxoplasmosis, tularemia, sporotrichosis, syphilis **neoplastic**: leukemia, lymphoma, metastasis, mycosis fungoides, Sezary s. **other**: amyloidosis, atopic dermatitis, exfoliative dermatitis, Gaucher's d., Kawasaki's d., Niemann-Pick d., phenytoin, Rosai-

Signs and Symptoms and Associated Conditions

Signs/Symptoms	Conditions
	Dorfman s., sarcoidosis, Schnitzler's s., serum sickness, Whipple's d.
lymphatic malformations	Klippel-Trenaunay-Weber s.
macrocephaly	proteus s., Riley-Smith s., Sanfilippo's s., Sotos' s.
macrodactyly	proteus s.
macroglossia	Beckwith-Wiedemann s., EMG s.
maculae ceruleae (sky blue spots)	blue to slate colored macules on lower trunk & upper thighs; Pthirus pubis infestation (crab lice)
macules, confetti	1-2 mm macules; vitiligo, chemical leukoderma, tuberous sclerosis
macules, genital	Ruvalcaba-Myhre-Smith s.
maculosquamous	flat lesion with fine scale; erythrasma, PR, tinea versicolor
malabsorption	collagen vascular d., dermatitis herpetiformis, dermatogenic enteropathy
malaise	Weber-Christian s.
malar rash	*see butterfly rash*
malignancy (internal)	bullous pemphigoid, Cowden's d., dermatitis herpetiformis, dermatomyositis, epidermolysis bullosa acquisita, erythema gyratum repens, erythema multiforme, erythroderma, Gardner's s., herpes gestationis, hypertrichosis lanuginosa acquisita, leukoderma, mucosal neuroma s., Muir-Torre s., necrolytic migratory erythema, neurofibromatosis, paraneoplastic acrokeratosis of Bazex, pemphigus vulgaris, Peutz-Jeghers s., porphyria cutanea tarda, Sweet's s., systemic amyloidosis, tuberous sclerosis, Wiskott-Aldrich s., xanthomas
mamillated	closely arranged pseudovesicular papules; Sweet's s.
marble cake pattern	whorled hypopigmentation; hypomelanosis of Ito
mastocytosis	**cardiopulmonary**: chest pain, dizziness, dyspnea, palpitations, syncope **cutaneous**: bullae, flushing, pruritus, urticaria **GI**: cramps, diarrhea, epigastric pain, N/V **neurologic**: H/A, cognitive disorder **other**: bone pain, fatigue, fever, malaise, weight loss
matchbox sign	patient presents with material (skin, lint, tissue) in small container; delusion of parasitosis
mechanic's hands	hyperkeratosis, fissuring, hyperpigmentation of hands; dermatomyositis (rare)
melanoma signs	**A B C D E: A**symmetry, **B**order irregularity, **C**olor mottling (brown, black, gray, red, white), **D**iameter, **E**levation, **E**nlargement history
menstruation (worsens)	cutaneous endometriosis, dermatitis herpetiformis
mental retardation	Baraitser's s., BIDS s., Bourneville's s., cardio-facio-cutaneous s., CHIME s., Christ-Siemens-Touraine s., Clouston's s., cri du chat s., cutis marmorata telangiectatica congenita, de Lange s., De Sanctis-Cacchione s., DeBarsy's s., Down s., Dubokowitz's s., EEC s., Elejalde s., epidermal nevus s., Fischer-Jacobsen-Clouston s., Gorlin's s., hypomelanosis of Ito, IBIDS s., Marinesco-Sjogren s.,

Signs and Symptoms and Associated Conditions

Signs/Symptoms	Conditions
	Moynahan's s., Netherton's s., Nicolaides-Baraitser s., Pallister-Killian s., phenylketonuria, proteus s., Richner-Hanhart s., Riyadh chromosome breakage s., Roberts phocomelia s., Rubinstein-Taybi s., Rud's s., Sabinas s., Sanfilippo's s., Schafer's s., Schimmelpenning-Feverstein-Mims s., Shokeir's s., Steijlen's s., Sturge-Weber s., Tay's s., trichomegaly, Vogt triad, Watson's s., Westerhof's s., Wyburn-Mason's s., Zinsser-Cole-Engman s.
metastases to skin late (>5 years)	breast, colon, melanoma, renal
metastasize	atypical fibroxanthoma, epithelioid sarcoma, leiomyosarcoma, malignant fibrous histiocytoma, malignant melanoma, neurofibrosarcoma, SCC
microcephaly	cri du chat s., DeBarsy's s., Neu-Laxova s., TORCH s.
micrognathia	progeria
microphthalmia	MIDAS s.
midline lesions	anterior cervical hypertrichosis, bronchogenic cysts, dermoid cysts, dimples, faun tails, hemangiomas, lipomas, pigmented macules, sinuses, skin tags, thyroglossal duct cysts
milia	bullous lichen planus, bullous pemphigoid, epidermolysis bullosa, lichen sclerosis, porphyria cutanea tarda, radiotherapy, trauma
mitral valve prolapse	cutis laxa, Ehlers-Danlos s. (type V), Marfan's s., osteogenesis imperfecta type I, PXE
mitral valve stenosis	Moynahan's s.
mitten deformity	pseudosyndactyly; recessive dystrophic EB
moccasin foot	erythema, hyperkeratosis, scale in moccasin distribution; tinea pedis (*T rubrum* usually)
mogul skier's palm	traumatic hypothenar ecchymosis from ski poles
molting	epidermal fragility leading to collarette-like scale; ichthyosis bullosa of Siemens
monkey facies	wrinkled face; marasmus
moon facies	rounded face; Cushing's s.
mosaic skin	fine desquamation with cracking along natural skin lines; kwashiorkor
mother patch	*see herald patch*
mulberry molars	abnormal teeth; congenital syphilis AKA Moon's molars
mutilations	carcinoma, leprosy, Raynaud's d., syphilis, tuberculosis
myalgia	toxic shock s.
myocardial infarction	progeria
myocarditis	Kawasaki d., SLE
myopathy	Chanarin-Dorfman s., polyarteritis nodosa
myositis	dermatomyositis, synergistic necrotizing myositis

Signs and Symptoms and Associated Conditions

Signs/Symptoms	Conditions
myxomas	Carney's s., LAMB s., NAME s.
neck webbing	de Lange s., Noonan's s., Turner's s.
necklace of Venus	see Venus' necklace in Eponym section
necklace sign	skin burns from cigarette ash falling on sleeping, intoxicated persons
necrolytic migratory erythema	glucagonoma (90%)
necrosis	**infectious**: bacterial (actinomycosis, anthrax, nocardia, Pseudomonas, RMSF, Streptococcus, typhus), fungal (blastomycosis, cryptococcosis, histoplasmosis, mucormycosis, sporotrichosis), viral (herpes zoster, vaccinia) **other**: DIC, medication, pyoderma gangrenosum, trauma, venom **vascular**: arteriosclerosis, Buerger's d, cryoglobulinemia, embolic, Kasabach-Merritt s., PAN, temporal arteritis, Wegener's granulomatosis
necrosis, distal extremities	arteriosclerosis, calciphylaxis, carcinoma, cholesterol emboli, CREST s., mixed connective tissue d., myeloid metaplasia, PAN, scleroderma, septic emboli, Sjögren's s., SLE
needle tracks	hyperpigmented linear scars along veins; intravenous drug injection
nephritis	serum sickness s.
neuralgia	benign cutaneous polyarteritis nodosa
neurocutaneous disease	acrodermatitis acidemica, adrenoleukodystrophy, albinism-deafness s., Björnstad's s., Brachmann-de Lange s., bullous dystrophy (Mendes da Costa type), CHILD s., CHIME d., Cockayne's s., Cross' s., DeBarsy s., Delleman's s., Down s., Elejalde's s., encephalocraniocutaneous lipomatosis, Goltz's s., Hartnup d., HID s., incontinentia pigmenti, Johnston's s., Kallmann's s., KID s., Klinefelter's s., Klippel-Trenaunay s., LEOPARD s., Lesch-Nyan s., Menkes d., MIDAS s., multiple sulfatase deficiency, nevoid basal cell carcinoma s., nevus comedonicus s., Nicolaides-Baraitser s., Noonan's s., OFD I s., Osler-Weber-Rendu d., Pallister-Killian s., Partington's s., phacomatosis pigmentokeratotica, piebald trait, pigmentary mosaicism of Ito, preaxial anonychia, proteus s, Satoyoshi's s., Schimmelpenning's s., Shapira's s., Steijlen's s., Sturge-Weber s., Tangier d., Ullrich-Turner s., Van Lohuizen's s., variegate porphyria, Verbov-Sharland s., Waardenburg's s., xeroderma pigmentosum
neurofibromas	NAME s., Watson's s.
neuropathy	acute intermittent porphyria, allergic granulomatosis, antimalarials, lymphomatoid granulomatosis, metronidazole administration, rheumatoid arthritis, Refsum's d., POEMS s., polyarteritis nodosa, primary neuritic leprosy, RA, SLE, thalidomide, vincristine
neutrophilia	pustular psoriasis (Von Zambusch), Sweet's s.
nevi, spider	alcoholics, familial, liver cirrhosis, normal persons (10%), OCPs, pregnancy, RA (on estrogen), thyrotoxicosis

Signs and Symptoms and Associated Conditions

Signs/Symptoms	Conditions
nevus flammeus	Klippel-Trenaunay s., normal, Sturge-Weber s., Wyburn-Mason s., AKA salmon patch, stork bite, port wine stain
nevus flammeus (trigeminal distribution)	Sturge-Weber s.
nicotine sign	yellow discoloration of distal fingers & fingernails; smokers
nipples, hyperkeratotic	acanthosis nigricans, Darier's d., ichthyosiform erythroderma, idiopathic, lymphoma, prostate cancer treated with estrogens
nodule	NERD s.
nodule, dermal	deep mycosis, DF, GA, lymphoma, metastases, syphilis, TB, xanthomatosis
nodule, dermal-subdermal	erythema nodosum, thrombophlebitis (superficial)
nodule, epidermal	BCC, KA, verruca vulgaris
nodule, epidermal-dermal	compound nevi, melanoma, MF, SCC
nodules, erythematous	**histiocytic**: AFX, DFSP, eosinophilic granuloma, eruptive xanthoma, foreign body granuloma, sarcoidosis **infectious**: abscess, atypical mycobacteria, KS, leishmaniasis, milker's nodule, myiasis, nodular scabies, orf, tularemia **inflammatory**: erythema induratum, erythema nodosum, insect bite reactions, Sweet's s., Weber-Christian d. **miscellaneous**: endometriosis **neoplasm**: clear cell acanthoma, clear cell hidradenoma, eccrine poroma, leiomyoma leukemia cutis, lymphoma cutis, metastasis **vascular**: angiokeratoma, angiosarcoma, hemangiopericytoma, periarteritis nodosa, pyogenic granuloma
nodules, inflammatory hand	atypical mycobacteria, cowpox, deep fungi, foreign body granuloma, furuncle, milker's nodule, orf, primary TB, tularemia
nodules, inflammatory leg	Buerger's d., deep fungi, embolism, erythema induratum, erythema nodosum, metastasis, nodular vasculitis, PAN, panniculitis, pyoderma, sarcoidosis, subcutaneous fat necrosis, Wegener's granulomatosis
numbness	leprosy, morphea, necrobiosis lipoidica diabeticorum, necrotizing fasciitis, primary neuritic leprosy, rhinoscleroma
nutmeg grater skin	hard nodules around hair follicles; starvation
nystagmus	Louis-Bar s., Wyburn-Mason's s.
obesity	acanthosis nigricans, acrochordons, candidiasis, hidradenitis suppurativa, intertrigo, melanocytic nevi, miliaria rubra, panniculitis of abdominal wall, psoriasis vulgaris (flexural), Rud's s., striae, subcutaneous arterial calcification, xerosis
ochronosis	yellow color; alkaptonuria, hydroquinone, phenol
ocular disease	atopic dermatitis, carcinoid s, Fabry d., homocystinuria, leprosy, Lyme borreliosis, Marfan's s., neurofibromatosis, onchocerciasis, pemphigus, PXE, PUVA-induced, retinoids, rosacea, sarcoidosis, syphilis, toxocariasis, tyrosinemia type II, vitamin A deficiency, vitiligo, xeroderma pigmentosum

Signs and Symptoms and Associated Conditions

Signs/Symptoms	Conditions
odoriferous skin	EHK
oil spot	yellow-brown subungual macule; psoriasis
oligomenorrhea	Stein-Leventhal s.
oligophrenia	Sjögren-Larsson s.
omphalocele	Beckwith-Wiedemann s.
onycholysis	drugs, fungal infections, hyperhidrosis, hyperthyroidism, hypothyroidism, impaired peripheral circulation, maceration, peeling skin s., psoriasis, shell nail s., solvents, trauma, yellow nail s., wetting
ophiasis	hair loss in a band around the lower occipital & temporal scalp (Greek; snake); alopecia areata
organomegaly	POEMS s.
osteitis	SAPHO s.
osteoma cutis	COPS s.,
osteomas	Gardner's s.
ovarian dysgenesis	Noonan's s., primary lymphedema, Turner's s.
oyster shell-like	black; pityriasis lichenoides ulceronecrotic (hyperacute)
pain & erythema	acrodynia, erythromelalgia, erythropoietic protoporphyria, palmar-plantar erythrodysesthesia s., photosensitivity, phototoxic reactions, Raynaud's s., SSSS, sunburn, TEN
pain & erythema, papules or plaques	arthropod assault, chilblains, dermatitis herpetiformis, nasociliary neuralgia, parapsoriasis, psoriasis, thermal injury, urticarial vasculitis
pain, bone	Schnitzler's s.
painful papules or nodules	adiposus dolorosa, angiolipoma, chondrodermatitis nodularis helices, clavi, eccrine spiradenoma, erythema nodosum, glomus tumor, granular cell tumor, leiomyoma, neuroma, nodulocystic acne, plantar warts
painful piezogenic pedal papules	transdermal fat herniations
painful skin lesions	blue rubber bleb nevus, dermatofibroma, endometriosis (cutaneous), granular cell tumor
painful subcutaneous nodules	angiolipoma, Dercum's d. (multiple painful lipomas), eccrine spiradenoma, glomus tumor, leiomyoma, neurilemmoma, neuroma
painful tumors	angiolipoma, chondrodermatitis nodularis helices, eccrine spiradenoma, glomus tumor, leiomyoma, neurilemmoma, neuroma, osteoma cutis
painless subcutaneous nodules	granular cell tumor, malignant fibrous histiocytoma
pallor	anemia, cold exposure, emotion, epinephrine, iron deficiency anemia, megaloblastic anemia, panhypopituitarism, shock

Signs and Symptoms and Associated Conditions

Signs/Symptoms	Conditions
palmar erythema	alcoholism, carcinoid, chemotherapy induced acral erythema, cirrhosis, DM, erythema palmare hereditorium, GVHD, Grave's d., hemochromatosis, Kawasaki's d., LE, leukemia, liver metastases, peeling skin s., pregnancy, rheumatoid arthritis, Wilson's d.
palmar hyperlinearity	ichthyosis vulgaris
palmar/plantar desquamation	Kawasaki's s., lamellar dyshidrosis, scarlet fever, toxic shock s.
palmoplantar keratoderma	acrokeratoelastoidosis of Costa, basal cell nevus s., bullous ichthyosiform erythroderma, Cantu's s., circumscribed keratoderma, Darier's d., dermal duct nevus, disseminate keratoderma with corneal dystrophy, dyskeratosis congenita (Zinsser-Cole-Engman s.), epidermolytic palmoplantar keratoderma (of Vorner), focal acral hyperkeratosis, glucan induced keratoderma in AIDS, hidrotic ectodermal dysplasia (Clouston's s.), Howell-Evans s., keratosis pilaris decalvans, keratosis punctata palmaris et plantaris, keratosis punctata of the palmar creases, keratoderma climactericum, keratoderma with deafness, lichen planus, Mal de Meleda, mutilating keratoderma of Vohwinkel, Naegeli's s., non-bullous ichthyosiform erythroderma, Olmstead s., pachydermoperiostosis, pachyonychia congenita, Papillion-Lefevre s., peeling skin s., PRP, porokeratosis plantaris discreta, pachyonychia congenita, progressive keratoderma (Greither's s.), punctate keratoderma (Buschke-Fischer s.), Richner-Hanhart s., Sezary s., Sjogren-Larson s., striate keratoderma, Unna-Thost s., yaws
palmoplantar pitting	basal cell nevus s., Darier's d., erythema multiforme, generalized follicular hamartoma, pneumonitis, reticulated acropigmentation of Kitamura
palmoplantar sign	yellow discoloration of palms & soles; typhoid fever, AKA Filipovitch's sign
pancreatic insufficiency	Schwachman's s.
paper money skin	thread-like telangiectasias similar to threads in US currency; alcoholism
papillomatosis, oral	Cowden's s.
papules, annular	alopecia mucinosa, arthropod bites, EED, elastosis perforans serpiginosa, GA, Jessner's lymphocytic infiltrate, leukemia cutis, lichen planus, lymphoma cutis, lymphocytoma cutis, Meischer's granuloma
papules, blue-black	blue nevus, nodular melanoma, angiokeratoma, Kaposi's sarcoma
papules, hemorrhagic	meningococcemia, vasculitis
papules, hyperkeratotic	acrokeratosis verruciformis of Hopf, confluent and reticulated papillomatosis, Darier's d., follicular LP, folliculitis, keratosis pilaris, keratosis punctata, Kyrle's d., lichen spinulosis, PRP
papules, lichenoid	lichen amyloidosis, lichen myxedematosus, lichen nitidus, lichenoid drug eruption, lichen simplex, lichen spinulosis, lichen striatus, LP, papular GA, sarcoidosis

Signs and Symptoms and Associated Conditions

Signs/Symptoms	Conditions
papules, linear	contact dermatitis, GA, insect bites, lichen striatus, linear epidermal nevus, linear porokeratosis, nevus verrucosus, verruca vulgaris
papules, yellow	xanthomatosis
papulosquamous	scaling papules; psoriasis
paraproteinemia	amyloidosis, angioedema, angioimmunoblastic LAD, edema, macroglossia, myeloma, necrobiotic xanthogranuloma, purpura, PG, Raynaud's phenomenon, scleroderma, Sneddon-Wilkinson s., xanthoma
parotid enlargement	AIDS (pediatric), alcoholism, ancyclosomiasis, DLE, Heerfordt s., pellagra, sarcoidosis, SSKI intake
pathergy	localization of disease to sights of trauma; Behçet's s., bowel associated dermatitis-arthritis s., pyoderma gangrenosum, Wegener's granulomatosis AKA Koebner phenomenon
peau d'orange	skin appears like an orange, thickened with minute dells; erysipelas, pretibial myxedema, PXE, scleredema, shagreen patch, traumatic fat necrosis, tuberous sclerosis AKA chicken skin
pebbling, scapular	Hunter's s.
pebbly skin (dorsal hand)	roughened like small pebbles; erythropoietic protoporphyria
pencil-in-cup deformity	radiographic finding; symmetric, conical osteolysis of proximal head; psoriatic arthritis (rare)
perianal dermatitis	Candida, contact dermatitis, cutaneous amebiasis, enterobiasis, Group B streptococcus, larva currens, psoriasis, psychogenic, seborrheic dermatitis, Sjögren's s., spice ingestion, TCN administration
periodontitis	cell associated glycoprotein deficiency, Hand-Schüller-Christian d., Letterer-Siwe d., Papillion-Lefevre s.
perioral eruption	acrodermatitis enteropathica, arteriovenous hemangioma, biotin responsive multiple carboxylase deficiency, blepharocholasis, chrysiasis, chronic bullous disease of childhood, Cowden's d. (trichilemmomas), essential fatty acid deficiency, glucagonoma, JEB-Herlitz, perioral dermatitis, primary amyloidosis, staphylococcal scalded skin s., zinc deficiency
perioral sparing	adenoma sebaceum, infantile atopic dermatitis, erythrose perubuccale pigmentaire of Brocq, perioral dermatitis, scarlet fever
periorbital edema	anticonvulsant hypersensitivity s., carcinoid, Chagas d. (Romaña's sign), contact dermatitis, cretinism, dermatomyositis, EBV infection, Fabry's d., Henoch-Schönlein purpura, myxedema, PSS, roseola, Sezary s., trichinosis
periorbital eruption	necrobiotic xanthogranuloma
peritonitis	familial Mediterranean fever
perleche	fissures at angle of the mouth; avitaminosis, dentures, idiopathic, moniliasis

Signs and Symptoms and Associated Conditions

Signs/Symptoms	Conditions
petechiae, newborn	congenital infection, hypoprothrombinemia (vitamin K deficiency), protein C deficiency, SLE, thrombocytopenia, trauma, von Willebrand's d., Wiskott-Aldrich s.
petechiae, non-palpable	**platelet alterations**: autoimmune thrombocytopenia, CLL, congestive splenomegaly, DIC, diet deficiency (B_{12}, folate, iron), drugs, lupus, lymphoma, marrow toxicity, May-Hegglin anomaly TTP, viral (CMV, EBV, rubella), Wiskott-Aldrich s. **non-platelet**: benign hypergammaglobulinemic purpura, chronic pigmented purpura, Hermansky-Pudlak s., intravascular venous pressure elevations
petechiae, perifollicular	scurvy
phakoma	asymptomatic nodular retinal mass; tuberous sclerosis
photoexacerbation	Darier's d., Grover's d., psoriasis, reticulated erythematous mucinosis
photophobia	acrodynia, acrodermatitis enteropathica, albinism Behçet's d., Chediak-Higashi s., chloroquine ingestion, Hermansky-Pudlak s., ichthyosis follicularis, IFAP s., interstitial keratitis of late congenital syphilis, juvenile xanthogranuloma, keratosis follicularis spinulosa decalvans, measles, oculocutaneous albinism, pretibial leptospirosis, Richner-Hanhart s., Sjögren's s., xeroderma pigmentosum
photosensitivity	amiodarone, Bloom's s., Cockayne's s., DLE, Darier's d., dermatomyositis, Hartnup's d., hereditary coproporphyria, INH treatment, lymphocytoma cutis, lymphogranuloma venereum, pellagra, pemphigus erythematosus, PIBIDS, porphyria, prolidase deficiency, reticular erythematous mucinosis, Rothmund-Thomson s., SCLE, SLE, trichothiodystrophy, xeroderma pigmentosum
photosensitivity, infants	**non telangiectatic**: erythropoietic porphyria, erythropoietic protoporphyria, xeroderma pigmentosum **telangiectatic**: Bloom's s., Cockayne's s., Rothmund-Thomson s.
phyrenoderma	hypothyroidism
phytophotodermatitis	*Compositae, Moraceae, Papilionaceae, Rutaceae, Umbelliferae*
phytosterolemia	betasitosterol, campestenol, stigmasterol
pigmentary demarcation lines	**type A**: Futcher's (Voigt's) lines **type B**: posteromedial lower extremities during pregnancy **type C**: mediosternal from clavicle to inferior sternum **type D**: posteromedian spine **type E**: bilateral symmetric periareolar hypopigmented macules
ping-pong patches	traumatic ecchymotic patches from ping-pong balls
pins and needles	follicular degeneration s. (scalp)
pitting scars of digits	PSS
pitting, lip	popliteal web s.
pitting, palms and soles	Darier's d., nevoid BCC s., pitted keratolysis
plaque primitive	herald patch of PR

Signs and Symptoms and Associated Conditions

Signs/Symptoms	Conditions
plaques, annular	alopecia mucinosa, deep fungus, DLE, EAC, fixed drug eruption, GA, granuloma faciale, Jessner's lymphocytic infiltrate, leprosy, leukemia cutis, lichen planus, lichen simplex, lues, lupus vulgaris, lymphocytoma cutis, lymphoma cutis, MF, necrobiosis lipoidica, nummular eczema, papular mucinosis, parapsoriasis, porokeratosis, psoriasis, sarcoid, tinea
plaques, erythematous	alopecia mucinosa, Bowen's d., DLE, eosinophilic granuloma, fixed drug eruption, Jessner's lymphocytic infiltrate, leishmaniasis, leprosy, leukemia cutis, lupus vulgaris, lymphoma cutis, MF, PMLE, pseudolymphoma, psoriasis, sarcoidosis
platyspondyly	Morquio's s.
plethoric facies	persistent facial erythema due to chronic vasodilatation & vasoregulatory loss; alcoholism
pleurisy	familial Mediterranean fever
pneumonia, recurrent	Churg-Strauss s.
poikiloderma	triad of atrophy, mottled pigmentation & telangiectasia; acrodermatitis chronica atrophicans, acrokeratotic poikiloderma, Bloom's s., **dermatomyositis**, COPS s., diffuse & macular atrophic dermatosis, drugs (arsenic, busulfan, steroids), dyskeratosis congenita, erythrokeratoderma viriabilis, Fanconi's anemia, GVHD (chronic), Hartnup d., heat/cold exposure, hereditary sclerosing poikiloderma, Kindler's s., large plaque parapsoriasis, **LE**, mycosis fungoides, parapsoriasis, **poikiloderma of Civatte**, radiodermatitis, Rothmund-Thomson s., Werner's s.
poliosis	Alezzandrini's s., alopecia areata, inflammatory processes, neurofibromatosis, piebaldism, poliosis with multiple malformations, prolidase deficiency, Tietze's s., tuberous sclerosis, vitiligo, Vogt-Koyanagi-Harada s., Waardenburg's s.
polygonal	shape of macules; idiopathic guttate hypomelanosis
polymorphous eruption	dermatitis herpetiformis, erythema multiforme, histiocytosis X, pityriasis lichenoides, PMLE
polyps	Cowden's d., Cronkhite-Canada s., Gardner's s., multiple hamartoma s., Muir-Torre s., multiple perifollicular fibromas, neurofibromatosis, Peutz-Jeghers s., Ruvalcaba-Myhre-Smith s., skin tags & polyps s.
pre-cancerous lesions	actinic keratosis, arsenical keratosis, Bowenoid papulosis, Bowen's d., chemical keratoses, cicatrix keratoses, cutaneous horn, erythroplasia of Queyrat, intraepidermal epithelioma, leukoplakia, radiation keratoses, tar keratosis, thermal keratoses
precocious puberty	McCune-Albright s., NAME s., tuberous sclerosis
pregnancy	herpes gestationis, impetigo herpetiformis, papular dermatitis of pregnancy, prurigo gestationis, pruritus gravidarum, PUPPP
pregnancy; exacerbates	acute intermittent porphyria, acrodermatitis enteropathica, aphthae, biological false positive for syphilis, chloasma, condylomata, cuta-

Signs and Symptoms and Associated Conditions

Signs/Symptoms	Conditions
	neous ciliated cysts, dermatomyositis, disseminated gonorrhea, dysplastic nevus, erythema nodosum, erythrokeratoderma viriabilis, estrogen receptor increase on nevus cells, familial cutaneous collagenomas, gonococcemia, granuloma inguinale hematogenous spread, hair thinning, herpes gestationis, hyperhidrosis, hyperpigmentation, hypertrichosis, keloids, lupus erythematosus, labial varicosities, linea nigra, Lofgren's s., malignant fibrous histiocytoma, melanoma(?), melasma, meralgia paresthetica, neurofibromatosis, onycholysis, palmar erythema, phlegmasia alba dolens, pityriasis rotunda, precipitation of primary lymphedema, progressive mesangiocapillary glomerulonephritis of partial lipodystrophy, purpuric "gloves & socks" s., pustular psoriasis, pyogenic granuloma, skin tags, SLE, spider angiomas, striae, telangiectasia, thrombotic thrombocytopenic purpura, tinea versicolor, unilateral nevoid telangiectasia s., varicosities, verruca, zinc deficiency
pregnancy; improves	alopecia areata, chilblains, dermatomyositis, nail growth, Fox-Fordyce d., hidradenitis suppurativa, lupus erythematosus, monilethrix, psoriasis, sarcoidosis
pregnancy; improves with delivery	herpes gestationis, PUPPPS, papular dermatitis of pregnancy
premature aging	acrogeria, Cockayne's s., diabetes mellitus, Down s., familial mandibulo-acral dysplasia, generalized lipodystrophy, metageria, neonatal progeroid s. of Wiedemann-Ratenstrauch, osteodysplastic xeroderma, pangeria, poikiloderma congenitale, progeria, prolidase deficiency
prenatal diagnosis	bullous ichthyosiform erythroderma, JEB-Herlitz, xeroderma pigmentosa
pretibial myxedema	non-pitting lower extremity edema; Graves' d., Hashimoto's thyroiditis, hypothyroidism
primary medallion	herald patch of PR
prostatitis	Reiter's s.
pruritus ani	*Candida*, contact dermatitis, dermatitis medicamentosa, leakage, lichen planus, penicillin allergy, pinworm, psoriasis, psychogenic, seborrheic dermatitis, spice ingestion, threadworm
pruritus, absent skin findings	AIDS, brain disease (abscess, infarct, tumor), carcinoid, hepatobiliary d., Hodgkin's d., hydroxyethyl starch infusion, hyperthyroidism, hypothyroidism, iron deficiency anemia, lymphoma, mastocytosis, MS, myeloma, paraproteinemia, polycythemia vera, Sjögren's s., uremia, visceral tumor
pruritus, after bathing	aquagenic pruritus, hypereosinophilic s., myelodysplasia, **polycythemia vera** AKA bath pruritus
pruritus, recurrent	onchocerciasis
pruritus, scalp	diabetic neuropathy

Signs and Symptoms and Associated Conditions

Signs/Symptoms	Conditions
pruritus, with cancer	carcinoid (upper trunk, legs, extensor arms), carcinoma (breast, pancreatic, lung, stomach), CNS tumors, Hodgkin's d., **leukemia**, lymphoma, multiple myeloma
pruritus, with infection	ascaris, candidiasis, hookworm, neurosyphilis, trichinosis
pruritus, with skin diseases, moderate	actinic reticuloid, bullous pemphigoid, chiggers, cutaneous larva migrans, eosinophilic pustular folliculitis, folliculitis, fungal infection, herpes gestationis, lichen simplex chronicus, linear IgA, miliaria, mycosis fungoides, pediculosis, pemphigus foliaceous, pityriasis lichenoides, pityriasis rosea, PMLE, progressive systemic sclerosis, psoriasis, psychogenic, PUPPP, seborrheic dermatitis, Sezary s., Sjögren's s., steroid acne, sunburn, sweat retention s., swimmer's itch, urticaria pigmentosa, xerosis
pruritus, with skin diseases, severe	acne necrotica miliaris, atopic dermatitis, contact dermatitis, dermatitis herpetiformis, dermographism, drug eruption, fiberglass dermatitis, Fox-Fordyce d., Grover's d., insect bites, lice, lichen planus, prickly heat, scabies, Sezary s., stasis dermatitis, urticaria
pruritus, with systemic diseases	AIDS, biliary disease/obstruction, cancer (breast, CNS, gastric, lung), diabetes insipidus (nasal tip), diabetes mellitus (scalp & candidal), hepatic cirrhosis, hepatitis C (30%), Hodgkin's d. (6%), hypereosinophilic s., hypertriglyceridemia (eruptive xanthomas), hyperthyroidism, hypothyroidism, intestinal parasites, intrahepatic cholestasis of pregnancy, leukemia, **lymphoma** (<5%), multiple myeloma, multiple sclerosis (paroxysmal), myelodysplastic s., neurological disorders, polycythemia vera (50%), SLE, Sjögren's s., thrombocytopenia (essential), **uremia** (90% of dialysis patients)
pseudoainhum	ancylostomiasis, burns, cholera, congenital ectodermal defects, diabetes mellitus, ergot poisoning, erythropoietic protoporphyria, frostbite, hereditary palmoplantar keratoderma, keratosis striata, leprosy, mal de Meleda, Olmsted's s., pachyonychia congenita, PRP, psoriasis, Raynaud's s., scleroderma, syringomyelia, spinal cord tumors, syphilis (tertiary), trauma, Vohwinkel's s.
pseudopelade	folliculitis decalvans, keratosis pilaris, lichen planus, lupus erythematosus, progressive systemic sclerosis
psoriasiform	psoriasis, SCLE
psychiatric symptoms	acute intermittent porphyria, autoerythrocyte sensitization s., basal cell nevus s., delusions of parasitosis, dysmorphic delusions, Dercum's d., factitial, Hartnup's d., hereditary coproporphyria, Klinefelter's s., Marshall-White s., neurotic excoriation, psychogenic pruritus, SLE, trigeminal trophic s.
ptosis	Noonan's s., Pallister-Killian s.
puberty exacerbates	cutis verticis gyrata, familial acanthosis nigricans, familial cylindroma, Koenen's tumors, pretibial dystrophic EB lesions, steatocystoma multiplex, syringocystadenoma papilliferum, unilateral nevoid telangiectasia s.

Signs and Symptoms and Associated Conditions

Signs/Symptoms	Conditions
puberty improves or initiates	EB albopapuloidea (Pasini), acatalesemia (Takahara's d.), EBS-Koebner, granulosis rubra nasi, erythrokeratoderma viriabilis, hydroa vacciniforme, pili torti, progressive symmetric erythrokeratoderma, tinea
puberty, precocious	McCune-Albright s., Rabson-Mendenhall s., Russell-Silver s.,
pulling boat hands	friction and damp cold with exposure create pernio-like condition
pulmonary disease	amyloidosis, blastomycosis, coccidioidomycosis, histoplasmosis, hypocomplementemic urticarial vasculitis s., Kaposi's sarcoma, Langerhan's histiocytosis, lipoid proteinosis, lymphomatoid granulomatosis, multicentric reticulohistiocytosis, Osler-Weber-Rendu s., paracoccidiodomycosis, scleroderma, Sweet's s., Wegener's granulomatosis, yellow nail s.
pulmonary fibrosis	Bruton's XLR agammaglobulinemia, chronic mucocutaneous candidiasis, dermatomyositis, MCTD, MTX, nitrofurantoin, PSS, sarcoid, vinyl chloride exposure
pulmonary infections	leukocyte alkaline phosphatase deficiency, Louis-Bar s.
pulmonary stenosis	LEOPARD s., multiple lentigines s., Noonan's s., Watson's s.
pup-tent sign	medial elevation of nail plate; lichen planus
purpura	amyloidosis, annularis telangiectoides, benzoates, cryoglobulins, cutaneous necrotizing venulitis, drugs, familial Mediterranean fever, Hodgkin's, leukemia, liver disease, lymphoma, measles, multiple myeloma, neoplasm (internal), purpura simplex, tartrazine
purpura fulminans	streptococcus, varicella
purpura, inflammatory retiform	benign cutaneous PAN, chilblains, Churg-Strauss s., leukocytoclastic vasculitis, livedoid vasculitis, PAN, PG, septic vasculitis, Wegener's granulomatosis
purpura, non-inflammatory retiform	**coagulation**: antiphospholipid antibody s., coumarin necrosis, DIC, paroxysmal nocturnal hemoglobinuria, livedoid vasculitis, protein C/S deficiency **cold-related**: cold agglutinins, cryofibrinogenemia, cryoglobulinemia **embolic**: cholesterol emboli, multiple myeloma, oxalate crystal deposition, thrombus (myxoma, endocarditis) **infection**: ecthyma gangrenosum, intra-vessel fungi (*Aspergillus, Cephalosporum, Mucormycosis*), strongyloidiasis **miscellaneous**: calciphylaxis, hypereosinophilic s., sickle cell anemia **occlusion**: heparin necrosis, myeloproliferative d., TTP
purpura, non-palpable	actinic, anticoagulants, benign hypergammaglobulinemic purpura, Cushing's d., DIC, drugs, Ehlers-Danlos s., Gardner-Diamond s., hemophilia, hepatic insufficiency, psychogenic purpura PXE, scurvy, systemic amyloidosis, thrombocythemia, vitamin K deficiency, Waldenstrom's macroglobulinemia **infections**: CMV, epidemic hemorrhagic fever, RMSF, rubella (congenital), SBE, toxoplasmosis, Weil's d.

Signs and Symptoms and Associated Conditions

Signs/Symptoms	Conditions
purpura, palpable	antiphospholipid antibody s., benign hypergammaglobulinemic purpura, Churg-Strauss s., cryoglobulins or cryofibrinogens, DIC, EM, emboli (cholesterol or arteriosclerotic), Henoch-Schönlein purpura, heparin necrosis, hypersensitivity vasculitis, **leukocytoclastic vasculitis**, myeloproliferative disease, PAN, PLEVA, protein C or protein S deficiency
purpura, pigmented	itching purpura, lichen aureus, pigmented purpuric lichenoid dermatosis of Gougerot & Blum, purpura annularis telangiectoides, Schamberg's d.
purpura, pinch	post traumatic periorbital purpura; amyloidosis
pustule	acne vulgaris, drug eruption (bromide, iodide), ecthyma, erythema toxicum neonatorum, fire ant bite, folliculitis, folliculitis barbae, impetigo, miliaria rubra, perleche, pustular psoriasis, Reiter's s., Ritter's d., rosacea, scabies, steroid acne, Sweet's s., tinea, transient neonatal pustular melanosis
pustules, neonate	acropustulosis of infancy, transient neonatal pustular melanosis
pustules, palms & soles	acrodermatitis continua of Hallopeau, infantile acropustulosis, pustulosis palmaris et plantaris
pustulosis	SAPHO s.
pyloric atresia	JEB
radii, absent	Rothmund-Thomson s.
radiotherapy; lesions arising in areas treated with	BCC, malignant fibrous histiocytoma, lymphangiectasia, angiosarcoma, leiomyosarcoma, SCC
ram's horn	onychogryphosis
rapidly evolving	atypical fibroxanthoma, keratoacanthoma, malignant granular cell tumor, merkel cell carcinoma, metastasis, nodular malignant melanoma, nodular pseudocarcinomatous fasciitis
recur after surgery	atypical fibroxanthoma, dermatofibrosarcoma protuberans, epithelioid sarcoma, lymphangioma circumscriptum, pyogenic granuloma
red man s.	exfoliative erythroderma
reflux, gastric	PSS
renal disease	Fabry's d., hypocomplementemic urticarial vasculitis s., polyarteritis nodosa, Wegener's granulomatosis
renal disease worsens	SSSS, *Vibrio vulnificus* infection
renal failure	half and half nails (Lindsay's nails), Kyrle's d.
reticular	net-like pattern; cutis marmorata, erythema ab igne, lichen planus (Wickham's striae), livedo reticularis
reticulated pigmentation	Dowling-Degos' d., Franceschetti-Jadassohn s., Kindler-Weary s.
retinal glistening dots	white macular dots; Sjögren-Larsson s. (pathognomonic)
retinitis pigmentosa	Cockayne's d., Refsum's d.

Signs and Symptoms and Associated Conditions

Signs/Symptoms	Conditions
rheumatoid nodules	idiopathic, rheumatic fever, rheumatoid arthritis, scleroderma, SLE (5%)
rose spots	2-3 mm blanching pink papules in crops on trunk, extremities; Salmonellosis-enteric fever (10-60%)
rower's rump	lichenification of buttock from friction
runner's nails	multiple Beau's lines, periodic nail plate shedding of toenails
runner's rump	ecchymoses of superior gluteal cleft
saber shins	orthopedic shin abnormality; congenital syphilis
sacroiliitis	Reiter's s.
saddle nose deformity	anhidrotic ectodermal dysplasia, Conradi's d., Hurler's s., late congenital lues, lepromatous leprosy, prolidase deficiency, relapsing polychondritis, Rothmund-Thomson s., SHORT s., syphilis (congenital)
salmon colored	large plaque parapsoriasis
salmon patch	fading macular stain
salt and pepper skin	hypopigmentation and hyperpigmentation; PSS
sandpaper skin	roughness due to minute papules; scarlet fever, TSS
satellite pustules	*Candida* intertrigo
sausage digit	appearance of fingers from swelling of PIP and DIP joints; MCTD, psoriatic arthritis
scale	arsenic dermatitis, atopic dermatitis, dermatophytosis (superficial), drug eruption, eczema, epidermolytic hyperkeratosis, exfoliative dermatitis, ichthyosis, keratoderma, keratosis pilaris, lichen planus, mycosis fungoides, parapsoriasis, pellagra, pityriasis alba, pityriasis rosea, pityriasis, PRP, psoriasis, scarlet fever, seborrheic dermatitis, secondary syphilis, xerosis
scale, double edged	Netherton's s. (ichthyosis linearis circumflexa)
scale, erythema superimposed	SCLE
scale, ostraceous	scale that appears like an oyster shell; psoriasis
scale, trailing	EAC
scalp lesions in adults	adenoid cystic carcinoma, arteriovenous fistulas, developmental anomalies, eccrine epithelioma, epidermal cysts, eosinophilic granuloma, heterotopic brain tissue, intracranial hemangioma, lipomas, meningioma, metastatic tumors, myeloma, osteomas, osteogenic sarcoma
scalp lesions in children	aplasia cutis congenita, cephalocele, cephalohematoma deformans, dermal sinus tumors, dermoid and epidermoid cysts, eosinophilic granuloma, hemangiomas, heterotropic brain tissue, leptomeningeal cysts, lipoma, meningioma, metastases, osteoma and osteogenic sarcoma, pilomatrixoma, sinus pericranii

Signs and Symptoms and Associated Conditions

Signs/Symptoms	Conditions
scapula lesions	elastofibroma dorsi, hereditary localized pruritus, hibernomas (interscapular), macular amyloidosis, notalgia paresthetica, pebbling of Hurler's s., pediculosis corporis, rheumatoid nodules, satellitosis with pyogenic granuloma
scarring	acne, brown recluse spider bite, cicatricial pemphigoid, deep infections, Degos' d., epidermolysis bullosa, folliculitis decalvans, herpes zoster, hidradenitis suppurativa, keratoacanthoma, leishmaniasis, lichen sclerosis, mixed connective tissue disease, morphea, nevus comedonicus, poikiloderma vasculare atrophicans, PCT, porphyria, sarcoidosis, syphilis, SLE, trauma, varicella
scars, lesions arising in	amyloidosis, BCC, Crohn's d., cutaneous endometriosis, generalized plane xanthoma, lichen planus, lichen sclerosis et atrophicus, milia, pityriasis rubra pilaris, psoriasis, sarcoidosis, SCC, verruca, xanthoma
sclera, blue-gray	nevus of Ota
scleroatrophy	Huriez s., Kindler-Weary s.
sclerodactyly	CREST s., Huriez s., Kindler-Weary s., MCTD, PACK s., PSS, scleroderma, SLE
sclerodermatous skin changes	acrogeria, amyloidosis, acrodermatitis atrophicans, ataxia telangiectasia, bleomycin, Borrelia infection, carbidopa, carcinoid, chloreythlene, dermatomyositis, diabetes mellitus, epoxy resins, GVH, gravitational edema, Hurlers s., hydrocarbons, hypothyroidism, IgA deficiency, industrial oil poisoning, Louis-Bar s., melorheostosis, PCT, PKU, POEMS s., pentazocine, perchlorethyelene and other organic solvents, pesticides, primary amyloid, progeria, rheumatoid arthritis, Rothmund-Thomson s., SLE, scurvy, scleroderma, Sheehan's s., shoulder-hand s., silica, silicon/paraffin implants, Sjögren's s., sodium valproate, toxic oil s., vinyl chloride exposure, Vitamin K administration, Werner's s., Winchester's s.
scleromalacia	RA
sclerosis	amyloidosis, carcinoid s., medication, GVHD (chronic), leprosy, lymphogranuloma venereum, morphea, myxedema, PCT, scleredema, scleroderma, scleromyxedema **congenital**; ataxia telangiectasia, congenital generalized fibromatosis, erythropoietic protoporphyria, Hunter's s., Hurler's s., lipoid proteinosis, phenylketonuria, progeria, Werner's s.
scoliosis	proteus s.
scutula	cup-shaped yellow crust surrounding hairs; favus (*Trichophyton schoenleinii*)
seal finger	erysipeloid-appearing finger after seal bite
seasonal	**spring worsens**: Kawaski's s., erythema multiforme **summer improves**: monilethrix, psoriasis **summer worsens**: Coxsackie infections, Hailey-Hailey d., itching purpura, PMLE, reactive perforating collagenosis
seborrheic distribution	Darier's d., **seborrheic dermatitis**

Signs and Symptoms and Associated Conditions

Signs/Symptoms	Conditions
seeds	thrombosed dermal capillaries from transepithelial elimination seen after paring lesion; clots, connective tissue chromoblastomycosis, fungal elements, wart AKA black dots
seizures	biotin deficiency, centrofacial lentiginosis, citrullinemia, cutis verticis gyrata, cystocercosis, Dupuytren's contracture, Elejalde s., epidermal nevus s., hypomelanosis of Ito, incontinentia pigmenti, knuckle pads, late congenital lues, midline nevus sebaceous, Moynahan's s., multiple carboxylase deficiency, neurofibromatosis, nevus sebaceous s., Pallister-Killian s., Partingtons s., Parry-Romberg s., partial unilateral lentiginosis, palmar/planter fibromatosis, phenylketonuria, Rud's s., SLE, seborrheic dermatitis, Sjögren-Larson s., Sturge-Weber s., toxocariasis, tuberous sclerosis, Wyburn-Mason's s.
serpiginous	snakelike lesions; larva migrans, lupus vulgaris, syphilis
shagreen patch	skin colored indurated plaque (collagenoma) usually on lumbosacral area; tuberous sclerosis
shin spots	macules or papules on anterior legs; diabetes, normal persons AKA diabetic dermopathy
siezures	biotin dependent carboxylase deficiency, tuberous sclerosis
sign of Leser-Trelat	*see Leser-Trelat sign in Eponym section*
signe de la bandera	flag sign of hair; kwashiorkor
simian crease	single palmar crease; de Lange s., cri du chat s., **Down s.**, Seckel's s., trisomy 13
sinuses	acne conglobata, hidradenitis suppurativa, kerion, lymphogranuloma venereum, mycetoma, onchocerciasis, paracoccidiodomycosis, pilonodal cyst, schistosomiasis **neck**: actinomycosis, branchial cleft cyst, dental sinus, scrofuloderma, thyroglossal duct cyst **rectal**: bowel carcinoma, Crohn's d., rectal abscess
skeletal abnormalities	hypomelanosis of Ito, Satoyoshi's s., Schimmelpenning-Feverstein-Mims s., Schwachman's s., Seckel's s., Sotos' s., Tay's s., Zinsser-Cole-Engman s.
skier's toe	subungual hematoma AKA tennis toe
skin lines	dermatomes, skin relaxation, Langer's lines of embryonic development, Voigt's lines, Futcher's lines (*see pigmentary demarcation lines*)
skin popping	atrophic, punched-out lesions; subcutaneous drug injection
skip areas	less involved areas between erythema; PRP
sky blue spots	*see maculae ceruleae*
slapped cheeks	bright erythema of cheeks in children; erythema infectiosum (5th disease)
smoking	arteriosclerosis obliterans, cancer (oral and lip), erythroplasia, leukoplakia, leukokeratosis nicotina palati, leukokeratosis nicotina glossi,

Signs and Symptoms and Associated Conditions

Signs/Symptoms	Conditions
	necrotizing ulcerative gingivitis (acute), melanoma (worse prognosis), palmoplantar pustulosis, psoriasis, Raynaud's d., SCC, skin metastases, thromboangiitis obliterans, wound healing (poor), wrinkles
soft skin	eunuchoid, hypopituitarism, hypothyroidism
sowdah	hyperpigmented areas; onchocerciasis (Arabic persons)
sphacelus	adherent, dry, dense necrotic membrane on ulcer bed; brown recluse spider bite, decubitus, diphtheritic, factitial, irradiation, ischemic
splenomegaly (*see HSM also*)	cardio-facio-cutaneous s., exfoliative erythroderma, Felty's s., Gunther's d., serum sickness s.
splinter hemorrhages	1 to 3 mm brown, red, or black linear discoloration beneath nail plate; dermatitis, hypertension, malignant neoplasms, mitral valve prolapse, mitral valve stenosis, peptic ulceration, psoriasis, rheumatoid arthritis, SLE, **subacute bacterial endocarditis**, trichinosis, trauma
sporotrichoid pattern	anthrax, bacterial lymphangitis, cat scratch disease, deep fungi inoculation site (blastomycosis, coccidioidomycosis, histoplasmosis), furunculosis, leishmaniasis, *Mycobacterium marinum, M. kansasii, M. scrofulaceum, M. cheloni, M. tuberculosis, Nocardia brasiliensis, Scopulariopsis blochi*, sporotrichosis, Staphylococcal angiitis, syphilis, tularemia
stable lesions	large plaque parapsoriasis, pagetoid reticulosis
stature	*see growth*
steatorrhea	acrodermatitis enteropathica, dermatitis herpetiformis (sprue), Whipple's d.
stellate abscesses	cat scratch d., lymphogranuloma venereum, tularemia
sterility	Silvestrini-Corda s.
sticky skin sensation	hypervitaminosis A s.
stinging skin sensation	erythropoietic protoporphyria
stomatitis, ulcerative	chronic granulomatous d., Hartnup's d., Reiter's s.
stork bite	fading macular stain of nuchae
strabismus	Hermansky-Pudlak s.
stress	acne, acne necrotica miliaris, acute necrotizing gingivitis, adrenergic urticaria, alopecia areata, aphthae, **atopic dermatitis**, cholinergic urticaria, DLE, dermatographism, dermatitis herpetiformis, distinctive exudative discoid and lichenoid dermatitis (oid-oid), dyshidrotic eczema, erythema nodosum leprosum, Fox-Fordyce d., furuncles/carbuncles, hereditary angioedema, **hyperhidrosis**, lichen simplex chronicus, PSS, pemphigus vulgaris, perioral dermatitis, pompholyx, prurigo nodularis, **psoriasis, seborrheic dermatitis**, SLE, sycosis, telogen effluvium, trichotillomania, Unna-Thost s., urticaria, vaginal candidiasis, vitiligo

Signs and Symptoms and Associated Conditions

Signs/Symptoms	Conditions
stretcher's scrotum	scrotal hematoma from aggressive stretching
striae	corticosteroid administration, Cushing's s., Marfan's s., normal in adolescent obesity, pregnancy, rapid growth, steroids, weight gain
string of pearls	papules along upper eyelid; lipoid proteinosis (pathognomonic)
stuck-on appearance	seborrheic keratoses
subcutaneous fat absence	Donohue's s.
sulfur flakes	yellow flakes of skin in facial follicular orifices; pellagra
summer sores	secondarily infected mosquito bites, usually in children
sunken veins	eosinophilic fasciitis
surfer's nodules	fibrous tissue mass or cystic lesion from trauma AKA athlete's nodules
swimmer's itch	non-human schistosome dermatitis
swimmer's lupus	AKA fish tank granuloma; *Mycobacterium marinum*
swimmer's shoulder	shoulder abrasion by beard during crawl stroke
syndactyly	Russell-Silver s.
synovitis	SAPHO s.
T zone	oiliness of nose, forehead, & central chin in combination skin
target lesion	concentric color change; erythema multiforme
tattoo reactions	granuloma annulare, lupus erythematosus reaction, photoallergy to pigments, sarcoid granuloma
teeth abnormalities	KID s.
teeth, natal	Jackson-Sertoli s.
telangiectasia	actinic damage, adenoma sebaceum, AIDS, angiokeratoma corporis diffusum, angioma serpiginosum, anhidrotic ectodermal dysplasia, ataxia telangiectasia, atrophie blanche, balanitis xerotica obliterans, basal cell carcinoma, blepharocholasis, Bloom's s., CREST s., carcinoma telangiectaticum, carcinoid, cirrhosis of the liver, Cockayne's s., dermatomyositis, DLE, essential telangiectasia, Fabry's d., Goltz's s., granuloma faciale, hereditary hemorrhagic telangiectasia, hereditary sclerosing poikiloderma, keloids, keratoacanthoma, large plaque parapsoriasis, LE, leprosy, Louis-Bar s., mastocytosis, miscellaneous genodermatosis, NLD, morphea, occupational melanosis, pangeria, poikiloderma, poikiloderma, poikiloderma congenitale, poikiloderma of Civatte, polycythemia rubra vera, pregnancy, prolidase deficiency, PSS, radiodermatitis, rosacea, Raynaud's d., sarcoid, scleroderma, SCLE, SLE, telangiectasia macularis eruptiva perstans, unilateral nevoid telangiectasia, varicose veins, variegate psoriasis, vinyl chloride, xeroderma pigmentosum, Zinsser-Cole-Engman s.
telangiectasia, chest wall	breast cancer
telangiectasia, facial	Bloom's s., Fabry's s., Rothmund-Thomson s.

Signs and Symptoms and Associated Conditions

Signs/Symptoms	Conditions
telangiectasia, many	**ataxia-telangiectasia, carcinoid s., Cushing's s., estrogen**, liver disease (alcoholic), PACK s., polycythemia, pregnancy, puberty, rosacea
telangiectasia, matted	PSS
telangiectasia, progressive	adenocarcinoma of bile duct, carcinoid
tennis shoe foot	red, shiny skin of toes & weight-bearing foot, may scale & fissure AKA juvenile plantar dermatosis
tent sign	1) pinching lesion leads to points within lesion; pilomatrixoma 2) medial elevation of nail plate; LP
thickened skin	diabetes (dorsal hands), Donohue's s., mucopolysaccharidoses, scleroderma
thrombocytopenia	Felty's s., Griscelli s., Kasabach-Merritt s., Letterer-Siwe d., lupus erythematosus, strawberry angiomas, Wiskott-Aldrich s.
thrombophlebitis	Behçet's d., cancer of pancreas, prostate, lung, liver, bowel, gallbladder, ovary; lymphoma, leukemia, Mondor's d.
thromboses	anticardiolipin Ab s., tumors
tinnitus	Ramsay-Hunt s.
tongue, burning	iron-deficiency anemia
tongue, fissured	Cowden's s., Melkersson's s.
tongue, painful	Plummer-Vinson s.
translucency	granulomas (sarcoid, deep fungal, tuberculosis, foreign body)
trauma	alpha-1 antitrypsin deficiency, aphthae, desert sore, DLE, dermatofibroma, dystrophia unguim mediana canaliformis, eosinophilic fasciitis, eosinophilic ulcer of the tongue, epidermolysis bullosa acquisita, fibrous epulis, fibrosarcoma, giant cell epulis, herpes simplex infection, Hailey-Hailey d., hereditary angioneurotic edema, keloid, keratoacanthoma, leiomyosarcoma, leg ulcers, leiomyosarcoma, leukonychia, leukoplakia, Mondor's d., morphea, onychauxis, onycholysis, onychotryphosis, onychoschizia, primary lymphedema (precipitates), PSS, protein C deficiency, psoriasis, pyogenic granuloma (fibroepithelial polyp), reactive perforating collagenosis, SLE, subacute nodular migratory panniculitis, trichorrhexis nodosa, tropical ulcer, yaws
trichrome lesions	dark complexion persons; vitiligo
tricuspid valve prolapse	Ehlers-Danlos s. (type V)
trident hands	hand defect; Seckel's s.
tripe palm	rugose pattern of palmar skin; acanthosis nigricans, carcinoma (stomach, lung), Gardner's s., KID s. AKA stippled keratoderma
triple response of Lewis	normal reaction to firm stroking of skin; wheal, flare, erythema
turban tumors	multiple cylindroma of scalp

Signs and Symptoms and Associated Conditions

Signs/Symptoms	Conditions
ulcer	arteriosclerosis obliterans, Arthus' reaction (purpura fulminans), brown recluse spider bite, cryoagglutinins, cryofibrinogenemia, cryoglobulinemia, decubitus ulcer, deep fungi, embolus, ergot poisoning, factitial, macroglobulinemia, MAGIC s., neoplasms, polyarteritis, polycythemia, PG, Raynaud's d., sepsis, syphilis, TB, thrombosis, TTP, Wegener's granulomatosis, yaws
ulcer, leg	**hematologic**: cryoagglutinins, cryofibrinogenemia, cryoglobulinemia, hypercoagulable states, leukemia, polycythemia vera, sickle cell anemia, thalassemia **infectious**: acid-fast bacteria, actinomycosis, anthrax, atypical myco-bacteria, blastomycosis, coccidioidomycosis, cryptococcus, ecthyma, histoplasmosis, leishmaniasis, leprosy, lues, Madura foot, pinta, *Pasteurella, Pseudomonas*, sporotrichosis, syphilis, tularemia, yaws **miscellaneous**: acrodermatitis chronica atrophicans, drugs, erythema induratum, Felty's s., neuropathic ulcers, nodular vasculitis, panniculitis, PG **neoplasia**: angiosarcoma, BCC, KS, melanoma, metastasis, MF, SCC **physical**: arthropod assault, burn, chemical, factitious, pressure, radiation, trauma **vascular**: atrophie blanche, arteriosclerosis obliterans, pernio, septic emboli, thromboangiitis obliterans, vasculitis, venous stasis
ulcer, painful	necrobiosis lipoidica, gout, calcinosis cutis, calciphylaxis, arteriosclerosis, thromboangiitis obliterans, atrophie blanche, hypertensive, pyoderma gangrenosum, Raynaud's d., vasculitis
umbilication	central depression in papule; molluscum contagiosum, sarcoid, sebaceous hyperplasia, varicella; AKA dell
upper respiratory infection	erythema nodosum, hypersensitivity angiitis, idiopathic thrombocytopenic purpura, IgA deficiency s., polyarteritis nodosa, purpura fulminans, scleredema, Sweet's s.
urethritis	Reiter's s.
urticaria	antigen sensitivity (allergens, caterpillar, drug, food, helminths, hymenoptera), atopy, autoimmune, drugs, erythropoietic protoporphyria, familial Mediterranean fever, hyper IgE s., idiopathic, infection, Muckle-Wells s., NERD s., physical urticaria, serum sickness, transfusion, urticarial vasculitis
UVA induced	PMLE, actinic prurigo, Henoch-Schönlein purpura, hydroa vacciniforme (hydroa estivale), phototoxicity, photoallergy, persistent light reactor, solar urticaria
UVB induced	PMLE, actinic prurigo, solar urticaria, hydroa vacciniforme
uveitis	Behçet's d., cobalt sensitivity, Heerfordt s., necrobiotic xanthogranuloma, psoriatic arthritis (juvenile), Reiter's s., sarcoidosis, vitiligo, Vogt-Koyanagi s.
varices	Klippel-Trenaunay-Weber s.
vascular malformations	von Hippel-Lindau d.

Signs and Symptoms and Associated Conditions

Signs/Symptoms	Conditions
velvety skin	Williams s.
venous malformations	Maffucci's s.
vermiculation	worm-like movements; smooth muscle hamartoma
verruga peruana	vascular papules & nodules developing in crops; Carrion's d. AKA Peruvian wart
vertigo	Ramsay-Hunt s., Vogt-Koyanagi-Harada s.
vesicles, hemorrhagic	gonococcemia, herpes zoster, HSV, meningococcemia
vesicles, neonate	candidiasis (congenital), erythema toxicum neonatorum, HSV (congenital), impetigo, incontinentia pigmenti, miliaria crystallina, miliaria rubra, scabies, syphilis (congenital)
volcanic border	raised, indurated lesion border; leishmaniasis
vomiting	Vogt-Koyanagi-Harada s.
warble	painful, swollen subdermal cavity containing a botfly larva; myiasis (*Dermatobia hominis*)
warmth	arthritis, cellulitis, erysipelas, hyperthyroidism, Paget's d. (of bone), sunburn
web neck	fetal hydantoin s., Klipper-Feil s., Noonan's s., Turner s.
white dermographism	stroking skin produces white line without red phase; atopy
wood grain	alternating bands of skin; erythema gyratum repens
wrinkling, premature	DeBarsy's s.
xanthoderma	yellow skin color; carotenemia, jaundice, quinacrine, xanthoma planum
xerophthalmia	dry eyes; Sjögren's s.
xerosis, congenital	Basan's s., Clouston's s., Sabinas s.
xerostomia	HIV infection, Sjögren's s.
yellow nails	lymphedema, smokers
yellow skin	carotenemia, diabetes mellitus, liver d.
zebra-like	alternating dark and light skin bands; erythema gyratum repens
zosteriform distribution	breast carcinoma (metastatic), connective tissue nevi, Darier's d., eccrine spiradenoma, epidermal nevi, herpes zoster, lichen planus, neurofibromas, nevus spilus, porokeratosis, zebra-like hyperpigmentation

Skin Diseases and Medications

Question	Yes	No	Do not know
1. Are there previous conclusive reports of this reaction?	+1	0	0
2. Did the adverse event appear after the suspected drug was administered?	+2	−1	0
3. Did the adverse reaction improve when the drug was discontinued or a specific antagonist was administered?	+1	0	0
4. Did the adverse reaction reappear when the drug was readministered?	+2	−1	0
5. Are there alternative causes (other than the drug) that could on their own have caused the reaction?	−1	+2	0
6. Did the reaction reappear when a placebo was given?	−1	+1	0
7. Was the drug detected in the blood (or other fluids) in concentrations known to be toxic?	+1	0	0
8. Was the reaction more severe when the dose was increased, or less severe when the dose was decreased?	+1	0	0
9. Did the patient have a similar reaction to the same or similar drugs in any previous exposure?	+1	0	0
10. Was the adverse event confirmed by any objective evidence?	+1	0	0

Definite association: score = or > 9

Probable association: score 5 to 8

Possible association: score 1 to 4

Doubtful association: score = or < 0

Adapted from Naranjo CA, Busto U, Sellers EM, et al. A method for estimating the probability of adverse drug reactions. Clin Pharmacol Ther 1981; 30 (2): 239-45.

Drug Reaction Classification

Classification of drug reactions

Type I: *immediate-type immunologic reaction*: IgE mediated urticaria/angioedema, anaphylactic shock ex: penicillin

Type II: *cytotoxic reaction*: 1) drug plus cytotoxic antibodies cause cell lysis (platelets and leukocytes) ex: cephalosporins, penicillin, rifampin, sulfonamides 2) drug plus antibodies form immune complexes and cause lysis or phagocytosis ex: chlorpromazine, isoniazid, quinidine, quinine, salicylamide, sulfonamides, sulfonylureas

Type III: *serum sickness, vasculitis*: IgG or IgM antibodies form to drug resulting in deposition of immune complexes in small vessels, activated by complement and recruitment of granulocytes; onset 5-7 days after drug introduction. Agranulocytosis, alveolitis, arthritis, hemolytic anemia, nephritis, thrombocytopenia, urticaria-like lesions, vasculitis

Skin Diseases and Medications

Drug Reaction Classification

	Type IV: *morbilliform exanthematous reactions*: cell-mediated immune reaction by sensitized lymphocytes reacting with drug, releasing cytokines
Type I reactions	angioedema, urticaria
Type III reactions	angioedema, exanthematous(?),fixed drug(?),Stevens-Johnson s., TEN, urticaria, vasculitis
Type IV reactions	bullous, exanthematous, fixed drug(?), lichenoid(?), photoallergic, Stevens-Johnson s.(?), TEN(?)
life threatening reaction signs & symptoms	**general**: arthralgias/arthritis, dyspnea, fever > 40° C, hypotension, lymphadenopathy, wheezing **laboratory**: abnormal LFTs, atypical lymphocytes, eosinophilia >1000/ul, lymphocytosis **skin**: angioedema, confluent erythema, laryngeal/glossal edema, mucous membrane erosions, necrosis, Nikolsky's sign, painful skin, palpable purpura, urticaria

Skin Disease	**Medication**
acanthosis nigricans	corticosteroids, diethylstilbestrol, estrogen, fusidic acid, hydantoin, INH, insulin, methyl testosterone, niacinamide, nicotinic acid, OCPs, pituitary extract, triazinate
acneiform eruption	ACTH, actinomycin D, amoxapine, androgens, azathioprine, corticosteroids, cyclosporine, dactinomycin, dilantin, ethambutol, ethionamide, fluoxymesterone, halogens, haloperidol, isoniazid, **lithium**, medroxyprogesterone, OCPs, phenobarbital, **phenytoin**, psoralen, quinine, tar, trimethadione, vinblastine, vitamin B12 (cyanocobalamin)
acral erythema	chemotherapeutics, cytosine arabinoside, doxorubicin, etoposide, fluorouracil, hydroxyurea, mercaptopurine, methotrexate, mitoxantrone
acrodynia	mercury
actinic keratoses (inflammation)	docetaxel, doxorubicin, **fluorouracil**, pentostatin, dactinomycin/vincristine/dacarbazine, doxorubicin/cytarabine/6-thioguanine, doxorubicin/vincristine, fluorouracil/cisplatin
allergic contact dermatitis	cisplatin, daunorubicin, doxorubicin, 5-fluorouracil (topical and IV), mechlorethamine, mitomycin
alopecia	allopurinol, anticoagulants, antithyroid drugs, β-blockers, bismuth, boric acid, bromocriptine, carbimazole, chemotherapeutics, chloramphenicol, cimetidine, clomiphene, colchicine, diazoxide, dilantin, ethionamide, fluorobutyrphenone, gentamicin, heavy metals, hydantoin, hypocholesterolemics, indomethacin, interferon-α, levodopa, methyldopa, metoprolol, NSAIDs, OCPs, piroxicam, potassium thiocyanates, propranolol, quinacrine, retinoids, Rozaxane, testosterone, thallium, thyroid drugs, trimethadione, thiouracil, triparanol, valproate, vitamin A

Skin Diseases and Medications

Skin Disease	Medication
alopecia, chemo-therapeutic agents	aminocamptothecin, amsacrine, bleomycin, carmustine, chlorambucil, cyclophosphamide, cytarabine, dacarbazine, dactinomycin, daunorubicin, doxorubicin, epirubicin, etoposide, fluorouracil, hydroxyurea, idarubicin, ifosfamide, irinotecan, mechlorethamine, melphalan, methotrexate, mitomycin, mitoxantrone, paclitaxel, teniposide, thiotepa, topotecan, vinblastine, vincristine, vindesine, vinorelbine
alopecia, permanent	busulfan (high dose)
anagen effluvium (inducers)	alkylating agents, antimetabolites, bleomycin, boron cyclophosphamide, mitotic inhibitors, thallium, thiouracil
anetoderma	penicillamine
basal cell carcinoma	arsenic
black hairy tongue	methyldopa, penicillin, tetracycline
Bowen's disease	arsenic
bullous eruptions	arsenic, barbiturates, bromides, halides, iodides, mercury, penicillin, phenolphthalein, salicylates
bullous pemphigoid	amoxicillin, dactinomycin/methotrexate, fluorouracil, furosemide, penicillin, PUVA, sulfasalazine
candidiasis	tetracyclines
capillaritis (purpura simplex)	aminoglutethimide
carcinogens, chemical	arsenic, 4,4'-bipyridyl, coal tar, immunosuppressants, nitrogen mustard, petroleum oils, PCB, pitch, psoralen, soot
cellulitis	antineoplastic agents, doxorubicin, 5-FU, mithramycin
ceruloderma	blue pigmentation; amiodarone, atabrine, bismuth, chloroquine, gold, iron lead, minocycline, mercury, silver
chilblains-like erythema	coumadin, phenindione, sulindac
color changes of skin due to chemical (*also see pigmentation*)	black: mercury, osmium trioxide blue: cobalt, indigo, oxalic acid (radiator cleaners), silver nitrate, silvadene brown: chrysarobin, anthralin, paraphenylenediamine, permanganates, phenothiazines green: copper dust orange: chlorine gas, phenothiazine, trinitrophenylmehtylnitramine red: soda ash, TNT yellow: dichromate, dinobuton, fluorescein dye, glutaraldehyde,
cutaneous reactions, most common	see *medications; most commonly causing cutaneous reactions*, in this section
cutaneous reactions, none or very rare	see *medications; rare (or no) cutaneous reaction*, in this section

Skin Diseases and Medications

Skin Disease	Medication
cutis laxa	
Darier's d.	ethyl chloride, lithium, phenol
delusion of parasitosis	atropine, methylphenidate, phenelzine
dermatitis herpetiformis (flare)	cyclophosphamide/doxorubicin/vincristine, iodides (exacerbate)
dermatomyositis-like	aspirin, diclofenac, hydroxyurea (long term), niflumic acid, penicillamine, practolol, tamoxifen, tegafur, tryptophan
discoid lupus erythematosus	penicillamine
drug reactions, common types	acanthosis nigricans, alopecia, annular erythema, bullous, dermatomyositis, eczematous, elastosis perforans serpiginosa, EM, erythema nodosum, erythrodermic/exfoliative, erythromelalgia, exanthematous (maculopapular), fixed, hidradenitis, hypertrichosis, ichthyosiform, lichenoid, lupus, lymphomatoid, panniculitis, pemphigoid, pemphigus, photosensitivity, pigmented, pityriasiform, porphyria, pseudoporphyria, psoriasiform, purpuric, pustular, sclerodermoid, Stevens-Johnson s., TEN, urticarial, vasculitic
eczema	aminophylline, antibiotics, antihistamines, arsenic, β-blockers, carbamazepine, chloral hydrate, disulfiram, diuretics, fluorouracil, gold, HMG-CoA reductase inhibitors, hypoglycemics, meprobamate, mercurials, minoxidil, neomycin, nystatin, penicillin, phenothiazines, procainamide, quinacrine, quinidine, resorcinol, streptomycin, sulfonamides, thiazide diuretics
elastosis perforans serpiginosa	penicillamine, thiopronine
eosinophilic fasciitis	L-tryptophan (contaminated)
eruption, exanthematous (chemotherapeutic agents)	bleomycin, carboplatin, cis-dichloro-trans-dihydroxy-bis-isopropylamine platinum (CHIP), chlorambucil, cytarabine, docetaxel, diethylstilbestrol, doxorubicin etoposide, 5-fluorouracil, hydroxyurea, methotrexate, mitomycin C, mitotane, mitoxantrone, paclitaxel, pentostatin, procarbazine, suramin, thiotepa
erythema annulare centrifugum	chloroquine, cimetidine, estrogens, penicillin, plaquenil, progesterone, salicylates
erythema multiforme	**allopurinol**, aminopenicillins, **anticonvulsants** (carbamazepine, diphenylhydantoin, phenobarbital, trimethadione), **barbiturates**, busulfan, bleomycin/cisplatin, bleomycin/cisplatin/vinblastine, carbamazepine, cephalosporin, chlorambucil, cimetidine, ciprofloxacin, codeine, cyclophosphamide, danazol, diethylstilbestrol, etoposide, furosemide, glutethimide, griseofulvin, **hydantoins**, hydroxyurea, lithium, mechlorethamine (IV), methotrexate, minoxidil, mitomycin C, mitotane, **NSAIDs**, oxyphenbutazone, paclitaxel, penicillamine, penicillin, phenobarbital, phenolphthalein, phenothiazines,

254

Skin Diseases and Medications

Skin Disease	Medication
	phenylbutazone, prazosin, pyritinol, rifampin, salazopyrin, salicylates, streptomycin, **sulfonamides**, sulfonylureas, suramin, **tetracycline**, trimethoprim
erythema multiforme-like	antihistamines, DNCB, DPCP, IPPD, rosewood, Rhus, sulfonamides
erythema multiforme, contactants	**chemicals**: brominated compounds, *N*-hydroxyphthalamide, phenyl sulfone derivatives, dinitrochlorobenzene **medications, topical**: econazole, ethylenediamine, idoxuridine, iodochlorhydroxyquin, mafenide acetate, mephenesin, neomycin, povidone iodine, proflavine, promethazine, pyrrolnitrin, scopolamine, sulfonamide, vitamin E **metals**: cobalt, nickel sulfate **plants**: poison ivy, primula, terpenes, St. John's wort **other**: epoxy resin, formaldehyde, isopropyl-*p*-phenylenediamine, soap, spray cologne, trichlorethylene, tropical wood (rio rosewood, pao ferro)
erythema nodosum	amidopyrine, bromides, busulfan, 13-*cis*-retinoic acid, diethylstilbestrol, **estrogen**, gold, halogens, isotretinoin, **OCPs, penicillin**, phenacetin, salicylates, **sulfonamides**, sulfones, sulfonylureas, **tetracycline**, thiazides, vaccines
erythema, acral	cisplatin, cyclophosphamide, **cytarabine**, daunorubicin, docetaxel, doxifluridine, **doxorubicin**, etoposide, floxuridine, **fluorouracil**, hydroxyurea, idarubicin, lomustine, melphalan, mercaptopurine, methotrexate, mitomycin, mitotane, paclitaxel, suramin, tegafur, vincristine
erythermalgia	bromocriptine, nicardipine, nifedipine, verapamil
erythroderma	acetylsalicylic acid, captopril, clofazimine, co-trimoxazole, etretinate, fenbufen, gentamicin, GM-CSF, ketoconazole, methotrexate, minoxidil, nystatin, oxytetracycline, phenobarbital, quinidine, sulfasalazine, sulfonamides, timolol
erythromelalgia	bromocriptine, nifedipine, pergolide
exanthematous eruption	**allopurinol**, amphotericin B, atropine, barbiturates, benzodiazepines, calcium channel blockers, captopril, **carbamazepine**, chloramphenicol, cisplatin, diltiazem, erythromycin, gentamicin, GM-CSF, gold, hydantoin, hypoglycemics, isoniazid, lithium, methazolamide, **nitrofurantoin**, NSAIDs, **penicillins**, phenothiazines, **phenylbutazone, phenytoin**, quinidine, **streptomycin, sulfonamides**, tetracyclines, thiazides, trazodone
exfoliative dermatitis (exfoliative erythroderma)	allopurinol, aminoglycosides, amiodarone, antimalarials, arsenic, aspirin, aztreonam, BAL, barbiturates, calcium channel blockers, captopril, **carbamazepine**, cefoxitin, cephalosporins, chlorambucil/busulfan, chloroquine, chlorpromazine, chlorpropamide, cimetidine, cisplatin, codeine, co-trimoxazole, dapsone, diltiazem, desipramine, diphenylhydantoin, ethylenediamine, fluorouracil, gold, griseofulvin, hydantoins, imipramine, indinavir, iodine, isoniazid, isotretinoin, lithium, mefloquine, mephenytoin, mercury, methotrexate, mexiletine, minocycline, neomycin, nifedip-

255

Skin Diseases and Medications

Skin Disease	Medication
	ine, nitrofurantoin, penicillin, phenindione, **phenobarbital**, phenothiazines, phenylbutazone, **phenytoin**, pyrazolone derivatives, quinacrine, quinidine, ranitidine, rifampin, streptomycin, sulfonamides, sulfonylureas, terbutaline, thalidomide, thiazides, trimethadione, trimethoprim, trazodone, vancomycin
fixed drug eruption	acetaminophen, **acetylsalicylic acid**, aminosalicylic acid, **ampicillin**, anticonvulsants, antifungals, antimalarials, arsenicals, **aspirin, barbiturates**, benzodiazepines, butazolidin-alka, chlordiazepoxide, ciprofloxacin, dacarbazine, dapsone, dextromethorphan, **diflunisal**, diphenhydramine, erythromycin, fiorinol, fluoroquinolones, gold, heroin, hydroxyurea, **ibuprofen**, methaqualone, meprobamate, metronidazole, minocycline, naproxen, norfloxacin, NSAIDs, nystatin, OCPs, opiates, oxyphenylbutazone, paclitaxel (bullous), paracetamol, penicillins, phenacetin, **phenolphthalein**, phenylbutazone, **piroxicam**, procarbazine, Quaalude, quinidine, quinine, salicylates, **sulfonamides**, sulindac, **tetracycline**, tolmetin, trimethoprim-sulfamethoxazole
flushing	alizapride, amyl nitrite, asparaginase, bleomycin, bromocriptine, butyl nitrite, capsaicin, carboplatin, carmustine, cholinergic drugs, cisplatin, cyclophosphamide, cyclosporine, cyproterone acetate, dacarbazine, didemnin B, diethylstilbestrol, diltiazem, docetaxel, doxorubicin, etoposide, fluorouracil (IV/topical), flutamide, interferons, leuprolide, lomustine, metoclopramide, mithramycin, morphine, niacin, nicotinic acid, nifedipine, opiates, paclitaxel, plicamycin, procarbazine, rifampin, suramin, tamoxifen, teniposide, thyrotropin-releasing hormone, trimetrexate, vancomycin, verapamil **EtOH following**: β-lactams, calcium carbamide, cefamandole, cefoperazone, chloramphenicol, chlorpropamide, disulfiram, griseofulvin, industrial chemicals (trichloroetylene, *N*-dimethylformamide, *N*-butyraldoxime), ketoconazole, metronidazole, moxalactam, phentolamine, quinacrine, sulfonylureas
flushing (pharmacologic menopause)	4-hydroxyandrostenedione, danazol, tamoxifen, clomiphene citrate, decapeptyl, leuprolide
folliculitis	dactinomycin, daunorubicin, fluorouracil, methotrexate, tar
furuncle	fluoxymesterone, methotrexate
gingival hyperplasia	cyclosporine, diltiazem, nifedipine, **phenytoin** (hydantoin derivatives), verapamil
hair color change	bleomycin (and combinations), cisplatin, cyclophosphamide (and combinations), methotrexate, tamoxifen
hair hyperpigmentation	actinomycin, bleomycin, cyclophosphamide, daunorubicin, doxorubicin, melphalan
hair pigment loss	bleomycin, chloroquine, haloperidol, mephenesin, nafoxidine
Henoch-Schönlein purpura	ampicillin, erythromycin, penicillin, quinidine, quinine

Skin Diseases and Medications

Skin Disease	Medication
hirsutism	ACTH, acetazolamide, corticosteroids, cyclosporin, diazoxide, diethylstilbestrol, dilantin, fluoxymesterone, hexachlorobenzene, minoxidil, penicillamine, phenytoin, tamoxifen
histamine-releasing	aspirin, bacteria toxins, chlortetracycline, codeine, compound 48/80, decamethonium, dextran, D-tubocurare, estrogen, EtOH, gallimine, gastrin, meperidine, morphine, NSAIDs, polymyxin antibiotics, quinine, radiocontrast media, scopolamine, snake venom, substance P, thiamin, vancomycin
hyperpigmentation, Addisonian	ACTH, busulfan (sun-exposed), 5-FU
hyperpigmentation, chemotherapeutic agents	bleomycin, brequinar sodium, busulfan, carmustine, cisplatin, cyclophosphamide, dactinomycin, daunorubicin, docetaxel, doxorubicin, fluorouracil, fotemustine, hydroxyurea, ifosfamide, mechlorethamine, methotrexate, mitoxantrone, plicamycin, procarbazine, tegafur, thiotepa, vinorelbine
hyperpigmentation, dermal	**melanotic**: fixed drug eruption **non-melanotic**: amiodarone, antimalarials, arsenic, bismuth, gold, iron, lead, mercury, minocycline, OCPs, PCB poisoning, phenothiazine, silver
hyperpigmentation, linear	bleomycin, zidovudine
hyperpigmentation, melasma-like	estrogen, mephenytoin, phenytoin
hyperpigmentation, mucosal	busulfan, cisplatin, cyclophosphamide, doxorubicin, fluorouracil, hydroxyurea, tegafur
hyperpigmentation, palms & soles	cyclophosphamide, dibromomannitol, doxorubicin, procarbazine
hypertrichosis	acetazolamide, anabolic steroids, bromocriptine, corticosteroids, cyclosporine, danazol, diazoxide, digoxin, diphenylhydantoin, dyazide, erythropoietin, estrogen, fenoterol, hydantoin, metyrapone, minoxidil, oxadiazolopyrimidine, penicillamine, phenothiazines, phenytoin, progesterone, psoralen, spironolactone, streptomycin, tacrolimus, testosterone, thyroid hormones
ichthyosiform, ichthyosis (acquired)	allopurinol, butyrophenone, cimetidine, clofazimine, dyrazine, ergocalciferol, hydrochlorothiazide, nafoxidine, nicotinic acid, retinoids, triparanol **hypocholesterolemics**: butyrophenones, diazacholesterol, dixyrazine, nicotinic acid, triparanol
intertrigo	amoxicillin, cefazolin, clindamycin, metronidazole
keloid	insulin
keratoderma	gold salts
lens opacities	chloroquine, chlorpromazine
lichenoid	ACE inhibitors, aminosalicylic acid, **antimalarials**, antimony, antipsychotics, anti-tuberculous agents, arsenic, β-blockers, bis-

Skin Diseases and Medications

Skin Disease	Medication
	muth, calcium channel blockers, captopril, carbamazepine, chloroquine, dapsone, demeclocycline, color film processors, **furosemide, gold**, hydroxyurea, hypoglycemics, iodide (contrast), isoniazid, ketoconazole, levamisole, lithium, mercury, methyldopa, NSAIDs, paraphenylenediamine, **penicillamine**, phenothiazines, phenytoin, propranolol, pyrimethamine, quinidine, quinine, **spironolactone**, streptomycin, sulfasalazine, sulfonylureas, tegafur, tetracycline, **thiazides**
lichenoid contact dermatitis	aminoglycosides, color film developer, dental restoration materials, gold, mercury, silver
lichenoid-oral	ACE inhibitors, allopurinol, cyanamide, dental restoration materials, gold salts, ketoconazole, methyldopa, NSAIDs, penicillamine, sulfonylureas
lichenoid-photodistributed	5-FU, carbamazepine, chlorpromazine, diazoxide, ethambutol, furosemide, pyritinol, quinidine, quinine, tetracyclines, thiazides
linear IgA d.	amiodarone, ampicillin, captopril, cefamandole, cyclosporine, diclofenac, glibenclamid, glucophage (?), IFN-γ, IL-2, iodine, lithium, penicillin G, phenytoin, somatostatin, trimethoprim/sulfamethoxasole, vancomycin, vigabatrin
lipoatrophy	insulin
livedo reticularis	amantadine, quinidine, quinine
lupus erythematosus	allopurinol, aminoglutethimide, β-blockers, captopril, carbamazepine, chlorthalidone, chlordiazepoxide, chlorpromazine, cimetidine, clofibrate, diethylstilbestrol, dilantin, ethosuximide, gold, griseofulvin, hydantoin, **hydralazine**, hydroxyurea, isoniazid, leuprolide, levodopa, lithium, lovastatin, methyldopa, methysergide, nitrofurantoin, OCPs, penicillamine, penicillin, phenothiazines, phenylbutazone, phenytoin, **procainamide** (25%), quinidine, reserpine, streptomycin, sulfonamides, tegafur, tetracycline, thiouracil, trimethadione
lupus erythematosus, subacute cutaneous	gold, photosensitizing medications, thiazides
mastocytosis, cutaneous	provoke; anticholinergic medications, EtOH, narcotics, polymyxin B sulfate, salicylates
medications; most commonly causing cutaneous reactions	amoxicillin 5%, trimethoprim-sulfamethoxazole 3%, ampicillin 3%, blood products 2%, semi-synthetic penicillins 2%, penicillin G 2%, acetylcysteine 0.9%, allopurinol 0.8%, gentamicin 0.5%, barbiturates 0.4%, metoclopramide 0.3%, atropine 0.2%, heparin 0.1%, furosemide 0.05%, diazepam 0.04%, potassium chloride 0.03%
medications; rare (or no) cutaneous reaction	acetaminophen, aminophylline, antacids, aspirin, codeine, digoxin, diphenhydramine, docusate sodium, ferrous sulfate, flurazepam, insulin, isosorbide dinitrate, magnesium, methyldopa, milk of Magnesia, nitroglycerin, potassium iodide, prednisone, prochlorperazine, promethazine, propranolol, spironolactone

Skin Diseases and Medications

Skin Disease	Medication
melanonychia	AZT, bleomycin, cyclophosphamide, ketoconazole, minocycline, psoralen
melasma	OCPs
morbilliform eruption	*see exanthematous eruption*
morphea	penicillamine
mucositis	retinoids
nail color change	**blue**: antimalarials, argyria, arsenic, chlorpromazine, ketoconazole, mercury, sulfa **yellow**: amphotericin B, beta-carotene, chromium salts, dinitrophenol, DNCB, fluorescein, penicillamine, tars, tetracycline
neutrophilic eccrine hidradenitis	bleomycin, chlorambucil, cyclophosphamide, cytarabine, doxorubicin, lomustine, mitoxantrone
ochronosis, exogenous	inhibition of sulfhydryl group of homogentisic acid oxidase; hydroquinone, mepacrine, phenol, quinacrine, resorcinol
onycholysis	doxycycline, 8-methoxypsoralen, minocycline, tetracycline, thiazides
panniculitis	bromine, iodine, penicillin, phenacetin, pyritinol, sulfathiazole
papules, keratotic	suramin
pellagra-like	anticonvulsants, antidepressants, chloramphenicol, 5-fluorouracil, isoniazid, 6-mercaptopurine, sulfapyridine
pemphigoid	ampicillin, captopril, **furosemide**, penicillamine, penicillin, phenacetin, psoralens, PUVA, sulfa drugs, thiol derivatives
pemphigus, drug-induced	aminophenazone, ampicillin, aminopyrine, aspirin (with ampicillin, indomethacin, penicillin, rifampin), aurothioglucose, azapropazone, captopril, cephalexin, ceftraxone sodium, digoxin, enalapril, ethambutol, 5-FU (topical), furosemide, gold sodium thiomalate, heroin, hydantoin, ibuprofen, indomethacin, interleukin 2, interferon β, isoniazid, levodopa, lysine acetylsalicylate, meprobamate, mercaptopropionylglycine, methimazole, nalidixic acid, nifedipine, optalidon, oxyphenylbutazone, pentachlorophenol, **penicillamine**, penicillin, phenacetin, phenylbutazone, phosphamide, phenobarbital, piroxicam, practolol, progesterone, propranolol, pyritinol, rifampin, sulfasalazine, thiopronine, thiopyridoxine, tincture of benzoin
pemphigus erythematosus	penicillamine
pemphigus vegetans	captopril
pemphigus vulgaris	penicillamine, penicillin, rifampin, thiopronine
persistent light reaction	musk ambrette, salicylanilides
petechiae, non-palpable	aspirin, heparin, quinine, quinidine
photoallergic drug reaction	amiodarone, antidepressants, antifungals, antimalarials, benzodiazepines, griseofulvin, hypoglycemics, musk ambrette, 6-methylcoumarin, NSAIDs, OCPs, PABA esters, phenothiazines, sulfonamides, sulfonylureas, thiazides, vinblastine

Skin Diseases and Medications

Skin Disease	Medication
photosensitizing	amiodarone, antidepressants, chloroquine, fluoroquinolones, fluorouracil, griseofulvin, methotrexate, nalidixic acid, NSAIDs, phenothiazines, sulfonamides, sulfonylureas, tetracyclines, thiazides, vinblastine (*also see following section*)
phototoxic drug eruption	**medications: amiodarone**, anthracene, benoxaprofen, brequinar sodium, chloroquine, chlorpromazine, dacarbazine, dactinomycin, demeclocycline, doxorubicin, doxycycline, 5-fluorouracil, furosemide, griseofulvin, HCTZ, hydroxyurea, methotrexate, mitomycin C, nalidixic acid, naproxen, **NSAIDs**, PABA, **phenothiazines**, piroxicam, porphyrins, procarbazine, psoralen, quinidine, sulfanilamide, **sulfonamides**, sulfonylureas, tegafur, tetracycline, thiazides, tolbutamide, vinblastine **other**: dye (eosin, methylene blue), fumocoumarins (fragrance, lime, celery, parsnip, fig), hemotroporphyrin, tar
phytophotodermatitis	bergamot, carrot (wild), cow parsnip, dill, fennel, gas plant, Persian lines, rue (common)
pigmentation-blue	**amiodarone**-slate blue, **argyria**-slate blue, **bismuth**-blue black on gingival margin, **bleomycin**-flagellate pigmentation, **chloroquine**-blue gray, **minocycline**-brown, gray, blue black in acne scar, **plaquenil**-blue black, **tetracycline**-blue cutaneous osteomas
pigmentation-brown	ACTH, arsenic, minocycline, OCPs, phenytoin
pigmentation-gray	chlorpromazine, minocycline
pigmentation-red	methysergide, rifampin-red man syndrome
pigmentation-yellow	cathaxanthin, phenazopyridine, quinacrine
pityriasiform, pityriasis rosea-like	acetylsalicylic acid, arsenic, barbiturates, β-blockers, bismuth, captopril, clonidine, gold, griseofulvin, isoniazid, isotretinoin, ketotifen, mercurials, methoxypromazine, metronidazole, NSAIDs, omeprazole, penicillamine, penicillin, pyribenzamine, salvarsan, tripelennamine
porphyria	cisplatin (*also see following section*)
porphyria cutanea tarda	androgens, busulfan, chloroquine, cyclophosphamide, dapsone, diethylstilbestrol, estrogen, EtOH, furosemide, griseofulvin, hexachlorobenzene, hydroxychloroquine, methotrexate, nalidixic acid, naproxen, OCPs, pyridoxine, quinidine, quinine, rifampin, sulfonylureas, tetracycline, 2,4,5-trichlorophenol (*also see following section*)
porphyria, acute intermittent	chlorambucil, cyclophosphamide (*also see following section*)
pruritus	**antimicrobials**: acyclovir, ampicillin, **antimalarials**, cephalosporins, chloroquine, colistin, **erythromycin**, halofantrine, ketoconazole, lomefloxacin, metronidazole, miconazole, polymyxin B, sulfonamides, suramin **cardiovascular**: amiodarone, beta-blockers, captopril, clonidine, diazoxide, diphenoxylate, dobutamine, enalapril, naftazone, **quinidine** **diuretics**: furosemide, HCTZ

Skin Diseases and Medications

Skin Disease	Medication
	hormones: anabolic steroids, dexamethasone, estrogen, **OCPs**, progesterone, testosterone **miscellaneous**: allopurinol, **aspirin**, bleomycin, **chlorpropamide**, colchicine, coumarin, heparin, imipramine, NSAIDs, **phenothiazines**, probenecid, **tolbutamide** **opiates**: butorphanol, cocaine, fentanyl, heroin, morphine **vitamins**: etretinate, isotretinoin, niacin, vitamin B complex
pseudolymphoma	ACE inhibitors, anticonvulsants, antidepressants, benzodiazepines, beta blockers, calcium channel blockers, dilantin, H1 & H2 antagonists, lipid-lowering agents, lithium, NSAIDs, phenothiazines, steroids
pseudoporphyria	furosemide, nalidixic acid, tetracycline (*also see following section*)
psoriasiform, induce or exacerbate	ACE inhibitors, acetylsalicylic acid, ampicillin, antimalarials, arsenic, chloroquine, codeine, cyclosporine, etretinate, gold, ibuprofen, interferons, interleukins, iodine, lithium, methoxsalen, morphine, penicillamine, pindolol, practolol, propranolol, quinidine
psoriasis, erythrodermic	**antimalarials, β-blockers**, captopril, chlorthalidone, clonidine, corticosteroids (withdrawal), digoxin, indomethacin, **lithium**, NSAIDs
psoriasis, exacerbation	antimalarials, β-blockers, lithium, steroid withdrawal
psoriasis, pustular	aminoglutethimide, lithium, OCPs, steroid withdrawal
purpura	anticonvulsants, aspirin, barbiturates, benzoate, carbamides, chloroquine, chlorothiazide, chlorpromazine, coumadin, gold, griseofulvin, heparin, iodides, methotrexate, NSAIDs, phenothiazines, phenylbutazone, quinidine, quinine, sedatives, sulfonamides, tartrazine, thiazides
purpura pigmentosa chronica	sedatives
pustular eruption	acetaminophen, amoxicillin, ampicillin, bromides, carbamazepine, cefaclor, erythromycin, imipenam, iodides, nifedipine, penicillin, quinidine
pustulosis, acute generalized exanthematous	**antibiotics**: azithromycin, cephalosporin, chloramphenicol, ciprofloxacin, doxycycline, erythromycin, isoniazid, itraconazole, norfloxacin, penicillin, streptomycin, sulfasalazine, terbinafine, trimethoprim, vancomycin, **others**: acetaminophen, allopurinol, carbamazepine, chromium picolinate, diclofenac, diltiazem, disulfiram, enalapril, furosemide, hydroxychloroquine, mercury, nifedipine, phenytoin, quinidine
pyoderma gangrenosum	bromides, GM-CSF, iodides, isotretinoin
pyogenic granuloma	isotretinoin
radiation enhancement	bleomycin, chlorambucil, cyclophosphamide (bleomycin, +dactinomycin, vincristine, doxorubicin, cisplatin, triazinate), dactinomycin, dactinomycin and amethopterin, doxorubicin, doxorubicin and cyclophosphamide, fluorouracil, fluorouracil and cisplatin, hydroxyurea, 6-mercaptopurine, methotrexate

261

Skin Diseases and Medications

Skin Disease	Medication
radiation recall	bleomycin, cyclophosphamide, cytarabine, **dactinomycin**, daunorubicin, **doxorubicin**, docetaxel, edatrexate, etoposide (VP-16), 5-fluorouracil, hydroxyurea, idarubicin, lomustine, melphalan, methotrexate, paclitaxel, tamoxifen, trimetrexate, vinblastine
rash, macular & papular	allopurinol, ampicillin, barbiturates, chloroquine, diflunisal, dilantin, gentamicin, gold salts, isoniazid, meclofenamate, penicillin, phenothiazines, phenylbutazone, piroxicam, quinidine, streptomycin, sulfonamides, thiazides, thiouracil, trimethoprim/sulfamethoxasole,
rash, morbilliform	ampicillin, aspirin, barbiturates, benzodiazepines, chlorpromazine, dapsone, erythromycin, gentamicin, gold salts, griseofulvin, isoniazid, phenothiazines, thiazides
Raynaud's d.	amphetamines, arsenic, β-adrenergic blockers, bleomycin (and combinations), clonidine, cyanamide, ergotamine, EtOH, heavy metals, methysergide, OCPs, tobacco, vincristine, vinyl chloride
"red man" s.	see exfoliate erythroderma
rosacea	aminophylline, amyl nitrite, cyclosporine, diazoxide, dipyridamole, EtOH, glutamate, hydralazine, iodides, isoprel, isordil, nicotinic acid, nitrate, papaverine, reserpine, theophylline, vasodilators
SCC, inflammation	fludarabine
SCLE	aldactone, chrysotherapy, griseofulvin, penicillamine, piroxicam, procainamide, sulfonylureas, thiazides
scleroderma-like	aliphatic hydrocarbons, aromatic hydrocarbons, bleomycin, carbidopa, cyclohexylamines, docetaxel, penicillamine, silica, trichlorethylene, valproic acid, vinyl chloride
sclerosis	bleomycin, polyvinylchloride, tryptophan, vitamin K (IM)
seborrheic dermatitis	arsenic, cimetidine, gold, methyldopa, neuroleptics, phenothiazines
seborrheic keratoses (inflammation)	cytarabine
serum sickness vasculitis	cephalosporins, penicillin, sulfa, thiazides
serum sickness-like	β-lactam antibiotics, cefaclor, dilantin, penicillin, sulfonamides
splinter hemorrhage	tetracycline
squamous cell carcinoma	arsenic
Stevens-Johnson s.	*see erythema multiforme*
stomatitis (chemotherapeutic agents)	amsacrine, bleomycin, cyclophosphamide, cytarabine, dactinomycin, daunorubicin, docetaxel, doxorubicin, edatrexate, epirubicin, floxuridine, fluorouracil, hydroxyurea (high-dose), idarubicin, mechlorethamine, 6-mercaptopurine, methotrexate, mithramycin, mitomycin, paclitaxel, procarbazine, tegafur, 6-thioguanine, tomudex, topotecan, vinblastine, vincristine
striae	corticosteroids, isoniazid
Sweet's s.	*all-trans*-retinoic acid, GM-CSF, minocycline, OCPs

Skin Diseases and Medications

Skin Disease	Medication
telangiectasia	carmustine, hydroxyurea, nifedipine, OCPs
thrombocytopenic purpura	NSAIDs, phenothiazines, quinidine, thiazides
toxic epidermal necrolysis	**allopurinol**, amoxapine, **ampicillin**, anti-tuberculosis drugs, asparaginase, **aspirin**, barbiturates, bleomycin, **carbamazepine**, cephalosporins, chlorambucil, chloramphenicol, chlorpropamide, ciprofloxacin, cladribine, cytarabine, dapsone, dicloxacillin, dilantin, disulfiram, doxorubicin, doxycycline, erythromycin, fansidar, 5-fluorouracil, gold, griseofulvin, hydantoin, hypoglycemics, imipramine, methotrexate, minipress, mithramycin, nitrofurantoin, NSAIDs, **oxicam derivatives**, penicillamine, penicillin, **phenobarbital**, phenolphthalein, phenybutazone, **phenytoin**, plicamycin, procarbazine, quinine, rifampin, streptomycin, **sulfonamides**, suramin, tetracycline, thiobendazole, trimethoprim/sulfadoxine, trimethoprim/sulfamethoxasole, valproic acid, vancomycin **With HIV infection**: clindamycin, erythromycin, fluconazole, phenobarbital, valproic acid, vancomycin
ulcer	barbiturates, ergotamine, halogens, methotrexate
ulcers, leg	hydroxyurea, methotrexate
ultraviolet recall	etoposide/cyclophosphamide, methotrexate, methotrexate/cyclophosphamide/fluorouracil, suramin
urticaria	ACE inhibitors, acetylsalicylic acid, ACTH, animal sera, azo dyes, barbiturates, benzoates, benzocaine, calcium channel blockers, cephalosporin, chloramphenicol, chlorpromazine, cimetidine, corticotropin, curare, dextran, enzymes, fluoxetine, griseofulvin, hormones, hydantoin, hydralazine, imipramine, indomethacin, insulin, mechlorethamine (nitrogen mustard), mesna, **NSAIDs, opiates, penicillin**, phenolphthalein, phenothiazines, phenylbutazone, pollen vaccines, polymyxin B, polypeptide procainamide, promethazine quinidine, **radiocontrast dye**, salicylates, streptomycin, sulfonamides, tetracycline, trazodone, trimethoprim
urticaria, non-allergic contact	acetic acid, alcohol, balsam of Peru, benzoic acid, caterpillar hair, cinnamic acid, cinnamic aldehyde, cobalt chloride, dimethyl sulfoxide, insect sting, methyl nicotinate, moth, sodium benzoate, sorbic acid, trafuril
urticaria, chemotherapeutic agents	amsacrine, L-asparaginase, bleomycin, busulfan, carboplatin, chlorambucil, cisplatin, cyclophosphamide, cytarabine, daunorubicin, diaziquone, didemnin B, diethylstilbestrol, docetaxel, doxorubicin, epirubicin, etoposide, 5-fluorouracil, mechlorethamine, melphalan, methotrexate, mitomycin C, mitotane, mitoxantrone, paclitaxel, pentostatin procarbazine, teniposide, thiotepa, trimetrexate, vincristine, zinostatin
urticaria (localized)	doxorubicin, epirubicin, idarubicin
vasculitis	ampicillin, chlorothiazide, phenytoin, thiouracil

Skin Diseases and Medications

Skin Disease	Medication
vasculitis, leukocytoclastic	allopurinol, aminosalicylic acid, busulfan, cimetidine, clindamycin, corticosteroids, cyclophosphamide, cytarabine, diltiazem, gold, griseofulvin, heparin, hexamethylene bisacetamide, hydantoins, hydralazine, hydroxyurea, indomethacin, insulin, iodides, ketocona-zole, levamisole, 6-mercaptopurine, methotrexate, mitoxantrone, nifedipine, NSAIDs, OCPs, penicillin, phenothiazines, phenylbuta-zone, procainamide, propylthiouracil, quinidine, quinine, serum, sotalol, streptokinase, streptomycin, sulfonamides, tamoxifen, tetra-cycline, thiazides, vaccine (influenza), vancomycin, vitamins
vesiculobullous eruption	amoxapine, arsenic, barbiturates, bromides, captopril, chemotherapeu-tic agents, dipyridamole, furosemide, griseofulvin, iodides, mercury, nalidixic acid, NSAIDs, penicillamine, penicillin, phenolphthalein, phenytoin, PUVA, salicylates, sulfonamides, thiazides, thioridazine
xanthoma (eruptive)	isotretinoin
xerostomia	anticholinergics, antihistamines, hypnotics, sedatives

Photosensitizing Medications, Categorical

anti-acne	isotretinoin, tretinoin
antibiotics	ciprofloxacin, clofazimine, erythromycin ethylsuccinate + sulfisoxa-zole, ethionamide, gentamicin, hexachlorophene, interferon α-2B, nalidixic acid, norfloxacin, pyrazinamide, trimethoprim, trimetho-prim +sulfamethoxasole (see sulfonamides and tetracyclines)
anticonvulsants	acetazolamide, carbamazepine, phenytoin
antidepressants (tricyclic and other)	amitripyline, amoxapine, chlordiazepoxide, +amitripyline, desipramine, doxepin, imipramine, isocarboxazid, maprotiline, nor-triptyline, perphenazine +amitripyline, protriptyline, trimipramine
antiemetics	*see antipsychotics*
antifungals	fentichlor, flucytosine, griseofulvin, jadit, multifungin
antihistamines	astemizole, azatadine, bromodipheyhydramine + codeine, brompheniramine, buclizine, carbinoxamine, chlorpheniramine, chlorpheniramine + D-pseudoephedrine, chlorpheniramine + phenyl-propanolamine, clemastine, cyclizine, cyclobenzaprine, cyprohepta-dine, dexchlorpheniramine, dimenhydrinate, diphenhydramine, diphenylpyraline, doxylamine, hydroxyzine, meclizine, methapyri-lene, methdilazine, orphenadrine, pheniramine, phenyl-propanolamine +chlorpheniramine, phenylpropanolamine + pheni-ramine + pyrilamine, promethazine, pyrilamine, terfenadine, trimeprazine, tripelennamine, triprolidine
antimalarial	quinine
antineoplastic	dacarbazine, floxuridine, fluorouracil, flutamide, methotrexate, vin-blastine
antiparkinsonian	selegiline

Skin Diseases and Medications

Photosensitizing Medications, Categorical

antipsychotics, tranquilizers, phenothiazines, and antiemetics	acetophenazine, butaperazine, carphenazine, chlorpromazine, chlorprothixene, ethopropazine, fluphenazine, haloperidol, mesoridazine, methdilazine, methotrimeprazine, nabilone, perphenazine, piperacetazine, prochlorperazine, promazine, promethazine, propiomazine, thiethylperazine, thioridazine, thiothixene, trifluoperazine, triflupromazine, trimeprazine
cardiac agents	*see hypertensive and cardiac agents*
cholesterol-lowering	lovastatin
estrogens	*see oral contraceptives*
glaucoma medication	methazolamide
gonadotropin inhibitor	danazol
hypertensive and cardiac agents	amiodarone, atenolol + chlorthalidone, captopril, clorthalidone +reserpine, diltiazem, enalapril, enalapril + hydrochlorothiazide, furosemide, guanethidine + hydrochlorothiazide, indapamide, labetalol, labetalol + hydrochlorothiazide, metoalazone, metoprolol, minoxidil, nadolol + bendrofumethiazide, nifedipine, propranolol + hydrochlorothiazide, quinethazone, quinidine gluconate, quinidine sulfate, timolol + hydrochlorothiazide, triamterene
hypoglycemics	*see sulfonylureas*
NSAIDs, antiarthritics, anti-inflammatory	auranofin, diclofenac, diflunisal, fenoprofen, flurbiprofen, gold compounds, ibuprofen, indomethacin, ketoprofen, meclofenamate, naproxen, phenylbutazone, piroxicam, sulindac, suprofen, tolmetin
oral contraceptives & estrogens	**estrogens**: chlorotrianisene, diethylstilbestrol, estradiol, estrogens (conjugated and esterified), estropipate **progesterones**: ethinyl estradiol, medroxyprogesterone, megestrol, norethindrone, norgestrel, quinestrol
phenothiazines	*see antipsychotics*
psoralens	methoxsalen, trioxsalen
sulfonamides	sulfacytine, sulfadiazine, sulfadoxine, sulfadoxine + pyrimethamine, sulfamethizole, sulfamethoxazole, sulfapyridine, sulfasalazine, sulfinpyrazone, sulfisoxazole, sulfone
sulfonylureas, oral hypoglycemics	acetohexamide, chlorpropamide, glipizide, glyburide, tolazamide, tolbutamide
sunscreen ingredients	6-acetoxy-2,4,-dimethyl-m dioxane, benzophenones, cinnamates, oxybenzone, paba esters
tetracyclines	chloretracycline, demeclocycline, docycycline, methacycline, minocycline, oxytetracycline, tetracycline
thiazide diuretics	bendroflumethiazide, benzthiazide, chlorothiazide, chlorthalidone, cyclothiazide, hydrochlorothiazide, hydroflumethiazide, poythiazide, rauwolfia serpentina + bendroflumenthiazide, reserpine + chlorothiazide, reserpine + hydralazine + hydrochlorothiazide, reserpine + hydrochlorothiazide, trichlormethiazide
tranquilizers	*see antipsychotics*

Skin Diseases and Medications

Photosensitizing Medications, Alphabetical

a   acetazolamide, acetohexamide, acetophenazine, amiodarone, amitripyline, amoxapine, astemizole, atenolol + chlorthalidone, auranofin, azatadine,

b   bendroflumethiazide, benzophenones, benzthiazide, bromodiphenhydramine + codeine, brompheniramine, buclizine, butaperazine,

c   captopril, carbamazepine, carbinoxamine, carphenazine, chlordiazepoxide + amitriptyline, chloretracycline, chlorothiazide, chlorotrianisene, chlorpheniramine, chlorpheniramine + phenylpropanolamine, chlorpheniramine + pseudoephedrine, chlorpromazine, chlorpropamide, chlorprothixene, chlorthalidone, cinnamates, ciprofloxacin, clemastine, clofazime, clorthalidone + reserpine, cyclobenzaprine, cyclizine, cyclothiazide, cyproheptadine

d   dacarbazine, danazol, demeclocycline, dexchlorpheniramine, diclofenac, diflunisal, diltiazem, dimenhydrinate, 6-Acetoxy-2,4,-dimethyl-m dioxane, diphenhydramine, diphenylpyraline, doxylamine, diethylstilbestrol, desipramine, doxepin, doxycycline

e   enalapril, enalapril + hydrochlorothiazide, erythromycin ethylsuccinate + sulfisoxazole, ethionamide, ethopropazine, estradiol, estrogens (conjugated and esterified), estropipate ethinyl estradiol

f   fentichlor, fenoprofen, floxuridine, flurbiprofen, flucytosine, fluorouracil, fluphenazine, flutamide, furosemide

g   gentamicin, glipizide, glyburide, gold compounds, griseofulvin, guanethidine + hydrochlorothiazide

h   haloperidol, hexachlorophene, hydrochlorothiazide, hydroflumethiazide, hydroxyzine

i   ibuprofen, imipramine, indapamide, indomethacin, interferon α-2B, isocarboxazid, isotretinoin

j   jadit

k   ketoprofen

l   labetalol, labetalol + hydrochlorothiazide, lovastatin

m   maprotiline, meclizine, meclofenamate, medroxyprogesterone, megestrol, mesoridazine, methacycline, methapyrilene, methazolamide, methdilazine, methotrexate, methotrimeprazine, methoxsalen, metoalazone, metoprolol, minocycline, minoxidil, multifungin

n   nabilone, nadolol + bendrofumethiazide, nalidixic acid, naproxen, nifedipine, norethindrone, norfloxacin, norgestrel, nortroptyline

o   orphenadrine, oxybenzone, oxytetracycline

p   PABA (para-aminobenzoic acid), perphenazine, perphenazine + amitriptyline, pheniramine, phenylbutazone, phenylpropanolamine + chlorpheniramine, phenylpropanolamine + pheniramine + pyrilamine, phenytoin, piperacetazine, piroxicam, polythiazide, prochlorperazine, promazine, promethazine, propiomazine, propranolol + hydrochlorothiazide, protriptyline, pyrazinamide, pyrilamine

q   quinestrol, quinethazone, quinidine gluconate, quinidine sulfate, quinine,

r   rauwolfia serpentina + bendroflumenthiazide, reserpine + chlorothiazide, reserpine +hydralazine +hydrochlorothiazide, reserpine + hydrochlorothiazide

s   selegiline, sulfacytine, sulfadiazine, sulfadoxine, sulfadoxine + pyrimethamine, sulfamethizole, sulfamethoxazole, sulfapyridine, sulfasalazine, sulfinpyrazone, sulfisoxazole, sulfone, sulindac, suprofen

Skin Diseases and Medications

Photosensitizing Medications, Alphabetical

t	terfenadine, tetracycline, thiethylperazine, thioridazine, thiothixene, timolol +hydrochlorothiazide, tolazamide, tolbutamide, tolmetin, tretinoin, triamterene, trichlormethiazide, trifluoperazine, triflupromazine, trimeprazine, trimethoprim, trimethoprim + sulfamethoxasole, trimipramine, trioxsalen, tripelennamine, triprolidine
v	vinblastine

*Modified from Levine JI. Medications that increase sensitivity to light; a 1990 listing. Rockville, Md; US Dept. of Health and Human Services

Porphyria: Drugs that May Precipitate Acute Porphyria

a	alcuronium, **alphaxalone, alphadolone**, alprazolam, aluminum preparations, amidopyrine, aminoglutethimide, aminophylline, **amitripyline, amylobarbitone**, amphetamines, antipyrine, apronalide, **auranofin, aurothiomalate**, azapropazone
b	baclofen, **barbiturates, bemegride**, bendrofluazide, benoxaprofen, benzbromarone, *benzylthiouracil, bepridil*, bromocriptine, busulphan, **butylscopolamine**
c	captopril, **carbamazepine, carbromal, carisoprodol**, cefuroxime, cephalexin, cephalosporins, cephradine, chlorambucil, **chloramphenicol, chlordiazepoxide, chlormezanone**, chloroform, chlorpropamide, cimetidine, cinnarizine, clemastine, clobazam, clomipramine HCL, clonazepam, **clorazepate**, cocaine, colistrin, co-trimoxazole, cyclophosphamide, cycloserine, cyclosporine
d	danazol, **dapsone**, dexfenfluramine, dextropropoxyphene, diazepam, dichloralphenazone, diclofenac NA, diethylpropion, dihydralazine, dihydroergotamine, **dimenhydrinate, diphenhydramine**, dothiepin HCL, doxycycline, **dydrogesterone**
e	**econazole, enalapril**, enflurane, ergometrine maleate, **ergot compounds**, ergotamine tartrate, **erythromycin, estramustine**, ethamsylate, **ethanol**, ethionamide, ethosuximide, **ethotoin**, etidocaine, etomidate
f	flufenamic acid, flunitrazepam, fluroxine, furosemide
g	glutethimide, gold preparations, griseofulvin
h	halothane, hydantoins (phenytoin, ethytoin, mephenytoin), hydralazine, hydrochlorothiazide, hyoscine N-butyl bromide
i	imipramine, isoniazid, isopropylmeprobamate
k	ketamine, ketoprofen
l	lead, lidocaine, lignocaine
m	mephenezine, meprobamate, mercury compounds, methoxyflurane, methsuximide, methyldopa, methyprylone, metoclopramide, metyrapone, metronidazole
n	nalidixic acid, nikethamide, novobiocin, nitrazepam, nitrofurantoin
o	oral contraceptives, oxazolidinediones (paramethadione and trimethadione), oxazepam
p	pancuronium, paraldehyde, pargyline, pentazocine, pentylenetetrazol, pethidine, phenoxybenzamine, phenylbutazone, phenylhydrazine, primidone, probenecid, progesterone, propanidid, pyrazinamide, pyrazolones (amidopyrine, antipyrine, isopropylantipyrine, dipyrone, sodium phenyl dimethyl pyrazolone), pyrimethamine

Skin Diseases and Medications

Porphyria: Drugs that May Precipitate Acute Porphyria

s	spironolactone, steroids, succinimides (ethosuximide, methsuximide, phensuximide), sulphonal, sulfonamides, sulfonylureas, sulthiame
t	tetracyclines, theophylline, tolazamide, tolbutamide, tranylcypromine, trional, troxidone
v	valproic acid, sodium valproate
x	Xylocaine

Porphyria: Drugs Thought to Be Safe in Acute Porphyria

a	acetazolamide, adrenaline, amethocaine, amytriptyline, aspirin, atropine
b	biguanides (phenformin, metformin), bromides, bumetanide, bupivicaine, buprenorphine
c	cephalexin, cephalosporins, chloral hydrate, chloramphenicol, chlormethiazole, chlorpheniramine, chloroquine, chlorpromazine, chlorothiazide, clofibrate, clonazepam, codeine, colchicine, corticosteroids, cyclizine
d	dexamethasone, diamorphine, diazepam, diazoxide, digitalis, diphenhydramine, dicoumarol anticoagulant, droperidol, digoxin
e	EDTA, ether (diethyl)
f	fentanyl, flurbiprofen,
g	gentamicin, glipizide, guanethidine
h	heparin, hydralazine, hyoscine
i	ibuprofen, imipramine, indomethacin, insulin
k	ketamine
l	labetalol, lithium
m	mecamylamine, meclizine, mefenamic acid, mersalyl, methadone, methylphenidate, morphine
n	naproxen, neostigmine, nitrofurantoin, nitrous oxide, nortriptyline
o	oxazepam
p	paracetamol, paraldehyde, penicillins, penicillamine, petinidine, phenoperidine, phenylbutazone, prednisolone, procaine, prisocaine, promethazine, propantheline bromide, propanidid, primaquine, prochlorperazine, promazine, propoxyphene, propranolol, prostigmine, pyrimethamine
q	quinine
r	rauwolfia alkaloids, reserpine, resorcinol, rifampicin
s	salicylates, streptomycin, succinylcholine
t	tetracycline, tetraethylammonium bromide, thiouracil, trifluoperazine, thiazides, tripelennamine, tubocurarine
v	valproate, vitamin B, vitamin C

Adapted from Michael R. Moore, Tschudy DP, Ann Intern Med 1975; 83: 851-64.

Skin Diseases and Medications

Pseudoporphyria: Associated Drugs, Categories

antiarrhythmics	amiodarone, quinidine
antibiotics	nalidixic acid, tetracycline, oxytetracycline
chemotherapy	5-fluorouracil, busulfan
diuretics	furosemide, chlorthalidone, butemide, triamterene/hydrochlorothiazide
foods	cola
hormones	estrogens/progesterones
immunosuppressants	cyclosporine, methotrexate
muscle relaxants	carisoprodol/aspirin
NSAIDs	naproxen, diflunisal, ketoprofen, nabumetone, oxaprozin
other	barbiturates, colchicine, chronic renal failure, hemodialysis, ultraviolet A radiation/sunbeds
sulfones	dapsone
sulfonylureas	tolbutamide
vitamin A derivatives	etretinate, isotretinoin
vitamins	brewer's yeast, pyridoxine, iron preparations

Pseudoporphyria: Associated Drugs, Alphabetical

a	amiodarone
b	barbiturates, brewer's yeast, busulfan, butemide
c	carisoprodol/aspirin, chlorthalidone, chronic renal failure, cola, colchicine, cyclosporine
d	dapsone, diflunisal
e	estrogens, etretinate
f	5-fluorouracil, furosemide
h	hemodialysis
i	iron preparations, isotretinoin
k	ketoprofen
m	methotrexate
n	nabumetone, nalidixic acid, naproxen
o	oxaprozin, oxytetracycline
p	progesterones, pyridoxine
q	quinidine
t	tetracycline, tolbutamide, triamterene/hydrochlorothiazide
u	ultraviolet A radiation/sunbeds

Skin Diseases and Medications

NSAIDs	diclofenac, indomethacin, sulindac

Adapted from Checketts SR, et al. Cutis 1999;63:223-5.

Surgery: Concepts and Definitions

advancement flap	tissue stretch from sides of wound
anesthetics, classification	**amides**: dibucaine hydrochloride (nupercaine), lidocaine **aminobenzoate esters**: benzocaine, benoxinate hydrochloride, tetracaine **benzoic acid esters**: cocaine, hxylcaine, piperocaine, proparacaine **miscellaneous**: cyclomethycaine, dimethisoquin, diperodon, dyclonine, prmoxine
basic surgical tray	#3 blade handle, Adson 1 × 2 delicate tip forceps, Iris scissors 4" curved serrated, 2 single prong skin hooks, 2 Halstead mosquito forceps 5" curved delicate tips, Webster needle holder 5" smooth jawed with tungsten-carbide inserts, Northbent suture scissors 4"
Burrow's triangle	triangle of tissue removed to facilitate rotation flap
clamp	chalazion: useful for stabilizing mobile mucosal surfaces
composite graft	graft of skin and other appendage (hair, cartilage) ex: hair transplant autograft donor sites: antihelix, inferior crus of ear helix, scalp, tragus
curette	1-10 mm, round or oval
dermatomes, electric	Brown (Zimmer): most common Padgett: cumbersome graft width adjustment, because uses shims Simon-Davol: light, but only one setting (0.015 thick and 1 5/16" wide)
dermatomes, free hand	Blue blade, Weck knife
digital nerve block	lidocaine without epinephrine, use < 2 cc, may use EMLA
dog ear	AKA redundant edge tissue, standing cutaneous cone, triangular redundant tissue
donor site—graft site	superior retroauricular area/upper eyelid—lower eyelid, lower retroauricular area—cheek/temple, preauricular area/lower lateral neck—mid cheek/chin, supraclavicular area-medial canthus/lower eyelid, upper lateral neck—helix, glabella—chin/forehead/nose inguinal fold/antecubital fold—hand, nasolabial fold—nose
EMLA	eutetic mixture of local anesthetics
epinephrine	1:100,000-1:300,000 avoid on fingers, ears, toes, nose, penis
forceps (pickups)	Adson: most common forcep, smooth, serrated, toothed (1 x 2), may have suturing platform Allis: tightly grasping tissue for mobilization (cyst removal) Bishop-Harmon: use for delicate tissue, 3 holes in handle, smooth, serrated, toothed (1 x 2) Brown Adson: 7-8 grasping teeth per side to grasp heavy tissue DeJardin: wide jaws, 8 teeth per side (horizontal) for cartilage Iris: narrow handle, delicate tissue, smooth, serrated or toothed (1 x 2)
forehead flap	may involve supratrochlear artery
freer elevator	instrument for use in nail removal
full thickness skin graft	ex: dog ear graft

Surgery: Concepts and Definitions

fusiform shape	3:1 ratio (except on back 1-1.5:1)
glabellar rotation flap	nose
gold handles	tungsten-carbide inserts in instruments
hemostats (snaps)	Halstead, Mosquito, Jacobsen
Hibiclens	avoid use around eyes, ear canal (use povodone/iodine)
island pedicle flap	near nasal ala
kite flap	*see island pedicle flap*
margins	BCC: 4 mm dysplastic nevus: 2 mm melanoma: 1–2 cm nevus: no margin
methylene blue	dye used to mark tumor margin, orientation
Mohs micrographic surgery	stepwise tumor removal with microscopic control allowing maximum preservation of normal tissue
Mohs micrographic surgery, indications	**BCC**: morpheaform, perineural, recurrent **embryonic fusion planes**: nasolabial fold, columella, preauricular, postauricular **size**: > 1 cm head & neck, > 2 cm trunk & extremities **tissue conservation**: ear, eyelid, genitalia, lips **tumor type**: malignant fibrous histiocytoma, microcystic adnexal carcinoma, dermatofibrosarcoma protuberans, merkel cell carcinoma **miscellaneous**: scar carcinoma, immunocompromised
m-plasty	30° angle to save tissue
mucosal advancement flap	no subcutaneous stitches, use silk
myocutaneous flap	nose
needle holders	Castroviejo: spring action, rotary clasp, very fine jaws for fine needles, occuloplastic surgery Crilewood: similar to Webster neuro-smooth: similar to Webster Derf: similar to Webster Halsey: similar to Webster Olsen-Hegar: scissors behind jaws for cutting suture Webster: most popular, variable length & fineness
O to H	eyebrow, rim of ear, (+/-)lip
O to Z	forehead, chin, large defects
recurrence, BCC	cryotherapy 7.5%, ED & C 8%, Mohs' 1%, radiation 9%
recurrence, recurrent BCC	ED & C 40%, excision 17.4%, Mohs' 5.6%, radiation 9.8%
recurrence, SCC	Mohs' <2cm: 1.9%, >2cm: 25.2%
rhomboid flap	120° and 60° angles, rotate around 60° angle
rotation flap	move adjacent tissue in arc
scalpel blade	#10 large blade, sharp belly, use for large lesions and thick tissue #11 sharp, pointed blade, use for incision & drainage, sharp angles, close margins #15 most versatile tip

Surgery: Concepts and Definitions

	#15C similar to #15 with narrower, more sharply tapered tip, use for small lesions or delicate tissue
scissors	bandage: heavy scissors with bulbous lower blade end to cut bandage Gradle: slightly curved short blade, delicate work iris: most commonly used scissors, used for dissection & undermining Metzenbaum: long handle & blade, useful for tissue undermining LaGrange: deeply curved sharp tips, handles with reverse curve, dissecting deep concave surfaces & removing hair transplant grafts Stevens tenotomy: similar to Gradle with longer blade suture: heavy blades, notch at end aid in suture removal Westcott: spring action, fine tips, eye lid work
skin hooks (rakes)	Frazier, Guthrie, Lahey
split thickness skin graft (STSG)	full thickness epidermis & partial thickness dermis ex: pinch graft donor sites: abdomen, anterior thigh, back, buttocks, scalp
subcutaneous suture	avoid on: ear, eyelid, (+/-)forehead
suture	absorptive: Vicryl slow absorptive: Maxon, PDS non-absorptive: Proline
tattoo pigments	**blue**: cobalt aluminate **blue/black**: carbon **brown**: ochre iron oxides **green**: chromic oxide/chromium sesquioxide **light blue**: cobaltous aluminate **red**: cinnabar & vegetable dyes, mercury, mercury sulfide (red cinnabar) **yellow**: cadmium sulfide
tip stitch	buried mattress suture
transposition flap	moves across tissue; bilobe, forehead, nasolabial, rhomboid

Therapy (Unusual and Regimens)

alpha methyldopa	Raynaud's s.
aluminum chloride	Hailey-Hailey d.
aminocaproic acid	angioedema
amphotericin B	mucocutaneous leishmaniasis
anthralin	alopecia areata
antidepressants	chronic urticaria (doxepin), paroxysmal pruritus, pruritus vulvae
antimalarials	dermatomyositis, hydroa vacciniforme, inflammatory morphea, PMLE, reticular erythematous mucinosis, solar urticaria,
aspirin	atrophie blanche, Degos' d., erythromelalgia, Kawasaki's d., polyarteritis nodosa
azathioprine	dermatomyositis, erythroderma, immunobullous disease, LE, leukocytoclastic vasculitis, livedo reticularis, pemphigus, persistent light reaction, PRP, PSS, pyoderma gangrenosum
azelic acid	acne
benzodiazepines	causalgia
β-carotene	DLE, erythropoietic protoporphyria
bleomycin	genital warts, keratoacanthoma
calcium gluconate	periungual chemical burns
cantharidin	molluscum, verrucae
capsaicin	post-herpetic neuralgia, pruritus
carbachol	Chediak-Higashi s.
carmustine (BCNU)	lymphomatoid papulosis, mycosis fungoides
charcoal	erythrocytic porphyria, pruritus of renal dialysis
chlorambucil	mucinoses
chloripramine	trichotillomania
chloroquine	PCT, REM s.
cholestyramine	biliary pruritus, circumileostomy eczema, PCT, primary biliary cirrhosis
cimetidine	chronic mucocutaneous candidiasis, Kaposi's sarcoma
clindamycin	Fox-Fordyce d., rosacea, vulvovaginal LP
clofazimine	DLE, pyoderma gangrenosum, Sweet's s.
clonidine	hyperhidrosis
colchicine	amyloidosis, aphthae, Behçet's disease, EBA, erythema nodosum, familial Mediterranean fever, idiopathic thrombocytopenic purpura, leukocytoclastic vasculitis, nodular vasculitis, palmoplantar pustular psoriasis, PG, pustular psoriasis, Sweet's s.
cyclophosphamide	allergic granulomatosis, dermatomyositis, erythroderma, immunobullous disease, leukocytoclastic vasculitis, mucinoses, pemphigus, polyarteritis nodosa, PSS, Wegener's granulomatosis

Therapy (Unusual and Regimens)

cyclosporin A	aphthous ulcers, atopic dermatitis, alopecia areata, Behçet's disease, dermatomyositis, EBA, erosive LP, generalized granuloma annulare, GVHD, pemphigus, pompholyx, psoriasis, pustulosis palmaris et plantaris, pyoderma gangrenosum, Reiter's s., scleroderma, urticaria/angioedema
cyproheptadine	acanthosis nigricans, acne, carcinoid s., cold urticaria
DMSO	lipoid proteinosis, primary amyloidosis, Raynaud's ulceration
dacarbazine	KS, melanoma
danazol	acne, angioedema, idiopathic thrombocytopenic purpura, premenstrual exacerbation of SLE, urticaria
dapsone	acropustulosis of infancy, acne conglobata, acne fulminans, actinomycosis, alopecia mucinosa, alpha-1-antitrypsin deficiency panniculitis, benign mucosal pemphigoid, brown recluse spider bites, bullous LE, bullous pemphigoid (young patients), chronic bullous disease of childhood, cicatricial pemphigoid, **dermatitis herpetiformis**, EED, GA, granuloma faciale, Hailey-Hailey d., Henoch-Schönlein purpura, LP/LE overlap, leishmaniasis, leprosy, leukocytoclastic vasculitis, linear IgA d., lymphomatoid papulosis, palmoplantar pustular psoriasis, pemphigus foliaceus, pemphigus vulgaris, pyoderma gangrenosum, relapsing polychondritis, SCLE, urticarial vasculitis
dexamethasone	hirsutism
dibutyl ester	alopecia areata
dilantin	DEB, JEB, glucagonoma, morphea
diltiazem	hyperhidrosis
dinitrochlorobenzene	alopecia areata
diphencyprone	alopecia areata
disodium cromoglycate	mastocytosis (relief of GI, skin & CNS symptoms)
disulfiram	nickel sensitivity
DMSO	hereditary localized pruritus
doxycycline	bullous pemphigoid
epinephrine	angioedema, mastocytosis
estrogens	hereditary hemorrhagic telangiectasia, rosacea
etoposide	Langerhan's cell histiocytosis
etretinate	keratoacanthoma, LP, PRP, psoriasis, pustular psoriasis, pustulosis palmaris et plantaris
evening primrose oil	atopic dermatitis
finasteride	androgenetic alopecia, hirsutism
fluoxetine	skin picking
flutamide	hirsutism
5-fluorouracil	actinic keratoses, basal cell epithelioma (superficial), condyloma, erythroplasia of Queyrat, KA (IL and topically), Paget's d., verrucae

Therapy (Unusual and Regimens)

fotemustine	melanoma
gentamicin	protothecosis
gold	DLE (Auranofin), pemphigus, psoriatic arthritis
grenz ray	lichen simplex chronicus
guanethidine	Raynaud's d.
hydroxychloroquine	DLE, PCT, REM s., subacute LE
IFN-α	episodic angioedema, hypereosinophilic s.
IFN-γ	atopic dermatitis
indomethacin	Reiter's s.
interferon (α & γ)	basal cell epithelioma, BCC, SCC, warts (genital), vulvodynia
isotretinoin	Darier's disease, DLE, ichthyoses, mucinoses, PRP, psoriasis (pustular, erythrodermic)
itraconazole	protothecosis
ketanserin	Raynaud's phenomenon
ketotifen	physical urticaria
KI	Sweet's s., erythema nodosum, subacute nodular migratory panniculitis, granuloma annulare, nodular vasculitis, blastomycosis, zygomycosis
levamisole	LP, SLE
masoprocol	actinic keratoses
melphalan	papular mucinoses, primary systemic amyloidosis
mercury	yellow oxide of mercury for eyelash pediculosus
metronidazole	acute necrotizing gingivitis, anaerobic infection of leg ulcers, rosacea
methotrexate	dermatomyositis, erythroderma, Hailey-Hailey d., immunobullous disease, keloids, keratoacanthoma, lymphomatoid papulosis, multicentric histiocytosis, scabies (crusted), PLEVA, PRP, psoriasis
minoxidil	alopecia areata
niacinamide	bullous pemphigoid, granuloma annulare, Hartnup d.
nifedipine	Raynaud's s.
nitrogen mustard	CTCL
OCPs	acne, hirsutism
papaverine	atopic dermatitis
pentoxyfylline	atrophie blanche, CNCH, leukocytoclastic vasculitis, livedo reticularis, PLEVA, Raynaud's s.
phlebotomy	PCT
photopheresis	CTCL, cutaneous sclerosis, GVH d.
pimozide	acarophobia, acne excoriee, dermatitis artefacta, delusion of parasitosis, monosynaptic hypochondriasis, onychotillomania, orodynia, total lipodystrophy

Therapy (Unusual and Regimens)

plasmapheresis	mucinoses, pemphigus
podofilox	condyloma
prazequantel	cysticercosis, schistosomiasis
prazosin	Raynaud's phenomenon
prolixin	acarophobia
propylene glycol	2:1 mixture with water for softening calluses/corns
psoralen + UVA (PUVA)	allergic contact dermatitis, alopecia areata, alopecia mucinosa, atopic dermatitis, CTCL, erythropoietic protoporphyria, granuloma annulare, Grover's d., GVH d., hydroa vacciniforme, LP, mastocytosis, morphea, persistent light reactor, pityriasis lichenoides chronica, lymphomatoid papulosis, parapsoriasis, pityriasis lichenoides, PLEVA, PMLE, polycythemia vera, pompholyx, PRP, psoriasis, pustulosis palmaris et plantaris, scleroderma, solar urticaria, urticaria pigmentosis, vitiligo
rePUVA	combination systemic retinoids plus PUVA for psoriasis
retinoids	aphthae, BCC, Darier's d., Grover's d., hidradenitis suppurativa, KA, keratodermas, LE, psoriasis, rosacea, SCC, XP
spironolactone	acne, hirsutism
squaric acid	alopecia areata
sulfur	scabies (pregnant women & infants <2 months old)
stanozolol	atrophie blanche, cryofibrinogen leg ulcers, cutaneous polyarteritis nodosa, NLD
thalidomide	actinic prurigo, aphthous ulcers (AIDS), chronic GVH, erythema nodosum leprosum, LE, PMLE, uremic pruritus
trimethoprim- sulfamethoxasole	chronic granulomatous d., nocardiosis
testosterone	lichen sclerosis
tetracycline	*Vibrio* infections, protothecosis
thalidomide	aphthae, Behçet's d., erythema nodosum leprosum, lupus profundus, prurigo nodularis, systemic nodular panniculitis (Weber-Christian)
thiabendazole	seabather's eruption
UVA/UVB	atopic dermatitis, pruritus
vinblastine	Kaposi's sarcoma
vitamin A	acneiform eruptions, acne, corns, Darier's d., Grover's d.
vitamin C	alkaptonuria, Chediak-Higashi s., Ehlers-Danlos type VI, miliaria
vitamin D	psoriasis, parapsoriasis
zinc sulfate	alopecia areata

Therapy (Unusual and Regimens)

Disease	Therapy
α-1 antitrypsin deficiency panniculitis	dapsone
acanthosis nigricans	cyproheptadine
acarophobia	pimozide, prolixin
acne	azelic acid, cyproterone, danazol, spironolactone, vitamin A
acne conglobata	dapsone
acne excoriee	pimozide
acne fulminans	dapsone
acneiform eruptions	vitamin A
acropustulosis of infancy	dapsone
actinomycosis	dapsone
acute necrotizing gingivitis	metronidazole
alkaptonuria	vitamin C
allergic granulomatosis	cyclophosphamide
alopecia areata	anthralin, cyclosporine A, dibutyl ester, dinitrochlorobenzene, diphencyprone, minoxidil, squaric acid, zinc sulfate
alopecia mucinosa	dapsone, psoralens
amyloidosis, primary	DMSO
angioedema	aminocaproic acid, danazol
aphthae	colchicine, thalidomide
atopic dermatitis	evening primrose oil, papaverine, psoralens
atopy	cyclosporine A
atrophie blanche	pentoxyfylline, stanozolol, aspirin
Behçet's d.	thalidomide
benign mucosal pemphigoid	dapsone
biliary pruritus	cholestyramine
blastomycosis	KI
brown recluse spider bite	dapsone
bullous LE	dapsone
bullous pemphigoid	dapsone, doxycycline, niacinamide
causalgia	benzodiazepines
Chediak-Higashi s.	carbachol, vitamin C
chronic bullous disease of childhood	dapsone
chronic granulomatous d.	trimethoprim-sulfamethoxazole

Therapy (Unusual and Regimens)

Disease	Therapy
chronic mucocutaneous candidiasis	cimetidine
CNCH	pentoxyfylline
cold urticaria	cyproheptadine
corns	vitamin A
corns/calluses	propylene glycol
cryofibrinogen leg ulcers	stanozolol
cutaneous polyarteritis nodosa	stanozolol
cysticercosis	praziquantel
Darier's d.	dermabrasion, laser, oral retinoids, oral vitamin A
DEB	dilantin
Dego's d.	aspirin
dermatitis artefacta	pimozide
dermatitis herpetiformis	dapsone
dermatomyositis	antimalarials, azathioprine, cyclophosphamide, methotrexate
DLE	beta-carotene, clofazimine, hydroxychloroquine, isotretinoin, gold
eczema, circumileostomy	cholestyramine
EED	dapsone
Ehlers-Danlos type VI	vitamin C
entomophthoromycosis	KI
erythema nodosum	colchicine, KI
erythema nodosum leprosum	thalidomide
erythrocytic porphyria	charcoal
erythroderma	azathioprine, cyclophosphamide, methotrexate
erythromelalgia	aspirin
familial Mediterranean fever	colchicine
glucagonoma	dilantin
Goeckerman regimen	treatment of psoriasis; UV plus crude coal tar
granuloma annulare	dapsone, KI, niacinamide
granuloma annulare, generalized	cyclosporine A
granuloma faciale	dapsone
Grover's d.	PUVA, retinoids (oral), steroids, vitamin A

Therapy (Unusual and Regimens)

Disease	Therapy
Hailey-Hailey d.	aluminum chloride hexahydrate 6.25%, dapsone, vitamin E, methotrexate, cyclosporin (topical)
harlequin fetus	oral retinoids
Hartnup d.	niacinamide
Henoch-Schönlein purpura	dapsone
hereditary hemorrhagic telangiectasia	estrogens
hirsutism	dexamethasone, finasteride, flutamide, OCPs, spironolactone
hydroa vacciniforme	antimalarials
hyperhidrosis	clonidine, diltiazem
idiopathic thrombo-cytopenic purpura	colchicine, danazol
inflammatory morphea	antimalarials
Ingram treatment	anthralin paste, UV & wraps; psoriasis treatment
JEB	dilantin
Kaposi's sarcoma	cimetidine
Kawasaki's d.	aspirin
keloids	methotrexate
keratoacanthoma	bleomycin, etretinate, 5-fluorouracil, methotrexate
keratoderma	biotin, salicylic acid, retinoids (oral), vitamin D3 analog
LE	azathioprine
leg ulcers, anaerobic infection	metronidazole
leishmaniasis	dapsone
leukocytoclastic vasculitis	colchicine, pentoxyfylline
lichen planus	levamisole
lichen planus, lupus erythematosus overlap	dapsone
lichen sclerosis	steroids
lichen simplex chronicus	grenz ray
linear IgA bullous dermatosis	dapsone
livedo reticularis	azathioprine
lupus profundus	thalidomide
lymphomatoid papulosis	carmustine (BCNU), dapsone, methotrexate
mastocytosis	psoralens

Therapy (Unusual and Regimens)

Disease	Therapy
miliaria	vitamin C
monosynaptic hypochondriasis	pimozide
morphea	dilantin
mucocutaneous leishmaniasis	amphotericin B
multicentric histiocytosis	methotrexate
mycosis fungoides	carmustine (BCNU)
necrobiosis lipoidica diabeticorum	stanozolol
nickel sensitivity	disulfiram
nocardiosis	trimethoprim-sulfamethoxasole
nodular vasculitis	colchicine
Norwegian scabies	methotrexate
onychotillomania	pimozide
orodynia	pimozide
palmoplantar pustular psoriasis	colchicine, dapsone
panniculitis, subacute nodular migratory	KI
parapsoriasis	psoralens, vitamin D
paroxysmal pruritus	amitryptiline
PCT	phlebotomy
pediculosis, eyelash	mercury, petrolatum
pemphigus foliaceus	dapsone
pemphigus vulgaris	dapsone
periungual chemical burns	calcium gluconate
persistent light reactor	azathioprine, psoralens
pityriasis lichenoides chronica	psoralens
PLEVA	methotrexate, pentoxyfylline, psoralens
PMLE	antimalarials, psoralens
polyarteritis nodosa	aspirin, cyclophosphamide
polycythemia vera	psoralens
pompholyx	psoralens (PUVA)
premenstrual exacerbation of SLE	danazol

Therapy (Unusual and Regimens)

Disease	Therapy
primary biliary cirrhosis	cholestyramine
protothecosis	gentamicin, itraconazole, tetracycline
PRP	azathioprine, etretinate, methotrexate
prurigo nodularis	thalidomide
pruritus	antihistamines, capsaicin, diphenhydramine, doxepin cream, pramoxine HCl
pruritus of renal dialysis	charcoal
pruritus vulvae	amitryptiline
pruritus, hereditary localized	DMSO
psoriasis	cyclosporine A, vitamin D
PSS	azathioprine, cyclophosphamide
pustular psoriasis	colchicine, etretinate
pyoderma gangrenosum	azathioprine, clofazimine, dapsone, mycophenolate mofetil
Raynaud's s.	alpha methyldopa, nifedipine
Raynaud's ulceration	DMSO
relapsing polychondritis	dapsone
reticular erythematous mucinosis	antimalarials
rosacea	azelaic acid, clonidine, estrogens, metronidazole, retinoids, spironolactone
schistosomiasis	praziquantel
SCLE	dapsone
seabather's eruption	thiobendazole
skin picking	fluoxetine
SLE	levamisole
solar urticaria	antimalarials, psoralens
Sweet's s	KI, colchicine, clofazimine
systemic nodular panniculitis (Webber-Christian)	thalidomide
total lipodystrophy	pimozide
urticaria pigmentosis	psoralens
urticaria, chronic	Doxepin
urticaria, physical	ketotifen
urticarial vasculitis	dapsone
vasculitis, nodular	KI

Therapy (Unusual and Regimens)

Disease	Therapy
Vibrio infections	tetracycline
Wegener's granulomatosis	cyclophosphamide
zygomycosis	KI

Herbal Therapy

acne	burdock root, tea tree oil, yellow dock
bruising	arnica, capsaicin, comfrey
burns	aloe vera, calendula
eczema	aloe vera, burdock, chamomile, evening primrose oil, witch hazel
herpes	lemon balm
onychomycosis	tea tree oil
pruritis	capsaicin, chamomile, chickweed
psoriasis	aloe vera, burdock root, capsaicin, milk thistle, red clover, yellow dock
shingle pain	capsaicin
tinea pedis	garlic, tea tree oil
ulcers, wounds	aloe vera, arnica, calendula, comfrey, echinacea, goldenseal, tea tree oil

Topical Steroid Potency

Group	Generic Name	Brand Name	Sizes Available
1 Most potent	Clobetasol propionate Betamethasone dipropionate Diflorasone diacetate Clobetasol propionate Halobetasol propionate	Cormax Cream & Ointment 0.05% Diprolene Gel & Ointment 0.05% Psorcon Ointment Temovate Cream & Ointment Ultravate Cream & Ointment 0.05%	15, 30, 45 gm 15, 45 gm 15, 30, 60 gm 15, 30, 45, 60 gm 15, 50 gm
2	Betamethasone dipropionate Triamcinolone acetonide Acetonide Betamethasone dipropionate Mometasone furoate Diflorasone diacetate Halcinonide Fluocinonide Diflorasone diacetate Fluocinonide Betamethasone dipropionate Diflorasone diacetate Desoximetason	Alphatrex Ointment 0.05% Aristocort Ointment 0.5% Cyclocort Ointment 0.1% Diprolene AF Cream & Ointment 0.05% Diprosone 0.05% Elocon Ointment 0.1% Florone Ointment 0.05% Halog, Halog-E Cream 0.1% Lidex Cream, Gel & Ointment 0.05% Lidex Solution 0.05% Maxiflor 0.05% Maxivate 0.05% Psorcon Cream 0.05% Topicort Cream & Ointment 0.25%	15, 45 gm 15 gm 15, 30, 60 gm 15, 45 gm 15, 45 gm 15, 30, 60 gm 15, 30, 60, 240 gm 15, 30, 60, 120 gm 30, 60 gm 20, 60 ml 45 gm 15, 30, 60 gm 15, 60 gm, 4 oz
3	Betamethasone dipropionate Triamcinolone acetonide Betamethasone valerate Fluticasone propionate Amcinonide Amcinonide Betamethasone dipropionate Diflorasone diacetate Halcinonide Halcinonide Fluocinonide Betamethasone diproprionate Desoximetasone Betamethasone valerate	Alphatrex Cream 0.05% Aristocort A Ointment 0.1% Betatrex Ointment 0.1% Cutivate Ointment 0.005% Cyclocort Cream 0.1% Cyclocort Lotion 0.1% Diprosone Cream 0.05% Florone Cream & E Cream 0.05% Halog Ointment 0.1% Halog Solution 0.1% Lidex E Cream 0.05% Maxivate Lotion 0.05% Topicort LP Cream 0.05% Valisone Ointment 0.1%	15, 45 gm 15, 60 gm 15, 45 gm 15, 30, 60 gm 15, 30, 60 gm 20, 60 ml 15, 45 gm 15, 30, 60 gm 15, 30, 60, 240 gm 20, 60 ml 15, 30, 60, 120 gm 60 ml 15, 60 gm 15, 45 gm
4	Triamcinolone acetonide Flurandrenolide Mometasone furoate Mometasone furoate Triamcinolone acetonide Fluocinolone acetonide Hydrocortisone valerate	Aristocort A Cream & Ointment 0.1% Cordran Ointment 0.05% Elocon Cream 0.1% Elocon Lotion 0.1% Kenalog Cream & Ointment 0.1% Synalar Ointment 0.025% Westcort Ointment 0.2%	15, 60, 240 gm 15, 30, 60 gm 15, 45 gm 30, 60 ml 15, 60, 80 gm 15, 30, 60 gm 15, 45, 60 gm
5	Betamethasone valerate Flurandrenolide Fluticasone propionate Prednicarbate Triamcinolone acetonide	Betatrex Cream 0.1% Cordran Cream 0.05% Cutivate Cream 0.05% Dermatop Cream 0.1% Kenalog Lotion 0.1%	15, 45 gm 15, 30, 60 gm 15, 30, 60 gm 15, 60 gm 15, 60 ml

Topical Steroid Potency

Group	Generic Name	Brand Name	Sizes Available
	Hydrocortisone butyrate	Locoid Cream & Ointment 0.1%	15, 45 gm
	Hydrocortisone butyrate	Locoid Solution 0.1%	20, 60 ml
	Fluocinolone acetonide	Synemol, Synalar Cream 0.025%	15, 30, 60 gm
	Desonide	Tridesilon 0.05%	15, 60 gm
	Betamethasone valerate	Valisone Cream 0.1%	15, 45 gm
	Hydrocortisone valerate	Westcort Cream 0.2%	15, 45, 60 gm
6	Aclometasone dipropionate	Aclovate cream & ointment 0.05%	15, 45, 60 gm
	Triamicinolone acetonide	Aristocort A 0.1 & 0.025	15, 60 gm
	Flurandrenooide	Cordran Cream & Ointment 0.025%	15, 30 gm
	Desonide	Desowen Cream & Ointment 0.05%	15, 60 gm
	Triamcinolone acetonide	Kenalog 0.025%	15, 80 gm
	Fluocinolone acetonide	Synalar Cream 0.01%	15, 30, 60 gm
	Desonide	Tridesilon Cream 0.05%	15, 60 gm
7 least potent	Hydrocortisone	Hytone Cream 2.5%	30, 60 gm
	Hydrocortisone	Hytone Lotion 1.0%	120 ml
	Hydrocortisone	Hytone Lotion 2.5%	60 ml
	Hydrocortisone, OTC	Hydrocortisone 1%	30, 60 gm